HEALTH SCIENCE FUNDAMENTALS

Exploring Career Pathways

Shirley A. Badasch, M.Ed, RN
Doreen S. Chesebro, B.Ed, LVN

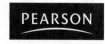

Upper Saddle River, New Jersey 07458

Notice: Care has been taken to confirm the accuracy of information presented in this book. The authors, editors, and the publisher, however, cannot accept any responsibility for errors or omissions or for consequences from application of the information in this book and make no warranty, express or implied, with respect to its contents.

The authors and publishers have exerted every effort to ensure that drug selections and dosages set forth in this text are in accord with current recommendations and practice at time of publication. However, in view of ongoing research, changes in government regulations, and the constant flow of information relating to drug therapy and drug reactions, the reader is urged to check the package inserts of all drugs for any change in indications of dosage and for added warnings and precautions. This is particularly important when the recommended agent is a new and/or infrequently employed drug.

Publisher: *Julie Alexander*
Publisher's Assistant: *Regina Bruno*
Executive Editor: *Joan Gill*
Associate Editor: *Bronwen Glowacki*
Media Product Manager: *John Jordan*
Media Project Manager: *Stephen Hartner*
Marketing Manager: *Harper Coles*
Marketing Specialist: *Michael Sirinides*
Marketing Assistant: *Lauren Castellano*
Senior Managing Editor: *Patrick Walsh*
Senior Operations Manager: *Ilene Sanford*
Cover Design: *Melissa Auciello-Brogan, Abshier House*
Cover Illustration/Photo: *Cover images used under license from Shutterstock.com, copyright Yuri Arcurs, Doug Stevens, iofoto, Pastushenko Taras, Julián Rovagnati.*
Director, Image Resource Center: *Melinda Patelli*
Manager, Rights and Permissions: *Zina Arabia*
Manager: *Visual Research: Beth Brenzel*
Manager, Cover Visual Research & Permissions: *Karen Sanatar*
Image Permission Coordinator: *Kathy Gavilanes*
Photo Researcher: *Alisa Alering*
Composition: *Melissa Auciello-Brogan, Abshier House*
Project Management and Developmental Editing: *Emergent Learning*
Editorial Production: *Claire Hunter and Michele Somody*
Printer/Binder: *Courier Printing, Westford, MA*
Typeface: *10/12 New Aster*

Pearson Prentice Hall™ is a trademark of Pearson Education, Inc.
Pearson® is a registered trademark of Pearson plc
Prentice Hall® is a registered trademark of Pearson Education, Inc.

Pearson Education Ltd., London
Pearson Education Singapore, Pte. Ltd
Pearson Education, Canada, Inc.
Pearson Education–Japan
Pearson Education, Upper Saddle River, New Jersey

Pearson Education Australia Pty, Limited
Pearson Education North Asia Ltd., Singapore
Pearson Educación de Mexico, S.A. de C.V.
Pearson Education Malaysia, Pte. Ltd.

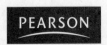

10 9 8 7 6 5 4
ISBN-13: 978-0-13-504372-1
ISBN-10: 0-13-504372-7

Contents

How to Use the Student Activity Guide

The Student Acitivty Guide is designed to help you develop new skills and the knowledge necessary to work in a health care environment. It is an addition to the textbook and guides you in learning to be a health care worker. Completing the worksheets, reports, and assignments reinforces your learning. Showing proficiency in skills gives you confidence when you begin your on-site training (on-site training may also be called community classroom or internship).

To use the Student Activity Guide most effectively:

- Carefully read each objective. Each objective tells you what you are expected to learn and to know.

- Follow the directions. If you are instructed to complete a worksheet before reading, for example, be certain to complete it in the suggested order. Completing it helps you understand the reading material.

- Use your text to help you complete each worksheet assignment. The knowledge that you gain on the worksheet is important for passing the unit or chapter evaluation.

- Your instructor has the key for each worksheet. Check your answers for accuracy. If you have difficulty with answers, return to the text and read the information again. Do not move on until you are certain that you understand all concepts. Each concept builds on another. If you do not learn one concept, the next is more difficult to learn.

- There are also skills that you must show proficiency in. Use the skills checkoff sheets, and practice until you can complete the skill. You need these skills when you begin your internship. Some of the skills check-off sheets are included in your activity guide. Ask your teacher for additional check-off sheets.

- When you feel confident that you can meet each objective, ask your instructor for the unit or chapter evaluation. The evaluation is a written test and may also include a demonstration of skills.

Successful completion of worksheets, the written evaluation, and demonstration of competency in skills are necessary before you can begin your internship.

To do this:

- Review your Student Activity Guide.

- Complete the worksheets in the order assigned. If a worksheet is assigned before reading the text, be certain to complete it first.

- Read the entire chapter.

- Complete all worksheets and skills demonstrations.

- Take the chapter evaluation.

It is very difficult to "play catch-up." Complete the worksheets and check-off sheets when they are assigned.

This Student Activity Guide and the text can be used in a self-paced program. As you complete each section or chapter and successfully pass the evaluations, you may proceed to the next section or chapter.

Your instructor may prefer to have all class members complete the assignments at the same time. In this case, be certain that you follow your instructor's directions.

When you have successfully completed the text and the Student Activity Guide, you will have gained a basic core of information. This information will be important in the health career you choose. We wish you success in any endeavor you choose to pursue in the health career field.

Survival Skills: Effective Study Habits

You can develop effective study habits and enjoy effective learning. There are some very important skills that help you study. When you learn them and use them, studying and remembering will be easier. These include:

- Planning where you study
- Planning your time
- Knowing your textbook
- Learning to read for key information
- Taking notes
- Preparing for tests and quizzes
- Taking tests and quizzes

PLANNING WHERE YOU STUDY

Choose a place to study that you find quiet and pleasant. Make this area the place you use to study, learn, and remember. Ask yourself:

- Is it quiet here?
- Do I have a desk or table that is large enough?
- Do I have the materials and equipment I need?
- Is my chair comfortable?
- Do I have enough light?
- Is my work space neat?

All of these questions are important. Plan your work area so you can answer yes to each question.

PLANNING YOUR TIME

Planning your time gives you a guideline. It keeps you from putting off what you need to do. It also gives you a way to schedule your fun time. Here are important things to remember:

- Study when you are most alert. People are alert at different times. Some are most productive in the morning, some in the evening or late at night.
- Choose when and where to study, and stick to the plan.
- Write exactly what you want to accomplish on your schedule—for example, write, "Learn the normal and abnormal reading of temperature, pulse, respirations, and blood pressure," not "do vital signs homework."
- Study 11/2 to 2 hours on any one subject. After this amount of time you tire easily and lose concentration. Take a break, and study another subject.

- Plan enough time to learn what you need to know.

- Study as soon after class as possible. Check your notes while they are fresh in your mind. Start the assignments while they are clear in your mind.

- Space your reviews. Review your notes weekly. Review from the beginning to refresh your memory. This helps you remember and improves your scores on tests and quizzes.

- Use "empty" hours during the day to study. Free periods between classes are good study times, and free you later for fun activities.

- Plan study make-up time. Immediately find time to make up study time when you miss a planned time. Adjust your written schedule also.

KNOWING YOUR TEXTBOOK

Your textbook is a guide to learning. Become familiar with your book. It is your friend.

- Think about the title. What is the book about?

- Read the Contents. It tells you what is in the book.

- Read the Preface. This is where the authors tell you about the book.

- Look at the Index. The more words you already know, the easier the text will be for you.

- Look for a glossary. It gives you important definitions of the words in the text.

- Look at a chapter in the book. All the chapters will look alike. Ask yourself:

- Is there a summary?

- Are there questions at the end?

- Write in the book if it belongs to you.

- Define words so you understand them.

- Write words in your native language if English is your second language.

- Highlight important information.

Use your book. It is your friend.

LEARNING TO READ FOR KEY INFORMATION

Frances P. Robinson, a psychologist at Ohio State University, developed the SQ3R method for reading your assignments. The SQ3R stands for survey/question/ read/recite/review:

- Survey to get the overall idea of what you are studying.

- Read the unit objectives carefully.

- Read headings to see what the units and topics are.

- Look at figures and tables.

- Read the summaries.

- Question to help you remember the information. Ask yourself:

- What does the word or phrase mean?
- Think about questions the author asks.
- Answer each objective.
- Read to get key information and answer questions.
- Read everything, including tables, figures, and illustrations.
- Think about what the author wants you to know. The objectives tell you what the author wants you to learn.
- Recite what you are learning. This helps you find out what you remember and understand. Stop as you read and try to tell yourself what you have read.
- Recall the main headings.
- What are the important ideas under each heading?
- Try to state what you have read without looking at the pages.
- Check for things you have left out and for errors.
- Review what you have read.
- Go back and review immediately after reading.
- Look at each heading and ask yourself what they mean.
- Recite the points under each heading.
- Check to see if you are right.
- Recite summaries.
- Reread the summaries.
- Review once or twice before your tests.
- Recite the information you must know for a test.

TAKING NOTES

Note taking helps you understand and remember. Your notes give you important information for reviewing. They should be clear and short and outline the most important parts.

- Read the assignment before the lecture.
- Look up unfamiliar terms.
- Listen for answers to material you do not understand.
- Ask questions in class.
- Keep separate sections for your classes.
- Use a new page for each lecture.
- Date your notes and number the pages.
- Use symbols and abbreviations (e.g., TPR, B/P, c–, s–; see medical terminology).
- Use phrases or words, not sentences, if possible.

- Put notes in your own words.

- Develop a code for your notes (e.g., ? = not clear; ! = important; * = assignment; Q = question; C = your own comments).

- Look for clues of important information:

  - Material on blackboard

  - Visual aids such as slides and overheads

  - Repeated information

  - Questions the instructor asks the class

- Go over notes as soon as possible after class and check them for errors.

- Be sure you understand your notes.

- Review your notes within 24 hours to help you remember

See the figure on page xv on taking notes for results.

PREPARING FOR TESTS AND QUIZZES

Taking tests and quizzes requires preparation. The preparation begins when you enter your class.

- Do your work daily.

- If you do not understand, ask.

- Take clear notes.

- Review daily.

- Test yourself.

- Study with others.

- Think about the instructor's point of view. What kinds of questions do you think will be asked?

- Go to the test with pencils, pens, and other needed supplies.

- Do not cram at the last minute.

- Go to class with a clear mind.

TAKING TESTS AND QUIZZES

When you are finally ready to take the test, follow these steps:

- Skim the whole test to help you know what is being asked and how it is organized.

- Be sure you understand the format. How do you answer? If you have questions, ask your instructor.

- Ask about items if you are not sure what is being asked.

- Budget your time. If a question is worth more points, give it more time.

- Do the easy items first.

- Begin working. Read carefully.

- Answer the question as it relates to class. For example, if you are asked about medical care in other cultures, answer from what you learned in class. Do not give information that you know but that was never discussed.

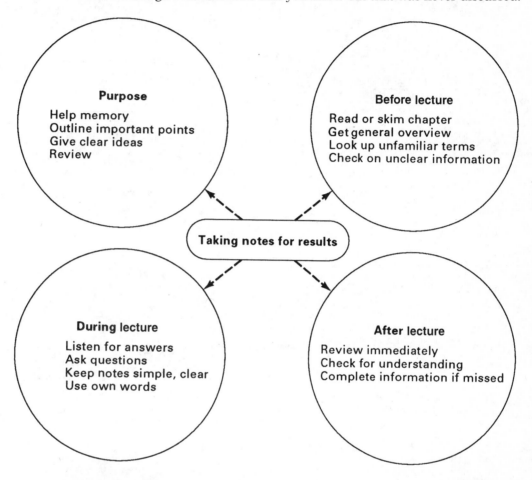

- Reread.

- Make changes or additions.

- Check to be sure you answered all the questions.

- Guess at items you are not sure of unless you are given other instructions.

Use these skills to help you be successful in your studies. Learn the information in your textbook carefully, and complete all assignments given in class and in your workbook. Effective study habits will help you become a successful health care worker.

Chapter 1 Introduction to Being a Health Care Worker

History of Health Care

- OBJECTIVES

When you have completed this section, you will be able to do the following:

- Match key terms with their correct meanings.

- Identify scientists and explain what they contributed to medicine.

- Choose one era in the history of health care and explain how health care technology changed.

- Discuss advances in medicine in the twentieth century.

- Research and report on possible advances in medicine for the twenty-first century.

- Explain the origin of medical ethics and the impact of medical advances on ethics.

- Compare health care in the past with health care in the twentieth and twenty-first centuries.

- Explain current trends in health care.

- DIRECTIONS

1. Complete vocabulary Worksheet 1.
2. Read this section.
3. Complete Worksheet 2 and Worksheet/Activity 3.
4. Ask your student for directions to complete Worksheets/Activities 4, 5, 6, and 7.
5. When you are confident that you can meet each objective listed above, ask your student for the section evaluation.

- ## EVALUATION METHODS
  - Worksheets/Activities
  - Class participation in activities
  - Written report
  - Written evaluation

- ## WORKSHEET 1

Match each definition in column B with the term in column A (18 points).

Column A

1. Accurate
2. Anesthesia
3. Asepsis
4. Antiseptic
5. Custodial
6. Dissection
7. Era
8. Geriatric
9. Observation
10. Microorganism
11. Monasteries
12. Noninvasive
13. Predators
14. Recipient
15. Stethoscope
16. Superstitious
17. Quackery
18. Exorcise

Column B

a. Organism so small that it can only be seen through a microscope.

b. Act of watching.

c. Loss of feeling or sensation.

d. Instrument used to hear sound in the body.

e. Not involving penetration of the skin.

f. Sterile condition; free from all germs.

g. One that receives.

h. Trusting in magic or chance.

i. Period of time.

j. Substance that slows or stops the growth of microorganisms.

k. Marked by watching and protecting rather than seeking to cure.

l. Organisms or beings that destroy.

m. Act or process of dividing, taking apart.

n. Homes for men following religious standards.

o. Practice of pretending to cure diseases.

p. Exact, correct, or precise.

q. Pertaining to old age.

r. To force out evil spirits.

There are 18 possible points in this worksheet.

• WORKSHEET 2

Identify nine scientists, and explain what they contributed to medicine (18 points).

1. _____
2. _____
3. _____
4. _____
5. _____
6. _____
7. _____
8. _____
9. _____

There are 18 possible points in this worksheet.

• WORKSHEET/ACTIVITY 3

Talk to an older person about diseases that affected past generations and that are no longer a primary threat. Ask them to describe how they tried to prevent illness caused by those same diseases. Write notes about your dialogue and prepare to report briefly to your classmates.

There are 20 possible points in this worksheet/activity.

• WORKSHEET/ACTIVITY 4

Choose one era in the history of health care, and write a short paper to explain how health care technology changed during that period (10 points). Use information learned in class, do research in the library, and/or use the Internet for your report. Follow these guidelines when preparing your report:

Type, word-process, or write neatly in ink.

Use 8.5-by-11-inch paper.

Use correct spelling and grammar.

There are 10 points in this worksheet/activity.

• WORKSHEET/ACTIVITY 5

In a small group of students, discuss the advances in medicine in the twentieth century. Answer the following questions during your discussion. Use information from your essay, class discussion, the textbook, and other classroom resources (25 points).

1. How did medical care for the injured and ill change from the time when patients were cared for in monasteries and homes?
2. Are these changes better for the patient?
3. Are more people cared for at home today than in the recent past?

4. How has the discovery of microorganisms affected research for AIDS, tuberculosis, and other serious diseases?

5. What do you feel are the greatest advances made in the twentieth century?

There are 25 points in this worksheet/activity.

● WORKSHEET/ACTIVITY 6

Bring to class an article from a newspaper, magazine, or Internet Web site that discusses current medical research. Give a report about the article to the class (25 points).

There are 25 points in this worksheet/activity.

● WORKSHEET/ACTIVITY 7

In a small group of students, dialogue about the following scenario.

A 55-year-old man and a 25-year-old man both need a new kidney or they will die. The 55-year-old man has a wife, children, and several grandchildren. He is a volunteer for many service organizations in his community and has received many awards for helping others. The 25year-old man is an alcoholic and has been in and out of jail since he was a child. He is not married and has no children. Assume that there is only one kidney available. Which person would you give the kidney to? Why?

There are 25 points in this worksheet/activity.

SECTION

1.2   Becoming a Health Care Worker

● OBJECTIVES

When you have completed this section, you will be able to do the following:

- Match key terms with their correct meanings.
- Discuss the importance of proper health care training.
- Describe the proper appearance for a health care worker.
- Discuss standards of behavior.
- Discuss the importance of confidentiality when working with patient records

● DIRECTIONS

1. Complete Worksheet 1.
2. Read the section.
3. Ask your teacher for directions to complete Worksheets 3 through 5.

4. When you are confident that you can meet each objective for this section, ask your teacher for the section evaluation.

5. Prepare responses to each item listed in Chapter Review.

6. Study your worksheets, activities, and section evaluations in preparation for the chapter evaluation.

● EVALUATION METHODS

- Worksheets/Activities
- Class participation in activities
- Written report
- Written evaluation

● WORKSHEET 1

Match each definition in column B with the correct term in column A (12 points).

Column A	Column B
1. Accredited	a. A pledge or promise.
2. Appearance	b. Keep up.
3. Commitment	c. Punished.
4. Confidentiality	d. A promise to keep certain information secret.
5. Converse	e. Attested and approved as meeting prescribed standards.
6. Hygiene	f. The way you stand.
7. Maintain	g. The way someone or something looks.
8. Polite	h. Talk, have a conversation.
9. Professional	i. The practice of keeping clean.
10. Recommendations	j. One who is paid for work.
11. Reprimanded	k. Suggestions.
12. Stance	l. Courteous

There are 12 possible points in this worksheet.

● WORKSHEET/ACTIVITY 2

Select two or three technical, community, or four-year colleges in your area. Find out if each one has an accredited health care program. Learn what type of degree is offered along with the requirements for earning that degree. (15 points).

● WORKSHEET 3

Underline the word or words that best complete the sentences about your professional appearance.

1. Dress according to your (personal style, facility's dress code).

2. Wear the (minimum, maximum) amount of jewelry.

3. Keep your name badge (out of sight, in view).

4. Wear your hair (up off your color, down and freely flowing).

5. Keep your nails (long or darkly polished, short and polished in light colors).

6. List four rules for good hygiene.

   a. _____

   b. _____

   c. _____

   d. _____

7. Describe at least two important practices for female healthcare providers.

   _____

   _____

8. Describe at least two important practices for male health providers.

   _____

   _____

There are 18 possible points in this worksheet.

● WORKSHEET 4

Describe why each of the following is a good standard of behavior when interacting with patients.

   a. Maintaining eye contact
   b. Smiling
   c. Maintaining an open stance
   d. Listening carefully
   e. Not gossiping

There are 15 possible points in this worksheet.

● WORKSHEET 5

You meet a patient who is complaining of severe leg pain and difficulty walking. She explains that she has been experiencing the pain for over six months and has had numerous tests, but physicians cannot find the cause of her condition. The patient tells you how her life has changed because she can no longer complete her daily activities. Write a paragraph explaining how the following personal characteristics could help you in your interaction with this patient. Be sure to define each characteristic as you describe it.

   ■ Competence

   ■ Dependability

   ■ Empathy

   ■ Honesty

   ■ Patience

   ■ Tact

There are 20 possible points in this worksheet.

Chapter 2 Understanding Health Care Systems

- ## OBJECTIVES

  When you have completed this section, you will be able to do the following:

  - Match key terms with their correct meanings.
  - Research a volunteer agency.
  - Define managed care.
  - Define ambulatory care.
  - Evaluate how managed care and ambulatory care meet the needs of the changing health care system.
  - Understand the role of government agencies in providing health care.
  - List six types of outpatient care and the type of treatment given.
  - Define wellness and preventive care.
  - Contrast the current trends with health care in the twentieth century.
  - Be able to use or read an organizational chart.
  - Give two reasons why the organization of health care facilities is important.
  - Explain a chain of command.
  - List and define the major services in health care.
  - Identify two departments in each major service.

- ## DIRECTIONS

  1. Complete vocabulary Worksheet 1 before beginning the reading.
  2. Read Chapter 2, Section 1.

3. Complete Worksheet 2.

4. Ask your teacher for directions to complete Worksheets/Activities 3, 4, and 5.

5. Complete Worksheet 6.

6. When you are confident that you can meet each objective for this section, ask your teacher for the section evaluation.

● EVALUATION METHODS

- Worksheets/Activities
- Class participation
- Written report
- Written evaluation

● WORKSHEET 1

1. Define the following key terms (8 points).

   a. Chronic _____

   b. Convalescence _____

   c. Rehabilitation _____

   d. Therapeutic _____

   e. Outpatient_____

   f. Chiropractic _____

   g. Hypertension _____

   h. Trend _____

Match each definition in column B with the correct key term in column A (8 points).

Column A

2. Diagnostic
3. Endowment
4. Psychiatric
5. Therapeutic
6. Immunization
7. Orthopedics
8. Specialties
9. Geriatric

Column B

a. Pertaining to the mind.

b. The medical specialty concerned with correcting problems with the skeletal system.

c. Fields of study or professional work.

d. A branch of medicine that deals with the problems and diseases of old age and aging people.

e. Pertaining to the determination of the

f. Substance given to make disease organisms

g. Gifts of property or money given to a group or organization.

h. Pertaining to the treatment of disease or injury

There are 18 possible points in this worksheet.

• WORKSHEET 2

Use the words listed below to complete the following statements (9 points).

facilities	hydrotherapy	communicable
maternal	prosthetics	surgical
referral	outpatient surgery	environmental sanitation

1. General hospitals, specialty hospitals, and clinics are examples of _____ that give patient care.

2. Reporting _____ diseases is one of the services provided by the public health department.

3. Rehabilitation centers often use _____ to treat patients.

4. The provider gave a _____ for the patient to see a heart specialist.

5. _____ are artificial parts made for the body.

6. Patients go for _____ when they do not need to stay in the hospital overnight.

7. A service that is related to the care of mothers is called _____ service.

8. The methods used to keep the environment clean and to promote health are _____ methods.

9. A procedure used to repair or remove a body part by cutting is a _____ procedure.

There are 9 possible points in this worksheet.

• WORKSHEET/ACTIVITY 3

Write a report on a volunteer agency using information from your textbook, the classroom, the library, or a local agency (25 points). Include the following information in your report:

- Goals of the agency
- Type of service it offers
- Number of active volunteers
- Number of paid workers
- How it is funded
- Who can be a volunteer

Follow these guidelines when preparing your report:

- Use 8.5-by-11-inch paper.
- Type, word-process, or write neatly in ink.
- Use correct spelling and grammar.

There are 25 possible points in this worksheet/activity.

• WORKSHEET/ACTIVITY 4

Follow your teacher's direction to tour a hospital, outpatient clinic, outpatient surgery, rehabilitation center, or inpatient hospital.

There are 10 points in this worksheet/activity.

● WORKSHEET/ACTIVITY 5

Gather articles, fliers, pamphlets, and so on about preventive health care. Create a bulletin board emphasizing a theme and giving guidelines that promote wellness. Example: Explain why proper diet, exercise, and socialization promote wellness or explain why immunization prevents illness.

There are 10 points in this worksheet/activity.

● WORKSHEET 6

1. Fill in this hospital organizational chart according to the information in your textbook (10 points).

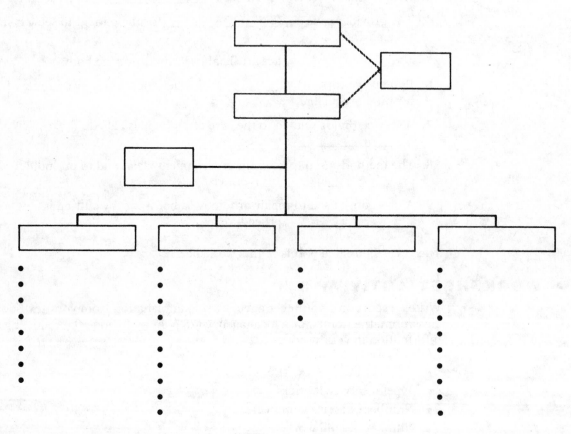

2. Give two reasons why the organization of health care facilities is important (2 points).

    a. _____

    b. _____

3. Name and define the four major health care services (8 points).

    a. _____

    b. _____

    c. _____

    d. _____

4. Identify the service for each of the following departments. In the space next to the department, write T for therapeutic, D for diagnostic, I for information, or E for environmental (11 points).

   a. Care management _____

   b. Central supply _____

   c. Audiology _____

   d. Cardiology _____

   e. Renal dialysis _____

   f. Utilization review _____

   g. Food service _____

   h. Imaging _____

   i. Nursing _____

   j. Health education _____

   k. Neurology _____

5. Explain a chain of command, and describe how it relates to you in the workplace (3 points). _____

There are 34 possible points in this worksheet.

SECTION

2.2

Health Care Systems

● OBJECTIVES

When you have completed this section, you will be able to do the following:

- Match key terms with their correct meanings.

- Explain how health care providers have modified their practices to provide patients quality health care at a lower cost.

- Explain the purpose of the Health Plan Employer Data and Information Set.

- Identify and differentiate the various health care systems.

- Compare and contrast health maintenance organizations and preferred provider organizations.

- Analyze and predict where and how certain factors such as cost, managed care, technology, an aging population, etc. may affect various health care delivery system models.

• DIRECTIONS

1. Complete Worksheet 1 before reading the section.
2. Complete Worksheet 2 and 5 as assigned.
3. Complete Worksheets/Activities 3 and 5.
4. Prepare responses to each item listed in Chapter Review.
5. When you are confident that you can meet each objective listed above, ask your teacher for the section evaluation.

• EVALUATION METHODS

- Worksheets/Activities
- Class participation
- Written report
- Written evaluation

• WORKSHEET 1

Match each definition in column B with the correct key term in column A (8 points).

Column A

1. Intervention
2. Co-payment
3. Benefits
4. Premium
5. Lawsuit
6. Preventative
7. Compensation
8. Legislation

Column B

a. The periodic payment to Medicare, an insurance company, or a health care plan for health care or prescription drug coverage.

b. A law or body of laws.

c. A set amount the subscriber pays for each medical service.

d. Intended to keep something from happening.

e. Payment.

f. Payment and assistance based on an agreement.

g. The act of getting involved to modify an outcome.

h. A legal action started by one person against another based on a complaint that the person failed to perform a legal duty.

There are possible points in this worksheet.

● WORKSHEET 2

1. Write a sentence explaining how each of the following practices might enable health care providers to lower costs for patients.

   a. Combining services

_____

_____

   b. Offering outpatient services

_____

_____

   c. Purchasing supplies in bulk

_____

_____

   d. Preventative care

_____

_____

2. Describe how government legislation aims to lower health care costs.

_____

_____

There are 10 possible points in this worksheet.

● WORKSHEET/ACTIVITY 3

On a sheet of paper, describe the purpose of the Health Plan Employer Data and Information Set (HEDIS). Use the Internet or other research materials to obtain a copy of the report. Identify the criteria used in the report.

There are 12 possible points in this worksheet/activity.

• WORKSHEET/ACTIVITY 4

A patient visits a doctor for her annual physical. Write a paragraph describing how she pays her bill to the health care provider and how her third-party payer is involved with her health insurance. Be sure to include the following terms in your paragraph:

- Co-payment
- Deductible
- Co-insurance
- Benefits
- Premium

Follow these guidelines when preparing your paragraph:

- Use 8.5-by-11-inch paper.
- Type, word-process, or write neatly in ink.
- Use correct spelling and grammar.
- Underline or highlight each term from the list above.

There are 20 possible points in this worksheet/activity.

• WORKSHEET 5

In the chart below, briefly summarize the main characteristics of each health-maintenance organization or provider.

Preferred Provider Organization	Medicaid	Medicare	Tricare

There are 8 possible points in this worksheet.

Cognitive Mapping Form

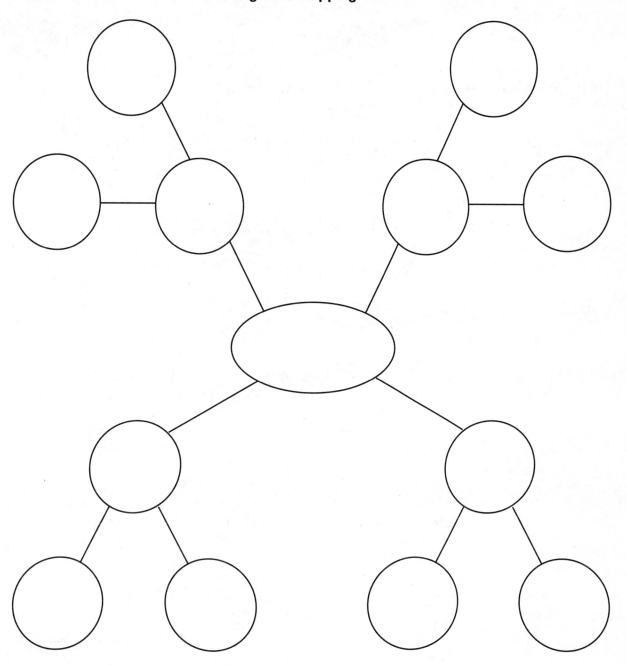

Chapter 3 Finding the Right Occupation for You

Career Search

• OBJECTIVES

When you have completed this section, you will be able to do the following:

- Define interests, values, and abilities.
- List five work-related values.
- Identify three resources for occupational research.
- Research three health careers.
- Explain the importance of a vocational portfolio.
- Complete an assignment addressing "What I Learned About Selecting a Career."

• DIRECTIONS

1. Read this section.
2. Complete Worksheets/Activities 1 and 2 as assigned.
3. Complete Worksheet 3 as assigned.
4. Complete Worksheets/Activities 4 through 6 as assigned.
5. Read the information about creating a Portfolio in Worksheet/Activity 7, then follow the instructions for beginning work on your Portfolio.
6. When you are confident that you can meet each objective listed above, ask your teacher for the section evaluation.

- ## EVALUATION METHODS
  - Worksheets/Activities
  - Class participation
  - Written report
  - Appearance and completeness of vocational portfolio
  - Written evaluation

- ## WORKSHEET/ACTIVITY 1

  Read the 10 values listed below. Think about each value, and decide which ones are most important to you.

  - *Job security.* Is it important that you find a job immediately upon the completion of your training program? How important is job availability?
  - *Leisure time.* Is it important for you to have extra time for leisure activities?
  - *Wages.* Is an average wage acceptable if you like your work, or do you require a very high wage?
  - *Recognition.* Is it important that the job you choose be respected by the people in your community?
  - *Creativity.* Do you like to come up with new ideas to solve problems, or do you prefer a job in which there is exactly one way to do things?
  - *Advancement.* Do you want a career that provides opportunities for promotion?
  - *Working environment.* Do you prefer to work indoors or outdoors?
  - *Home life.* Do you want to work a daytime schedule (9 A.M. to 5 P.M.), with some overtime and with weekends and holidays off, or are you willing to do shift work (all hours, any day of the week)?
  - *Responsibility.* Do you want a job that requires you to make a number of decisions?
  - *Management.* Do you want to be responsible for supervising the work of other people or for organizing many tasks at once?

  1. Think about each value and decide which values are most important to you. Put your most important value as 1, the next most important as 2, and the least important as 10.

  Original Values List

  1. _____
  2. _____
  3. _____
  4. _____
  5. _____
  6. _____
  7. _____
  8. _____
  9. _____
  10. _____

2. Use the following values grid to compare each pair of values in column A through I. Compare the value that you identified as 1 against the value that you identified as 2. Circle the number of the value that means more to you.

   Then compare value 1 against value 3, 1 against 4, and so on. Circle the important value in each pair. When you have completed column A, do the same with the other columns, using the grid.

Values Grid

Columns	A	B	C	D	E	F	G	H	I
	1 2								
	1 3	2 3							
	1 4	2 4	3 4						
	1 5	2 5	3 5	4 5					
	1 6	2 6	3 6	4 6	5 6				
	1 7	2 7	3 7	4 7	5 7	6 7			
	1 8	2 8	3 8	4 8	5 8	6 8	7 8		
	1 9	2 9	3 9	4 9	5 9	6 9	7 9	8 9	
	1 10	2 10	3 10	4 10	5 10	6 10	7 10	8 10	9 10

3. When you finish comparing your values, total the times you circled each number. Count the number of 1s, 2s, and 3s, and so on that are circled. Enter the totals for each value here.

   1.____ 2.____ 3.____ 4.____ 5.____ 6.____ 7.____ 8.____ 9.____ 10.____

4. Recopy your original list below.

5. Fill in the prioritized values list, beginning with the value that you circled most often.

6. Have your values changed? Are you surprised by the results? Knowing your work values will help you decide on a satisfying career.

Values

Original List	Prioritized List
1. _____	1. _____
2. _____	2. _____
3. _____	3. _____
4. _____	4. _____
5. _____	5. _____
6. _____	6. _____
7. _____	7. _____
8. _____	8. _____
9. _____	9. _____
10. _____	10. _____

There are 40 possible points in this worksheet/activity.

● WORKSHEET/ACTIVITY 2

From the following list, choose the 15 abilities that bring you the greatest satisfaction and that you would like to use in a job.

____ Accepting others

____ Adjusting things

____ Advising, coaching

____ Appreciating beauty

____ Arranging, scheduling

____ Assembling, producing

____ Assigning tasks

____ Assisting others to see themselves

____ Attention to detail

____ Budget preparation, financial planning

____ Building, constructing

____ Calculating

____ Cataloging

____ Clerical ability

____ Collecting things

____ Comparing

____ Compiling

____ Composing

____ Conveying warmth

____ Coordinating, organizing

____ Counseling

____ Creating products

____ Cultivating, growing

____ Curing, nursing

____ Decorating

____ Delegating responsibility

____ Demonstrating

____ Designing

____ Developing rapport, relationship building

____ Discovering, detecting

____ Distributing, delivering

____ Drafting, making layouts

____ Dramatizing, acting

____ Drawing, illustrating

____ Ear for languages, accents

____ Empathizing

____ Encouraging, raising others' self-esteem

____ Estimating

____ Evaluating

____ Experimenting, testing

____ Explaining

____ Finding shortcuts

____ Finger or manual dexterity

____ Generating ideas

____ Identifying, defining

____ Imagining, fantasizing

____ Influencing, persuading, selling

____ Informing, teaching, training

____ Installing

____ Lifting, pushing, balancing

____ Listening

____ Maintaining

____ Managing

____ Measuring

____ Mechanical reasoning

____ Memory for detail

____ Molding, shaping

____ Money management

____ Motivating

____ Musical ability

____ Numerical ability

____ Observing, examining, monitoring

____ Offering support, serving others

____ Operating tools or machinery

____ Ordering, purchasing

____ Organizing, putting in order

____ Organizing outdoor activities

____ Setting up equipment

____ Photography

____ Physical coordination, agility

____ Planning, developing programs, formulating ideas

____ Precision working

____ Preparing reports

____ Public speaking

____ Questioning

____ Record keeping

____ Rehabilitating	____ Supervising
____ Repairing, fixing	____ Taking inventory
____ Researching	____ Talking easily with strangers
____ Responding to feelings	____ Teamwork
____ Retrieving	____ Tending animals
____ Reviewing, screening	____ Transcribing
____ Risk taking	____ Troubleshooting
____ Sensitivity to others' needs	____ Verbal ability
____ Setting up equipment	____ Visualizing
____ Sports ability	____ Writing ability

There are 15 possible points in this worksheet/activity.

● WORKSHEET 3

Choose a career that interests you, and use Section 2 of this chapter in your textbook and other resources to answer the following questions (25 points).

- What is the name of the career?
- What type of work is done in this career?
- What personal qualities and abilities are needed for success in this career?
- What are the educational requirements? High school graduation? Four years of college?
- Is licensure, certification, or registration required?
- What are the working conditions?
- Are there advancement opportunities?
- What wages and benefits are usually offered?
- What is the job outlook for the future?
- Where can you get further information about the career?
- Are at least seven of the abilities you marked on Worksheet 2 needed for this career?

There are 25 possible points in this worksheet.

● WORKSHEET/ACTIVITY 4

Interview an employee who works in an occupation that interests you. You may do the interviews by phone, by mail, by e-mail, or in person. Make contact ahead of time to obtain consent for the interview. Here are some sample questions that you might ask (100 points).

- How did you select this occupation?
- What are the educational requirements?
- What are the opportunities for advancement?
- What do you like about your job?
- What are the hours? Do you have any control over your work schedule?
- Is there job security?
- Are you satisfied with the salary you receive?
- Is the job structured, or is there flexibility?
- Do you feel that you are respected in your position?
- What are your major responsibilities in the job?

There are 100 possible points in this worksheet/activity.

• WORKSHEET/ACTIVITY 5

Visit a career center or library, and answer the following questions on a separate sheet of paper (100 points).

1. What materials are available to help you learn about specific careers?

2. Use the Internet to research one career that interests you, and write a brief discussion of what you found out about the occupation.

There are 100 possible points in this worksheet/activity.

• WORKSHEET/ACTIVITY 6

Write a paper titled "What I Learned About Selecting a Career" (75 points). Include the following in your paper:

- How interests affect career choice.

- How abilities affect career choice.

- How work values affect career choice.

- What you have learned about your interests, abilities, and work values and how they will affect your career choice.

Follow these guidelines when preparing your report:

- Use 8.5-by-11-inch paper.

- Type, word-process, or write neatly in ink.

- Use correct spelling and grammar.

There are 75 possible points in this worksheet/activity.

• WORKSHEET/ACTIVITY 7

A portfolio contains documents that show your knowledge of a subject. A vocational portfolio shows the abilities, knowledge, and skills that you have learned in your vocational area. It is a valuable collection of documents that demonstrate to a possible employer the various skills you have gained and professional experiences you have had. You are responsible for putting your portfolio together in a professional manner.

Your portfolio should also include a private section that you use for valuable career hints. This section should be removed before the portfolio is given to others for review. You may use this section for tips to yourself and informal documentation of useful information.

Purpose of Your Portfolio

Your portfolio shows your mastery of the required knowledge, skills, and abilities in your vocational area. It is also a resource that enables you to provide possible employers, a college, or another training program with information about you. Once you have completed your portfolio, you will feel a sense of satisfaction in the work you have accomplished.

Complete the title page with the words "Vocational Portfolio" and your name. Place Worksheets 3 through 7 in your Vocational Portfolio (200 points).

There are 200 possible points in this worksheet/activity.

Section

3.2 Overview of Careers

● OBJECTIVES

When you have completed this section, you will be able to do the following:

- Define the key terms.

- Compare and differentiate the services performed by the therapeutic, diagnostic, information, and environmental services.

- Explain the meaning of therapeutic, diagnostic, information, and environmental services.

● DIRECTIONS

1. Complete Worksheet 1.

2. Read this section.

3. Complete Worksheets 2 and 3 as assigned.

4. Complete Worksheets/Activities 4 and 5.

5. Prepare responses to each item listed in the Chapter Review.

6. When you are confident that you can meet each objective listed above, ask your teacher for the section evaluation.

● EVALUATION METHOD

- Worksheets

- Class participation

- Written evaluation

● WORKSHEET 1

Fill in the crossword puzzle with the terms below (38 points).

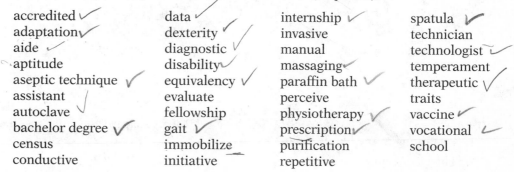

accredited   data   internship   spatula
adaptation   dexterity   invasive   technician
aide   diagnostic   manual   technologist
aptitude   disability   massaging   temperament
aseptic technique equivalency paraffin bath   therapeutic
assistant   evaluate   perceive   traits
autoclave   fellowship   physiotherapy   vaccine
bachelor degree gait   prescription   vocational
census   immobilize   purification   school
conductive   initiative   repetitive

Note: ▢ indicates a blank space between two words or at the end of a word.

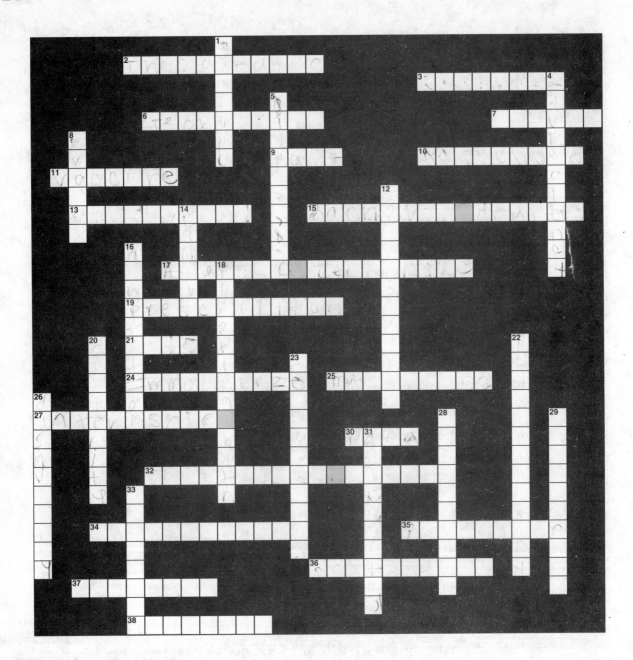

Clues

Across

2. Relating to the treatment of disease or injury.

3. Involving penetration of the body during a test.

6. Able to transfer electrical current.

7. Pertaining to the hand.

9. The way an individual walks.

10. A type of sterilizer.

11. A fluid that protects against a given disease.

13. A worker who is knowledgeable about the details of a particular job.

15. A degree given by a college or university after the successful completion of four years of study.

17. The method used to make the environment, the worker, and the patient as germ-free as possible.

19. A written direction for preparing and giving treatment.

21. An assistant or helper.

24. To cause a body part to be immovable.

25. The therapeutic rubbing, kneading, or stroking of the body.

27. A program in which students study with a professional to develop skills they have learned in a classroom.

30. The plural of datum.

32. A school that trains people with special aptitudes in specific trades or occupations.

34. The act of eliminating foreign or harmful elements.

35. An aide or a helper.

36. Taking the first step; thinking and acting without being told.

37. A natural or acquired talent or ability.

38. To examine, judge, appraise, or estimate.

Down

1. A knifelike tool with a broad, flat blade.

4. Equality in substance, degree, value, force, or meaning.

5. Relating to the determination of the nature of a disease or injury by examination.

8. The qualities one needs to be successful in a certain type of job.

12. A specialist in the study of a technical field.

14. The number of patients in a hospital.

16. A change or adjustment to meet a need.

18. A procedure involving a warm, waxy liquid that becomes hard as it cools; frequently used to ease the pain of arthritis in the hands.

20. Skill in using one's hands.

22. Physical therapy.

23. The traits or qualities of one's nature.

26. Limitation.

28. A scholarship or grant awarded to a graduate student in a college or university.

29. Repeating the same thing over and over.

31. Authorized, licensed, or certified.

33. To become aware of through any of the senses.

There are 38 possible points in this worksheet.

● WORKSHEET 2

Compare the services performed by the therapeutic, diagnostic, information, and environmental services (12 points).

Department	Service	Contribution to Team Goal for Patient
Example:		
Nursing	Therapeutic	Treats patient by performing procedures
_____	_____	_____
_____	_____	_____
_____	_____	_____

There are 12 possible points in this worksheet.

26

WORKSHEET 3

Identify one health occupation in each of the health services (diagnostic, therapeutic, information, and environmental), and explain why it is found in that service (16 points).

Occupation	Service	Duty
Example:		
Electrocardiography tech	Diagnostic	Tests to help determine the condition of the heart in order to make a diagnosis
1. _____	_____	_____
2. _____	_____	_____
3. _____	_____	_____
4. _____	_____	_____

There are 16 possible points in this worksheet.

WORKSHEET/ACTIVITY 4

Part A

Find the National Health Care Skills Standards. They can be located at the following Web site: http://www.wested.org/nhcssp/nhcss03.htm. Prepare a poster that summarizes the core and cluster standards. Select a core standard and prepare a brief oral presentation describing the knowledge and skills required for it.

Part B

Visit the States' Career Clusters Initiative (SCCI) Web site at http://www.careerclusters.org/. Identify and list the 16 major occupational categories. Discuss how the clusters can be helpful to both students and teachers.

There are 30 possible points in this worksheet/activity.

Ask your instructor to help you seek a job shadowing opportunity in one health occupation of your choice. Then, complete the job sharing contract after you are assigned a time, place, and person to shadow.

• WORKSHEET/ACTIVITY 5 JOB SHADOWING CONTRACT

Student Name: _____

Class Title: _____   **Time:** _____

Job Shadowing Assignment: _____

Street Address: _____

City: _____

Date(s): _____   **Time(s):** _____

Purpose: To observe a work setting in an occupational area of interest as part of the student decision-making process leading to vocational training.

Student Agrees to:
- Dress in clothes/uniform as described by the instructor.
- Communicate in an ethical, professional manner, reflecting the values described in Chapter 3 of this text.
- Be an interested observer, without interrupting the work process.

There are 25 possible points in this worksheet/activity.

Chapter **4** Employability and Leadership

Job-Seeking Skills

● OBJECTIVES

When you have completed this section, you will be able to do the following:

- Match key terms with their correct meanings.

- List seven places to seek employment opportunities and explain the benefits of each.

- Explain four ways to contact an employer.

- Name three occasions when a cover letter is used.

- List eight items required on a résumé.

- Identify seven items generally requested on a job application form.

- Write a cover letter and a résumé.

- Complete a job application.

- List five dos and five don'ts of job interviewing.

- Write a thank-you letter to a prospective employer.

● DIRECTIONS

1. Read this section.
2. Complete Worksheet 1.
3. Ask your teacher for directions to complete Worksheets/Activities 2 through 7.
4. When you are confident that you can meet each objective for this section, ask your teacher for the section evaluation.

- **EVALUATION METHODS**
  - Worksheets/Activities
  - Class participation
  - Mock interview
  - Vocational Portfolio

- **WORKSHEET 1**

  1. Explain why a vocational portfolio is important (5 points). _____

  2. List seven places to seek employment opportunities, and explain the benefits of each (14 points).

     a. _____

     b. _____

     c. _____

     d. _____

     e. _____

     f. _____

     g. _____

  3. List four ways to contact an employer (4 points).

     a. _____
     _____

     b. _____

     c. _____

     d. _____

  4. Name three occasions when a cover letter is used (3 points).

     a. _____

     b. _____

     c. _____

  5. List eight items required on a résumé (8 points).

     a. _____

     b. _____

     c. _____

     d. _____

     e. _____

     f. _____

     g. _____

     h. _____

6. Identify seven items generally requested on a job application form (7 points).

a. _____

b. _____

c. _____

d. _____

e. _____

f. _____

g. _____

There are 41 possible points in this worksheet.

• WORKSHEET/ACTIVITY 2

Write a cover letter following the guidelines in your text in Section 4.1, "Ways to Contact an Employer." Figure 4.2 is an example of a block letter format. See the Vocational Portfolio for additional examples.

- Use 8.5-by-11-inch paper.

- Type, word-process, or write with ink on one side only.

- Use correct grammar and spell correctly.

There are 100 possible points in this worksheet/activity:

- Format 5

- Spelling 10

- Neatness 10

- Grammar 25

- Composition 25

- Content 25

• WORKSHEET/ACTIVITY 3

Write a résumé following the guidelines in your text in Section 4.1, "Ways to Contact an Employer." Figure 4.3 is an example résumé.

- Use 8.5-by-11-inch paper.

- Type, word-process, or write with ink on one side only.

- Use correct grammar and spell correctly.

There are 100 possible points in this worksheet/activity:

- Format 5

- Spelling 10

- Neatness 10

- Grammar 25

- Composition 25

- Content 25

• WORKSHEET/ACTIVITY 4

Complete a job application provided by your teacher.

- Use a black pen.

- Fill in every line or answer every question.

- Spell correctly.

- Print neatly.

There are 75 possible points in this worksheet/activity:

- Spelling 25

- Neatness 25

- Completeness 25

• WORKSHEET/ACTIVITY 5

1. List five dos and five don'ts of job interviewing (10 points).

Dos	Don'ts
a. _____	_____
b. _____	_____
c. _____	_____
d. _____	_____
e. _____	_____

2. Participate in a mock interview. Be able to answer the following questions (10 points).

a. What do you enjoy about working in health care?

b. What are your strengths?

c. What are your weaknesses?

d. What would you do if the client started yelling at you and complaining about you?

e. As a health care worker, what is the most important part of your job?

f. Why do you want to work for [name of company]?

g. Is there any reason why you cannot be here on a regular basis?

h. The position requires lifting. Is there any reason why you cannot do it?

i. If you had an opportunity to go to the beach but were scheduled for work, what would you do?

j. This position requires weekend work. Is there any reason why you cannot work on weekends?

Class Critique of Mock Interview

Directions: Pretend you are interviewing a prospective employee for your own business. Answer the following questions, using your best judgment concerning the interviewee. Make a check next to Yes or No to indicate your answer.

1. Is the interviewee dressed appropriately?   Yes   No

2. Did the interviewee greet the interviewer by name?   Yes   No

3. Did the interviewee's handshake appear to be firm?   Yes   No

4. Did the interviewee wait for an invitation to be seated before sitting down?
   Yes   No

5. Did the interviewee's answers leave a question in your mind about
   truthfulness and sincerity?   Yes   No

   Helpful comments: _____

6. Did the interviewee show enthusiasm?   Yes   No

7. Was the interviewee prepared with good answers to each question?
   Yes   No

   If not, give examples. _____

8. What would you recommend the interviewee do differently for the next
   interview? _____

There are 20 possible points in this worksheet/activity.

● WORKSHEET/ACTIVITY 6

Compile corrected, perfectly typed or word-processed, well-formatted,
professional-looking documents that reflect the results of your own job search,
including a sample resume and cover letter to three different potential employers.

Your teacher will explain how you will be graded.

● WORKSHEET/ACTIVITY 7

Work with your teacher and the whole class to create a bulletin board with
classified advertising information.

Everyone in the class must bring in at least one ad from a classified newspaper,
a Web site, the Yellow Pages, or another regional advertising source, such as a
business journal.

Prepare a bulletin board with ad samples. Be sure to include employment
agencies, area hospitals, nursing homes, and medical offices.

Keep the board updated as you find new listings.

Each listing brought in will earn a point and participation in the preparation of
the board will earn points at the teacher's discretion.

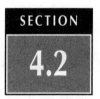

SECTION

4.2   Keeping a Job

● OBJECTIVES

When you have completed this section, you will be able to do the following:

- Match key terms with their correct meanings.

- List four employer responsibilities.

- List four responsibilities of a good employee.

34

• DIRECTIONS

1. Complete Worksheet 1 before beginning the reading.
2. Read this section.
3. Ask your teacher for directions to complete Worksheet/Activity 2.
4. When you are confident that you can meet each objective listed above, ask your teacher for the section evaluation.

• EVALUATION METHODS

- Worksheets/Activities
- Class participation
- Written evaluation

• WORKSHEET 1

1. List four employer responsibilities identified with the appropriate value (4 points).

   a. Dignity _____

   b. Excellence _____

   c. Service _____

   d. Fairness and Justice _____

2. List the responsibilities of a good employee identified with the appropriate value (11 points).

   - Dignity

     a. _____

     b. _____

     c. _____

   - Excellence

     a. _____

     b. _____

     c. _____

     d. _____

   - Service

     a. _____

     b. _____

   - Fairness and Justice

     a. _____

     b. _____

There are 15 possible points in this worksheet.

- **WORKSHEET 2**

  Write a one-or-two-page, double-spaced paper explaining what you consider your most important responsibility as an employee. Follow these guidelines when preparing your paper:

  - Use 8.5-by-11-inch paper.

  - Type, word-process, or write neatly in ink.

  - Use correct spelling and grammar.

  There are 100 possible points in this worksheet:

  - Format 5

  - Spelling 10

  - Neatness 10

  - Grammar 25

  - Composition 25

  - Content 25

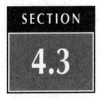

SECTION

4.3 Becoming a Professional Leader

- **OBJECTIVES**

  When you have completed this section, you will be able to do the following:

  - Match key terms with their correct meanings.

  - Name the three main benefits of being a member of a student health vocational organization.

  - Name six benefits of being a member of a professional organization.

  - Identify ways to find a professional organization.

  - Identify steps to becoming a leader.

  - Describe the goals and role of HOSA.

  - Summarize why you plan to participate in a student and professional organization.

- **DIRECTIONS**

  1. Complete Worksheet 1.

  2. Ask your teacher for directions to complete Worksheet/Activity 2.

  3. When you are confident that you can meet each objective for this section, ask your teacher for the section evaluation.

- **EVALUATION METHODS**

  - Worksheets/Activities

  - Class participation

  - Written evaluation

• WORKSHEET 1

1. Define the following terms (3 points).

a. Leadership _____

b. Priority_____

c. Extemporaneous _____

2. Name the three main benefits of being a member of a student health vocational organization (3 points).

a. _____

b. _____

c. _____

3. Name six benefits of being a member of a professional organization (5 points).

a. _____

b. _____

c. _____

d. _____

e. _____

f. _____

4. Identify six ways to find a professional organization (6 points).

a. _____

b. _____

c. _____

d. _____

e. _____

f. _____

5. Which of the following exhibit leadership qualities? Write an *X* in the appropriate spaces (5 points).

____ a. Coach	____ f. Clown	____ k. Police Officer
____ b. Enthusiast	____ g. Naysayer	____ l. Nurturer
____ c. Referee	____ h. Friend	____ m. Cheerleader
____ d. Gossip	____ i. Facilitator	____ n. Devil's advocate
____ e. Boss	____ j. Joiner	____ o. Zealot

There are 22 possible points in this worksheet.

• WORKSHEET/ACTIVITY 2

Summarize in a one-page, double-spaced paper why you plan to participate in student and professional organizations.

- Use 8.5-by-11-inch paper.
- Type, word-process, or write neatly in ink.
- Spell correctly.
- Use proper grammar.

There are 75 possible points in this worksheet:

- Spelling 10
- Neatness 10
- Grammar 28
- Composition 27

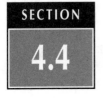

SECTION 4.4

Professional Development

• OBJECTIVES

When you have completed this section, you will be able to do the following:

- Match key terms with their correct meanings.
- Explain the importance of maintaining professional competency.
- List five reasons why professionals need to learn and grow.
- Describe five resources for professional development.
- Explain how to research a health science career path,
- List the important features to research about each career.
- Explain how to revise a career plan.
- List three reasons people change careers.

• DIRECTIONS

1. Complete Worksheet 1 and 2 as assigned.
2. Complete Worksheets/Activities 3 and 4.
3. When you are confident that you can meet each objective for this section, as your teacher for the section evaluation.

• EVALUATION METHODS

- Worksheets/Activities
- Class participation
- Written evaluation

• WORKSHEET 1

Choose from the following terms to complete each sentence. (4 points)

accredited

career plan

mentor

professional development

1. A _____ is an experienced person who can offer advice and guidance.

2. _____ is education for people who have already begun their careers to help them continue to grow.

3. A program is _____ if it has been approved and recognized by a governing body.

4. You have a _____ if you have a strategy for a growth as a professional.

There are 4 possible points in this worksheet.

• WORKSHEET 2

Think about the importance of maintaining professional competency. Consider what this means to you.

1. List five reasons why a professional needs to learn and grow.

   a. _____

   b. _____

   c. _____

   d. _____

   e. _____

2. List five resources for professional development.

   a. _____

   b. _____

   c. _____

   d. _____

   e. _____

There are 20 possible points in this worksheet.

● WORKSHEET/ACTIVITY 3

Select a health science career path. (You may wish to look back at Chapter 3 for ideas.) Use various resources to research the career path you selected.

Write a one-page, double-spaced paper naming the career you selected and describing the features you researched. Explain why you considered those features to be important. Describe the methods you used to research the career path. Tell how and why you might revise your career plan over time.

- Use 8.5-by-11-inch paper.

- Type, word-process, or write neatly in ink.

- Spell correctly.

- Use proper grammar.

There are 75 possible points in this worksheet:

- Spelling 10

- Neatness 10

- Grammar 28

- Composition 27

● WORKSHEET/ACTIVITY 4

Work with another student. Pretend that you are an employee and your partner is a career counselor. Have a discussion in which you explain the reasons why you have decided to change your career path. The "counselor" should describe other reasons why people change careers. Explain how you plan to go about changing your career path.

There are 25 possible points in this worksheet.

Chapter 5 Understanding Legal Obligations

5.1 Understanding the Patient's Rights

• OBJECTIVES

When you have completed this section, you will be able to do the following:

- Explain the importance of the Patient's/Client's Bill of Rights.
- Understand the rights to which a patient is entitled.
- Measure the rights of the patient against the needs of the health care facility.
- Understand the responsibilities of the patient in the health care process.

• DIRECTIONS

1. Complete Worksheet 1.
2. Read the section.
3. Complete Worksheets 2, 3, and 4.
4. When you are confident that you can meet each objective listed above, ask your teacher for the section evaluation.

• EVALUATION METHODS

- Worksheets/Activities
- Class participation
- Written evaluation

● WORKSHEET 1

Define each of the following terms in your own words. Then use each term in a complete sentence. (10 points)

1. living will

_____

_____

2. durable power of attorney

_____

_____

_____

3. continuity of care

_____

_____

_____

There are 10 possible points in this worksheet.

● WORKSHEET 2

1. Explain the importance of the Patient's/Client's Bill of Rights (5 points).

_____

_____

_____

2. Answer the following questions, using the Bill of Rights as your guide.

a. Mrs. Rodriguez is admitted to the hospital and told that he requires a surgical procedure. He was unconscious during examination and wants to know the doctor who performed it and her qualifications. The doctor prefers not to interact with patients. What will you do, and why (5 points)?

_____

_____

_____

b. Mr. McDonnell wants you to mail a letter to his family for him. Your supervisor tells you to read the letter before you send it because she doesn't want him to complain. What will you do, and why (5 points)?

_____

_____

_____

There are 15 possible points in this worksheet.

● WORKSHEET 3

In a well-developed paragraph, explain the significance of the Omnibus Budget Reconciliation Act of 1987. Tell how the Resident's Bill of Rights is similar to and different from the Patient's Bill of Rights.

There are 25 possible points in this worksheet.

● WORKSHEET 4

A patient is meeting with a physician to discuss a possible treatment for an injury. List and describe three responsibilities of the patient.

There are 15 possible points in this worksheet.

SECTION

5.2

Understanding Your Legal Responsibilities

● OBJECTIVES

When you have completed this section, you will be able to do the following:

- Match key terms with their correct meanings.
- Explain why understanding legal responsibilities is important.
- Explain the importance of licensure, certification, and registration in helping improve quality health care.
- Summarize the importance of confidentiality in health care.
- Identify a law that helps ensure the confidentiality of medical information.
- Identify resources that can help you report illegal or unethical behavior.
- Understand elements of a contract.
- Explain the role of natural death guidelines and declarations.
- Describe the purpose and types of advance directives.

● DIRECTIONS

1. Complete Worksheet 1 after reading the section.
2. Complete Worksheets/Activities 2 and 3.
3. Ask your teacher for directions to complete Worksheets 4 through 6.
4. When you are confident that you can meet each objective listed above, ask your teacher for the section evaluation.

● EVALUATION METHODS

- Worksheets/Activities
- Class participation
- Written evaluation

• WORKSHEET 1

Match each term in Column A to the correct definition in Column B.

A

_____ agent

_____ certification

_____ contract

_____ directive

_____ exempt

_____ expressed contract

_____ implied contract

_____ licensure

_____ ombudsman

_____ recognition

_____ registration

_____ relevant

B

a. A social worker, nurse, or trained volunteer who ensures that patients are properly cared for and respected.

b. The quality of being acknowledged or seen.

c. An agreement in which some of the terms are not expressed in words.

d. A process by which a person is made able to do a job, and recognized as such.

e. A list of individuals on an official record who meet the qualifications for an occupation.

f. Pertaining to, or having to do with, the patient/client.

g. A person or business authorized to act on another's behalf.

h. A legal documents that is often used to define the terms of patient care.

i. An agreement in which the terms are presented in written form.

j. Something that serves to guide or impel towards an action or goal.

k. A process by which a governmental authority gives permission to a person or health care organization to operate or to work in a profession.

l. To be free or released from some liability or requirement to which others are subject.

There are 12 possible points in this worksheet.

• WORKSHEET/ACTIVITY 2

Work with a partner. Together discuss why it is important for health care workers to understand legal responsibilities. Refer to the Patient's/Client's Bill of Rights in Section 5.1 if necessary.

There are 10 possible points in this worksheet/activity.

• WORKSHEET/ACTIVITY 3

Discuss how licensure, certification, and registration help improve the quality of health care. Think about the importance of verifying this information. Interview someone from a local hospital or other healthcare facility. Before you contact the person, write a list of questions you might ask about the importance of these systems and the need to verify such information. Share your findings.

There are 25 possible points in this worksheet/activity.

● **WORKSHEET 4**

Read each of the following situations and answer the questions that follow.

1. Your day has been busy and you are short on time. You run into a coworker in an elevator and decide to quickly discuss Mrs. Henderson's hysterectomy scheduled for the following day. How might this compromise confidentiality (5 points)?

_____

_____

2. A 65-year-old man has a heart attack and is admitted to the hospital with a poor prognosis. He asks you not to share his medical information with his wife because he thinks she will be overwhelmed by the news. His wife then sees you in the hall and asks about her husband's prognosis. Should you tell her (5 points)?

_____

_____

3. A mentally ill woman is admitted to the hospital with a severe injury. While you are changing the bandages, she tells you that she plans to kill her ex-boyfriend when she is released. She tells you that you cannot tell anyone. What should you do (5 points)?

_____

_____

There are 15 possible points in this worksheet.

● **WORKSHEET 5**

List four kinds of information that are protected by HIPPA.

1. _____
2. _____
3. _____
4. _____

There are 8 possible points in this worksheet.

● **WORKSHEET 6**

1. Explain what natural death guidelines and declarations do (5 points).

_____

_____

2. Describe the purpose of an advance directive and name two forms of advance directives (8 points).

_____

_____

_____

3. Define living will (2 points). _____

There are 15 possible points in this worksheet.

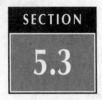

SECTION 5.3   Medical Liability

- ● **OBJECTIVES**

    When you have completed this section, you will be able to do the following:

    - Match key terms with their correct meanings.

    - Explain the difference between civil law and criminal law.

    - Explain medical liability.

    - Explain medical malpractice.

    - List six common categories of medical malpractice.

    - Provide examples of behaviors that are infractions of medical torts.

- ● **DIRECTIONS**

    1. Complete Worksheet 1.

    2. Read the section.

    3. Complete Worksheet 2 and 3.

    4. Ask your teacher for directions to complete Worksheet/Activity 4.

    5. When you are confident that you can meet each objective for this section, ask your teacher for the section evaluation.

    6. Prepare responses to each item listed in Chapter Review.

- ● **EVALUATION METHODS**

    - Worksheets/Activities

    - Class participation

    - Written evaluation

- ● **WORKSHEET 1**

    Write each word listed below in the space next to the statement that best defines it (20 points).

Defamatory	Misrepresentations
Diagnosis	Obligation
Informed consent	Prudent
Liable	Resultant
Malpractice	Tort

    _____ a. Failure of a professional person, as a physician, to render proper services through reprehensible ignorance or negligence or through criminal intent, especially when injury or loss follows.

    _____ b. An event that is caused by some action.

_____ c. Untruths; lies.

_____ d. Under civil law, a wrong committed by one person against another.

_____ e. Does what a reasonable and careful person who do in the specific situation.

_____ f. The legal condition in which a person agrees to something, after he or she understands all the facts and implications of an action or event.

_____ g. Moral responsibility.

_____ h. The identification of a medical condition.

_____ i. A statement that causes injury to another's reputation.

_____ j. Legally responsible.

There are 20 possible points for this worksheet.

• WORKSHEET 2

Explain the difference between civil law and criminal law. Give an example of a health care situation that would fall into each category. (10 points)

_____

_____

_____

_____

There are 10 possible points for this worksheet.

• WORKSHEET 3

1. Explain medical liability (2 points)

_____

2. Explain medical malpractice (2 points)

_____

3. List six common categories of medical malpractice (6 points).

_____

_____

_____

_____

_____

_____

There are 10 possible points in this worksheet.

● WORKSHEET/ACTIVITY 4

Select one of the following terms:

Libel	Reportable conditions
Slander	Negligence
False imprisonment	Reasonable care
Invasion of privacy	Sexual harassment

Research examples related to the term from the healthcare industry. Select and describe the example. Challenge your classmates to identify the term you selected.

There are 20 possible points in this worksheet/activity.

Chapter **6** Medical Ethics

Ethical Roles and Responsibilities of a Health Care Worker

- **OBJECTIVES**

    When you have completed this section, you will be able to do the following:

    - Match key terms with their correct meanings.
    - Summarize the code of ethics that every health care worker follows.
    - Explain why following a code of ethics is important.
    - Use the value indicators to explain the employee's responsibilities to his or her employer.
    - Explain how each health care worker affects the health care team.
    - Demonstrate communication objectives that promote patient satisfaction.

- **DIRECTIONS**

    1. Complete Worksheets 1 and 2 as assigned.
    2. Your teacher will provide you with directions to complete Worksheet/Activity 3.
    3. Complete Worksheets 4 and 5 as assigned.
    4. When you are confident that you can meet each objective listed above, ask your teacher for the section evaluation.

- **EVALUATION METHODS**

    - Worksheets/Activities
    - Class participation in Activities
    - Role play
    - Written evaluation

• WORKSHEET 1

Write each word listed below in the space next to the statement that best defines it. Some words may be used more than once (10 points).

appropriate   ethics   project (verb)
confidential   justice   responsibility

_____ 1. Private, restricted, secret.

_____ 2. Treating others with fairness.

_____ 3. Told in trust that it will not be repeated.

_____ 4. To display or show.

_____ 5. Rules of conduct of a given profession.

_____ 6. One's answerability to an employer in areas such as dependability and honesty.

_____ 7. To give off an attitude

_____ 8. A code of conduct representing ideal behavior for a group of people.

_____ 9. Suitable.

_____ 10. Correct.

There are 10 possible points in this worksheet.

• WORKSHEET 2

There are many ways to express the values discussed in this section. Explain in your own words and expand the value indicators identified in the Code of Ethics (Table 6.1) to describe attitudes and actions that are not mentioned in the text (24 points). Be prepared to share your answers in class.

1. Dignity

_____

_____

_____

2. Service

_____

_____

_____

3. Excellence

_____

_____

_____

4. Fairness/Justice

_____

_____

_____

Explain in your own words and expand the value indicators identified in Table 6.2, Responsibilities of an Employee, to describe attitudes and actions that are not mentioned in the text.

5. Dignity

_____
_____
_____

6. Service

_____
_____
_____

7. Excellence

_____
_____
_____

8. Fairness/Justice

_____
_____
_____

There are 24 possible points in this worksheet.

• WORKSHEET/ACTIVITY 3

Your teacher will give you a role to play. Working with three other students, develop a skit from the information your teacher gives you. Show the right way and the wrong way to respond to the situation in the role-play. Ask the class to tell you what values or code of ethics you are representing (25 points).

There are 25 possible points in this worksheet/activity.

• WORKSHEET 4

Summarize the code of ethics that every health care worker follows (12 points).

_____
_____
_____
_____
_____
_____

There are 12 possible points in this worksheet.

• WORKSHEET 5

Write each word or phrase listed below in the space next to the statement that best illustrates it (6 points).

attitude   grooming   rules and regulations
dependability   honesty   team concept

_____ **1.** No gum chewing allowed; cleanliness required.

_____ **2.** Every worker doing his or her part to care for patients.

_____ **3.** Doing your job to the best of your ability.

_____ **4.** Willingness to do a good job; always being positive.

_____ **5.** Never saying you have completed a task when you have not.

_____ **6.** Following the policy and procedure manual.

7. Explain how each health care worker affects the health care team (6 points).

_____

_____

_____

_____

_____

_____

There are 12 possible points in this worksheet.

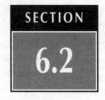

SECTION 6.2
Recognizing and Reporting Illegal and Unethical Behavior

• OBJECTIVES

When you have completed this section, you will be able to do the following:

- Match key terms with their correct meanings.
- Explain the importance of reporting illegal and unethical incidents.
- Identify three expectations of every employee, regarding the treatment of others.
- Identify three resources that can help you report illegal or unethical behavior.

• DIRECTIONS

1. Complete Worksheets 1 and 3 as assigned.
2. Complete Worksheets/Activities 2 and 4 as assigned.
3. When you are confident that you can meet each objective listed above, ask your teacher for the section evaluation.
4. Prepare responses to each item listed in Chapter Review.

● EVALUATION METHODS

- ■ Worksheets/Activities
- ■ Class participation in Activities
- ■ Written evaluation

● WORKSHEET 1

Circle the letter of the best answer.

1. What does it mean to *recognize* that a negative incident has occurred?

    a. You correct it.

    b. You observe it.

    c. You cause it.

    d. You report it.

2. How does a person feel if they are being *harassed*?

    a. Annoyed

    b. Helped.

    c. Pleased.

    d. Thankful.

3. To *report* an incident means to

    a. cover it up.

    b. cause it.

    c. tell someone about it.

    d. think about it.

4. An *illegal* action is one that is

    a. helpful to another person.

    b. considered ethical behavior.

    c. outlined in an employee manual.

    d. prohibited by law.

There are 8 possible points in this worksheet.

● WORKSHEET/ACTIVITY 2

Describe an example that supports the following statement:

It is important to report illegal and unethical incidents.

Explain how reporting the incident protects people.

There are 12 possible points in this worksheet.

• WORKSHEET 3

List three expectations of every employee, regarding the treatment of others.

1. _____

2. _____

3. _____

List three resources that can help you report illegal or unethical behavior.

4. _____

5. _____

6. _____

There are 12 possible points in this worksheet.

• WORKSHEET/ACTIVITY 4

Reporting incidents can sometimes be difficult. Work with a partner to discuss the following case studies.

1. You and a friend attended nursing school together. You share an apartment near your place of employment. One day, you happen to notice that your friend is rushing to measure doses of medicine. As a result, some patients receive an incorrect dosage. Discuss your ethical responsibility as well as your loyalty to your friend.

2. While collecting medicine for a patient, you observe a coworker placing pain medication from the hospital pharmacy in his pocket. When you confront him, he explains that he has an old knee injury and does not have time to have it checked out. Discuss what course of action you should take.

3. You have developed a great working relationship with a doctor at your health care facility. Your communication is always professional and productive. However, the doctor does not have the same relationship with another co-worker. The doctor constantly speaks to your co-worker in a critical and demeaning manner. You do not want to hurt your relationship with the doctor, but you have observed the harassment on many occasions. Discuss how you should handle this situation.

There are 25 possible points in this worksheet/activity.

Chapter **7** Wellness

7.1 Holistic Health

- **OBJECTIVES**

  When you have completed this section, you will be able to do the following:

  - Match key terms with their correct meaning.
  - List three parts of holistic health.
  - Explain wellness and preventive care.
  - Compare holistic health to disease oriented care.

- **DIRECTIONS**

  1. Complete vocabulary Worksheet 1.
  2. Read this section.
  3. Complete Worksheets 2 and 3 as assigned.
  4. When you are confident that you can meet each objective for this section, ask your teacher for the section evaluation.

- **EVALUATION METHODS**

  - Worksheets
  - Class participation
  - Written evaluation

- **WORKSHEET 1**

  Define the following vocabulary words (5 points).

  1. Holistic _____
  2. Infirmity _____
  3. Elimination _____

4. Aerobic _____

5. Self-esteem _____

There are 5 possible points in this worksheet.

● WORKSHEET 2

1. List five ways to achieve physical fitness (5 points).

a. _____

b. _____

c. _____

d. _____

e. _____

2. Mental fitness allows us to _____ effectively and feel balanced (1 point).

3. Spiritual fitness allows us to experience (a) _____ and (b) _____ in life (2 points).

4. Explain wellness and preventive care (3 points). _____

5. List three parts of holistic health (3 points).

a. _____

b. _____

c. _____

There are 14 possible points in this worksheet.

● WORKSHEET 3

1. Choose one thing about yourself that you want to improve—for example, physical fitness, social skills, or self-esteem.

2. Begin a journal, and write in it every day. For example, if you decide to exercise more, include the following:

- How you feel about exercising
- If you skip a day, why
- Whether you feel good about yourself when you exercise
- Any observations that you feel are important

3. Set a goal—for example, to do 20 abdominal crunches.

4. Develop a plan to reach your goal. For example, "During the next month, I will do abdominal crunches every day, starting with one the first day and adding one more each day until I can do 20."

5. Reward yourself when you reach the halfway mark and when you reach your goal. For example, buy a new pair of workout shorts when you can do 10 crunches.

6. When you have reached your goal, write a one-page paper describing how the experience has affected you. Answer the following in your paper:

- Does keeping a journal help you follow the necessary steps to reach your goal?
- Is it easier to work toward a goal when you have a plan?
- If you did not reach your goal, what happened?

Include any additional observations you have about this exercise.

There are 50 possible points in this worksheet.

Sample Plan to Achieve a Goal

Goal: To be able to do 20 abdominal crunches daily in one month.

Plan: Begin with one crunch and add one additional crunch each day.

MONTH	DAY	TIME	NO. OF CRUNCHES	REWARD
May	1	9 A.M.	1	
	10	9 A.M.	11	Buy new shorts
	30	8 P.M.	30	Weekend vacation

SECTION 7.2 Understanding Human Needs

● OBJECTIVES

When you have completed this section, you will be able to do the following:

- Match key terms with their correct meanings.
- Name four physiological needs that must be met to maintain stability.
- Name four psychological needs that must be met to maintain stability.
- Explain five benefits of pet-facilitated therapy.
- Match five defense mechanisms with the correct descriptions.
- Explain how you use defense mechanisms daily.

● DIRECTIONS

1. Complete vocabulary Worksheet 1.
2. Read this section.
3. Complete Worksheets/Activities 2 and 3 as assigned.
4. Complete Worksheets 4 and 5.
5. Ask your teacher for directions to complete Worksheet/Activity 6.
6. When you are confident that you can meet each objective for this section, ask your student for the section evaluation.

● EVALUATION METHODS

- Worksheets/Activities
- Class participation
- Written report
- Written evaluation

• WORKSHEET 1

Define the following terms (16 points).

1. Idolizing _____
2. Rapport _____
3. Sensory _____
4. Anxiety_____
5. Impaired _____
6. Aggressiveness _____
7. Friction _____
8. Procedures _____
9. Psychological _____
10. Stability_____
11. Recognition _____
12. Physiological _____
13. Hostility_____
14. Therapies_____
15. Frustration _____
16. Value_____

There are 16 possible points in this worksheet.

• WORKSHEET/ACTIVITY 2

Go to the library, and research Maslow's hierarchy. Write a paper with the following information (250 points):

- Who is Maslow?
- What is his hierarchy?
- Why is it important to understand Maslow's hierarchy as an individual? As a health care worker?

Follow these guidelines when preparing your report:

- Use 8.5-by-11-inch paper.
- Type, word-process, or write neatly in ink.
- Use correct spelling and grammar.

There are 250 possible points in this worksheet/activity.

• WORKSHEET/ACTIVITY 3

In a small group of students, discuss the following questions. Use this worksheet to take notes, and be prepared to participate in a class discussion (100 points).

1. How are patients' needs affected when they require medical tests or are ill or injured? Give at least three examples that are not in the text. _____
2. How are your needs met at home, in school, and in the workplace? _____
3. What are the benefits of having a pet in the home or taking a pet to visit in a long-term care facility? Do you think this is a good idea? Why? _____

There are 100 possible points in this worksheet/activity.

● WORKSHEET 4

1. Name four physiological needs that must be met to maintain stability (4 points).

   a. _____

   b. _____

   c. _____

   d. _____

2. Name the four biological needs that maintain life (4 points).

   a. _____

   b. _____

   c. _____

   d. _____

3. Name four psychological needs that must be met to maintain stability (4 points).

   a. _____

   b. _____

   c. _____

   d. _____

4. List the five physical changes that occur with pet-facilitated therapy (5 points).

   a. _____

   b. _____

   c. _____

   d. _____

   e. _____

There are 17 possible points in this worksheet.

● WORKSHEET 5

1. Write each defense mechanism listed below in the space next to the statement that best illustrates it (5 points).

   identification   projection   rationalization
   compensation   sublimation

   _____ a. Mary arranges her hair exactly as her favorite teacher does.

   _____ b. I couldn't afford the dress, but I bought it because it will cost more tomorrow.

   _____ c. Jim's dad yells at him, and Jim gets really mad at you.

   _____ d. Jerry took his anger out on the basketball.

   _____ e. I wanted to play the piano but didn't do well, but I did do outstanding work in biology.

2. Mark each of the following statements *T* for true or *F* for false (7 points).

_____ a. Understanding defense mechanisms helps you to understand behavior.

_____ b. Many people do not use defense mechanisms.

_____ c. As a health care worker, it is important to realize that people use defense mechanisms to protect themselves.

_____ d. If all psychological needs are met, you can assume that all physiological needs have also been met.

_____ e. When individuals enter the hospital, they experience a change in routine.

_____ f. Studies show that pets do not have an effect on the body.

_____ g. Hospitals are only one place where pet-facilitated therapy is being used.

3. Mr. Levine is going for surgery in the morning. He is frightened and thinks that he may die. What basic need is threatened (1 point)? _____

4. Mrs. White is an elderly lady who lives alone. Her daughter found her very confused. She had not had anything to eat or drink for two days. What basic need does this represent (1 point)? _____

5. Ms. Garcia had a stroke one year ago. She is unable to read, taste, or hear well. She also has severe loss of sensation in her hands. What basic need is threatened (1 point)? _____

6. Mr. Desqi has a severe droop in his left eyelid and stutters. People always look at him and have trouble understanding him. He was a public speaker before this happened. What basic need is threatened (1 point)?_____

7. Mary Kandel's small daughter has asthma and is in the hospital. Mary has several children at home and feels torn about where she should spend her time. Everything feels out of control. What basic need is threatened (1 point)? _____

There are 17 possible points in this worksheet.

● WORKSHEET/ACTIVITY 6

In a small group of students, develop a role-play that represents the defense mechanism your teacher assigns you. Present the role-play to the class, and ask your classmates to guess which defense mechanism you are demonstrating (150 points).

There are 150 possible points in this worksheet/activity.

7.3 Cross-Cultural Terms and Principles

● OBJECTIVES

When you have completed this section, you will be able to do the following:

- Explain how culture influences behavior.

- Identify culturally acceptable and effective gestures, terms, and behaviors.

- Recognize communication techniques that create a positive exchange of information.

- Identify common folk medicine practices.

- Compare and contrast cultural differences.

- Explain how understanding cultural beliefs affects you as a health care worker.

● DIRECTIONS

1. Read this section.

2. Complete Worksheets/Activities 1 and 2 as assigned.

3. Complete Worksheets 3 and 4 as assigned.

4. Complete Worksheet/Activity 5 and Worksheet 6.

5. When you are confident that you can meet each objective for this section, ask your teacher for the section evaluation.

● EVALUATION METHODS

- Worksheets/Activities

- Class participation

- Written report

- Verbal report

- Written evaluation

● WORKSHEET/ACTIVITY 1

Your teacher has placed sheets of paper on the walls. The sheets are labeled with the names of different cultures. Walk around the room, and write on each sheet something that you have heard or believe about each culture. Discuss the students' beliefs about these cultures. Are they true? Is it possible to make assumptions about a person based on his or her culture?

There are 25 possible points in this worksheet/activity.

62

• WORKSHEET/ACTIVITY 2

Work in teams of four to research a culture of your choice (50 points).

1. Use National Geographic, the Internet, or other resources for your research.

2. As a team, decide each team member's responsibility.

3. Include the following in your report:

- Language
- Religious beliefs
- Medical practices
- Feasts and celebrations
- Costumes

4. Prepare a 10-minute presentation about the culture that your group researched. Present it to the class.

There are 50 possible points in this worksheet/activity.

• WORKSHEET 3

1. Write each culture listed below in the space next to the relevant statement. Use only those that apply. Some cultures may be used more than once (6 points).

Cambodian	Anglo-American	Vietnamese
African-American	Navajo	Japanese
Southeast Persian	Mexican-American	Laotian

_____ a. This culture only allows a parent to touch the head of a child.

_____ b. This culture only allows the elderly to touch the head of a child.

_____ c. The people of this culture avoid eye contact as a form of respect.

_____ d. The people of this culture use peripheral vision instead of direct eye contact.

_____ e. In this culture, people do not shake hands in greeting.

_____ f. In this culture, people greet one another with a salute.

2. Mark each of the following cultures with an *X* if it is a close-contact culture or an *O* if it is a more-distant culture (9 points).

_____ a. Latin American

_____ b. American

_____ c. Canadian

_____ d. Mediterranean

_____ e. Northern European

_____ f. African

_____ g. Southern European

_____ h. English

_____ i. Indonesian

There are 15 possible points in this worksheet.

• WORKSHEET 4

1. Which of the following statements help develop positive opinions about other cultures? Mark each statement *T* for true if it helps or *F* for false if it does not help (10 points).

    _____ a. Keep an open mind.

    _____ b. Take only the opinion of a trusted friend.

    _____ c. One piece of information about a specific culture is enough to form a true opinion.

    _____ d. Your behavior sends a message to others.

    _____ e. When more than one culture is present, the definition of a behavior is often different.

    _____ f. Health care workers do not need to adapt their behavior when working with people of another culture.

    _____ g. Behavior is developed by people, places, and experiences.

    _____ h. Prejudices are difficult to form.

    _____ i. Voice tones cause positive or negative reactions.

    _____ j. Adapting your voice when speaking to others who are learning English will make them feel uneasy.

2. Write each culture listed below in the space next to the relevant statement about folk medicine. Some cultures may be used more than once (10 points).

    Armenian   Koreans   Iranian

    Chinese   Hmong and Mien Tribes   Vietnamese

    Cambodian   Native American Indian Central and South American

    _____ a. Cupping is used to relieve head pain.

    _____ b. One week after a baby is born, the mother is given a party.

    _____ c. Acupuncture is practiced.

    _____ d. The color white is a sign of bad luck.

    _____ e. Spiritual ceremonies are performed to please the spirits that cause illness.

    _____ f. The "evil eye" is believed to cause sudden illness.

    _____ g. Menstruating women are afraid to get their heads wet.

    _____ h. Poor health is accepted in a spirit of fatalism.

    _____ i. Shamen are sometimes called to remove pain.

    _____ j. Coining is used to relieve pain.

3. Choose two cultures and compare and contrast cultural differences (50 points).

There are 70 possible points in this worksheet.

● WORKSHEET/ACTIVITY 5

Write a one-paragraph paper explaining how understanding cultural beliefs affects you as a health care worker (200 points). Follow these guidelines when preparing your report:

- Use 8.5-by-11-inch paper.
- Type, word-process, or write neatly in ink.
- Use correct spelling and grammar.

There are 200 possible points in this worksheet/activity.

● WORKSHEET/ACTIVITY 6

Conduct an Internet search for information on one or more topics covered in Chapter 7 related to wellness and meeting your needs and the needs of others. For example:

- Language, religion, medical practices, or feasts and celebrations of any culture or nationality
- Nutrition
- Exercise
- Biofeedback

When you have identified some good information, print it out for your portfolio. Prepare a brief, one-paragraph explanation of why you chose to print out and keep the information you did. Why did you consider that Web site a trustworthy source of information? Why did you think other Web sites were not so good? Be prepared to explain to your classmates your thoughts on doing research on the Internet.

There are 100 possible points in this worksheet/activity.

Chapter **8** Teamwork

SECTION

8.1 Teamwork

• OBJECTIVES

When you have completed this section, you will be able to do the following:

- Match key terms with their correct meanings.
- Identify types of health care teams.
- Explain how a team builds cohesiveness and productivity.
- Recognize characteristics of effective teams.
- Explain the roles and responsibilities of team members.
- Recognize underlying factors and situations that may lead to conflict.
- Apply verbal and nonverbal communication skills in a team setting.
- Apply conflict resolution strategies in a team setting.

• DIRECTIONS

1. Complete Worksheets 1 and 2 as assigned.
2. Ask your teacher for directions to complete Worksheets/Activities 3 and 4.
3. Complete Worksheets/Activities 5 and 6.
4. When you are confident that you can meet each objective for this section, ask your teacher for the section evaluation.
5. Prepare responses to each item listed in Chapter Review.

● EVALUATION METHODS

- Worksheets/Activities
- Class participation in Activities
- Role play
- Written evaluation

● WORKSHEET 1

Match each of the definitions in Column B to the correct term in Column A.

A

_____ **1.** feedback

_____ **2.** interdisciplinary

_____ **3.** dynamics

_____ **4.** mission statement

_____ **5.** goals

_____ **6.** cohesiveness

_____ **7.** facilitator

_____ **8.** task

_____ **9.** compromise

_____ **10.** prioritize

_____ **11.** productivity

_____ **12.** interdependent

_____ **13.** discipline

_____ **14.** teamwork

_____ **15.** conflict

_____ **16.** delegate

_____ **17.** role

_____ **18.** collaborate

B

a. Motivating or driving forces.

b. Cooperative effort from a group of people working together for a common purpose.

c. The power to reach goals and get results.

d. Involving two or more subject areas.

e. A function to be performed; job.

f. To work together.

g. Aims, purposes, or intentions.

h. A branch of instruction or learning, such as cardiology.

i. State of being well-integrated or unified.

j. A contradiction, fight, or disagreement.

k. Information received as a result of something done or said.

l. To give another person responsibility for doing specific task.

m. A position, responsibility, or duty.

n. A settlement of differences between parties by each party agreeing to give up something that it wants.

o. Depending on each other.

p. A summary describing the aims, values, and overall plan of an organization or individual.

q. To arrange or deal with in the order of importance.

r. A person responsible for leading or coordinating a group.

There are 18 possible points in this worksheet.

● WORKSHEET 2

1. List and define the five rights of delegation (20 points).

a. Right_____

b. Right_____

c. Right_____

d. Right_____

e. Right_____

2. Briefly describe each of the following types of health care teams (20 points):

a. Ad hoc group

_____

_____

b. Nominal care group

_____

_____

c. Unidisciplinary group

_____

_____

d. Multidisciplinary team

_____

_____

e. Interdisciplinary team

_____

_____

There are 40 possible points in this worksheet.

● WORKSHEET/ACTIVITY 3

Plan an interview with a member or several members of a health care team at a local nursing home facility. Before your interview, write a list of at least 10 questions you will ask. Consider such concepts as the organization of the team, the goals they strive to achieve, as well as the procedures they have in place to increase productivity and avoid conflict.

1. _____

2. _____

3. _____

4. _____

5. _____

68

6. _____

7. _____

8. _____

9. _____

10. _____

Discuss with your teacher options for conducting your interview.

There are 25 possible points in this worksheet/activity.

● WORKSHEET/ACTIVITY 4

Form a team with three to five other students assigned by your teacher. Work together to decide what type of health care team you are. Then form a mission statement. Define the roles and tasks of your team members. Decide if your team has a leader. Identify issues that may lead to conflict among the members of your team.

Assume the roles you outlined for your team. Present your team to the class by reading the mission statement you prepared and summarizing your goals and roles.

There are 50 possible points in this worksheet/activity.

● WORKSHEET/ACTIVITY 5

Draw or paste a picture of yourself on a sheet of posterboard. Write "Team Leader" at the top of your poster. Around your picture, write words or phrases that describe the traits of a good leader. Include as many as you can.

There are 30 possible points in this worksheet/activity.

● WORKSHEET/ACTIVITY 6

In a well-developed paragraph, describe some reasons why conflicts might arise among the members of a health care team. Discuss ways that conflicts can be resolved. Create an example to use in your explanation. Work with a group of students to role play the example you have created.

Type your paragraph on 8.5 x 11 sheet of paper. Double space the text of your paragraph. Proofread your paragraph to check for grammar and spelling.

There are 40 possible points in this worksheet/activity.

Chapter **9** Effective Communication

SECTION
9.1 Interpersonal Communication for All Ages

● OBJECTIVES

When you have completed this section, you will be able to do the following:

- Match key terms with their correct meanings.
- Explain why communication is important.
- Name four elements that influence our relationship with others.
- List three barriers to communication.
- Identify your communication assertiveness level.
- List four elements necessary for communication to take place.
- Describe three things that a good listener does.
- Differentiate between verbal and nonverbal communication.

● DIRECTIONS

1. Complete Worksheet 1.
2. Ask your teacher for directions to complete Worksheet/Activity 2.
3. Complete Worksheet 3.
4. Ask your teacher for directions to complete Worksheet/Activity 4.
5. Complete Worksheets 5 and 6.
6. When you are confident that you can meet each objective listed, ask your teacher for the section evaluation.

• EVALUATION METHODS

- Worksheets/activities
- Class participation
- Written evaluation

• WORKSHEET 1

Match each definition in column B with the correct vocabulary word in column A (13 points).

Column A	Column B
_____ **1.** Annoyance	a. To communicate or make known.
_____ **2.** Biases	b. Unwillingness to tolerate.
_____ **3.** Convey	c. Showing pinking or reddening of the skin.
_____ **4.** Courteous	d. Below; lower.
_____ **5.** Discretion	e. Describing a person with a word that limits him or her.
_____ **6.** Flushed	f. Polite; considerate toward others.
_____ **7.** Gesture	g. Influences; prejudices.
_____ **8.** Impatience	h. Written in a manner that can easily be read.
_____ **9.** Inferior	i. Concern about what one says and does.
_____ **10.** Labeling	j. Motion of a part of the body to express feelings or emotions.
_____ **11.** Legible	k. Exchange of information.
_____ **12.** Prejudices	l. Irritation.
_____ **13.** Communication	m. Judgments or opinions formed before the facts are known.

There are 13 possible points in this worksheet.

• WORKSHEET/ACTIVITY 2

In this activity you will:

- Wear glass that blurs your vision.
- Put cotton in your ears to experience loss of hearing.
- Wear heavy rubber gloves to experience loss of feeling while trying to count change or pick up paper.

At the end of this activity be prepared to dialogue about the experience and discuss ways you as a health care worker can make a difference when caring for people with disabilities.

There are 10 possible points in this worksheet/activity.

• WORKSHEET 3

1. Explain why communication is important (1 point).

   _____

   _____

   _____

   _____

2. Name four elements that influence our relationship with others (4 points).

   a. _____

   b. _____

   c. _____

   d. _____

3. List three barriers to communication (3 points).

   a. _____

   b. _____

   c. _____

There are 8 possible points in this worksheet/activity.

• WORKSHEET/ACTIVITY 4

This communication game will help you:

- Discover that words mean different things to different people.

- Identify words that indicate clear directions.

Note to teacher: In groups of two, have students sit back to back. Give each student an identical set of colored squares, circles, triangles, and so on. Have one student put the pieces down one by one to create a design. Ask that student to describe the design clearly enough so that the other student will replicate it exactly. No questions may be asked! How well did the communication go? Are the designs alike? Were directions exact and clear? Change the communicator and receiver, and repeat the activity.

There are 10 possible points in this worksheet/activity.

● WORKSHEET 5

Directions: Mark each statement below by placing a check (✓) in the true or false column indicating your feelings about the statement.

Assertiveness Inventory

TRUE	FALSE	STATEMENT
		1. I know what my good points are and I tell others what they are.
		2. I like to make myself look good and sometimes tell others unrealistic stories to make me look better than I am.
		3. Defending myself and expressing my feelings makes me feel uncomfortable.
		4. Sometimes I make other people feel unimportant, afraid, or stupid.
		5. I let others get their way because I don't like to make a scene.
		6. I usually feel that my views and feelings are not important to others.
		7. Others' rights are not important to me.
		8. I am careful not to abuse or be cruel when telling others that I do not agree with them.
		9. I usually take as much as I can from others even when it is unfair.
		10. I receive compliments and thank the other person for the comment.
		11. It is easier to say yes than no, even when I'd really like to say no.
		12. Other people tell me I make unreasonable requests of them.
		13. I defend my rights, and I let others do the same.
		14. I usually try to be the center of conversation.
		15. I don't like to ask others to do things.
		16. I start and carry on conversations without discomfort.
		17. It is difficult for me to tell others what my good points are.
		18. I usually do not insist that my rights be respected.
		19. I usually ask for what is mine.
		20. I listen to criticism without acting defensive.
		21. When I am angry or criticizing others, I tend to assault them physically or verbally to get my point across.
		22. It is easy for me to say positive things about others.
		23. When I know I'm right it doesn't matter if I hurt someone's feelings.
		24. When I get my way in a conversation I usually feel good, but later I feel guilty.

To evaluate your Assertiveness Inventory, do the following:

1. On the chart below, place a circle around the number of each statement you marked true.

2. Add the number of circles in each column. (If all numbers in a column are circled, the total will be 8.)

3. The column with the highest number indicates your preferred form of communication.

	UNASSERTIVE	ASSERTIVE	AGGRESSIVE
	3	1	2
	5	8	4
	6	10	7
	11	13	9
	15	16	12
	17	19	14
	18	20	21
	24	22	23
Total			

There are 24 possible points in this worksheet.

• WORKSHEET 6

1. List three elements necessary for communication to take place (3 points).

   a. _____

   b. _____

   c. _____

2. Describe three things that a good listener does (3 points).

   a. _____

   b. _____

   c. _____

3. Differentiate between verbal and nonverbal communication (10 points).

   _____

   _____

   _____

   _____

There are 16 possible points in this worksheet.

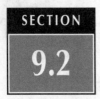

Communication Technologies

● OBJECTIVES

When you have completed this section, you will be able to do the following:

- Match key terms with their correct meanings.

- Demonstrate responding, transferring a caller, and taking a message.

- Apply basic listening skills.

- Use communication technology such as a fax machine, e-mail, or Internet to access and distribute data and other information.

● DIRECTIONS

1. Complete Worksheets 1 and 2.

2. Ask your teacher for directions to complete Worksheets/Activitise 3, 4, and 5.

3. Complete Worksheet/Activity 6.

4. When you are confident that you can meet each objective listed, ask your teacher for the section evaluation.

● EVALUATION METHODS

- Worksheets/activities

- Class participation

- Written evaluation

- Role-play

● WORKSHEET 1

Write the term that matches each description on the line.

attachment	etiquette	pertinent
blind copy	fax machine	recipient
carbon copy	Internet	reliable
cover page	memorandum	username
credible		Web site

_____ 1. The first page of a fax.

_____ 2. A short note written to help a person remember something or to remind a person to do something.

_____ 3. Professional behavior.

_____ 4. Relating directly to the matter at hand; relevant.

_____ **5.** A unique identifier composed of alphanumeric characters, used as a means of initial identification to gain access to a computer system or Internet Service Provider.

_____ **6.** A device that sends and receives printed pages or images as electronic signals over telephone lines.

_____ **7.** A file linked to an e-mail message.

_____ **8.** An e-mail feature that allows a person to send a copy of an e-mail to another person.

_____ **9.** An e-mail feature that allows a person to send an e-mail to multiple people without them seeing the other receivers' e-mail addresses.

_____ **10.** A worldwide computer network with information on many subjects.

_____ **11.** Worthy of belief or confidence; trustworthy.

_____ **12.** Dependable, accurate, honest.

_____ **13.** A person or thing that receives.

_____ **14.** A group of pages on the Internet developed by a person or organization about a topic.

There are 14 possible points in this worksheet.

• WORKSHEET 2

1. What are three ways to demonstrate open, honest, and respectful communication when using the telephone? (3 points)

a. _____

b. _____

c. _____

2. Each of the following questions is inappropriate. Rewrite the questions to improve them. (5 points)

a. What's your name? _____

b. What did you say? _____

c. Can't you speak up? _____

d. What do you want? _____

e. Huh? _____

3. What are two materials you should have when answering the telephone? (2 points)

a. _____

b. _____

4. What are two important pieces of information you should share with a caller when you need to transfer a call? (2 points)

a. _____

b. _____

5. List four pieces of information you should include whenever leaving a telephone message. (5 points)

a. _____

b. _____

c. _____

d. _____

There are 17 possible points in this worksheet.

• WORKSHEET/ACTIVITY 3

You will be divided into groups of three. Role-play a situation where two people will have a telephone conversation, while the third person will observe the interaction. At the end of the role-play, the observer will give helpful feedback about what was observed. This activity will help you:

- Identify how others perceive you.

- Create ideas about how to improve your telephone communication skills.

There are 25 possible points in this worksheet/activity.

• WORKSHEET/ACTIVITY 4

Prepare a fax that is ready to send to a health care facility to request a patient's medical records. Make up the details of the records as well as the names of the patient, facility, and physicians. Include an appropriate cover page. Exchange faxes with a partner. Critique each other's papers to identify any missing information.

There are 20 possible points in this worksheet/activity.

• WORKSHEET/ACTIVITY 5

As a group, brainstorm a topic that requires an e-mail to be written to a health care facility. Pretend that your teacher is that facility. Write an e-mail about the topic discussed. Be sure to include all of the elements of a professional e-mail. Carbon copy another student in the class as a physician involved in the situation.

Be sure to check your e-mail before sending it. Check your grammar and spelling. Check that you have included your contact information. Make sure your e-mail describes the situation and why you are writing in a pleasant, but clear, manner.

There are 20 possible points in this worksheet/activity.

• WORKSHEET/ACTIVITY 6

Choose a topic of medical research that interests you. Use the Internet to find five credible Web sites that provide information about the topic. Make a list of the domain names of each of the Web sites you visited. Decide if some Web sites are more reliable than others. Describe reasons you used to evaluate the sites.

There are 10 possible points in this worksheet/activity.

9.3 Computers in Health Care

• OBJECTIVES

When you have completed this section, you will be able to do the following:

- Match key terms with their correct meanings.
- List and explain how four computerized diagnostic tests help diagnose disease or illness.
- State how environmental services use computers.
- Describe ways that information services use computers.
- Discuss ethics and confidentiality as they relate to computers.

• DIRECTIONS

1. Complete vocabulary Worksheet 1.
2. Read this section.
3. Complete Worksheets 2 and 3 as assigned.
4. When you are confident that you can meet each objective listed above, ask your teacher for the section evaluation.

• EVALUATION METHODS

- Worksheets
- Class participation
- Written evaluation

• WORKSHEET 1

Match each definition in column B with the correct vocabulary word in column A.

Column A	Column B
_____ 1. Antagonist	a. Changing from one form to another.
_____ 2. Contingency	b. Health Plan Employer Data Information System.
_____ 3. Converting	c. One who works against.
_____ 4. HEDIS	d. Involving entering or puncturing the body.
_____ 5. Homeostasis	e. Constant balance within the body.
_____ 6. Invasive	f. X-ray technique that produces film of detailed cross section of tissue.
_____ 7. Tomography	g. Event that may occur but is not intended or likely to happen.

There are 7 possible points in this worksheet.

• WORKSHEET 2

1. Name four computerized diagnostic tests, and explain how they help diagnose disease or illness (8 points).

a. _____

b. _____

c. _____

d. _____

2. Give three examples of how environmental services use computers (3 points).

a. _____

b. _____

c. _____

3. Give three examples of how information services use computers (3 points).

a. _____

b. _____

c. _____

4. Discuss ethics and confidentiality as they relate to health care (10 points).

_____

_____

_____

There are 24 possible points in this worksheet.

• WORKSHEET 3

Respond to the following scenarios.

1. While completing your assigned work on the computer, you notice that a co-worker had an appointment for a repeat biopsy. You wonder if something is wrong, and you feel very concerned about her health. How will you handle your concern?

2. Your brother knows that a friend is in the hospital, but he doesn't know why. He asks you to find out by looking it up on the computer when you are at work. What will you say or do?

There are 10 possible points in this worksheet.

SECTION

9.4 **Charting and Observation**

● OBJECTIVES

- When you have completed this section, you will be able to do the following:
- Match key terms with their correct meanings.
- Explain the difference between subjective and objective observations.
- Explain which type of reporting allows immediate feedback and action.
- List information that must be on all health records.
- Apply five general charting guidelines.

● DIRECTIONS

1. Read this section.
2. Complete Worksheet 1 as assigned.
3. Complete Worksheet 2 as assigned.
4. When you are confident that you can meet each objective listed, ask your teacher for the section evaluation.

● EVALUATION METHOD

- Worksheet
- Class participation
- Written evaluation

● WORKSHEET 1

Write the term that correctly completes each statement on the lines provided.

chart	flushed	objective
confidential	legible	observation
distress	narrative	subjective
documentation	notation	

1. She made an _____ that the patient was becoming depressed.
2. The patient made a _____ assessment of his condition.
3. The doctor's analysis of the patient's condition is considered to be an _____ assessment.
4. The patient's face appeared _____ after completing the stress test.
5. The burn patient was in great _____ for weeks after the accident, even after receiving pain medication.

6. The nurse continued to maintain written _____ of the patient's progress.

7. He wasn't sure if the patient's nervousness was significant, but he made a _____ just in case it proved to be pertinent to his condition.

8. It is essential that the physician _____ the patient's treatment throughout her hospital stay.

9. Medical notes must be _____ so other people are able to read them.

10. In addition to statistics, the physician includes a _____ of the events that occurred with the patient.

11. The information in the patient's chart is _____, which is why the chart is not left where other people would have access to it.

There are 11 possible points in this worksheet.

• WORKSHEET 2

1. List four senses used for making observations (4 points).

   a. _____

   b. _____

   c. _____

   d. _____

2. Explain the difference between subjective and objective observations (6 points).

   a. Subjective: _____

   b. Example 1: _____

   c. Example 2: _____

   d. Objective: _____

   e. Example 1: _____

   f. Example 2: _____

3. Which type of reporting allows immediate feedback and action? Give two examples of situations requiring immediate reporting (3 points).

   a. Type of reporting: _____

   b. Example 1: _____

   c. Example 2: _____

4. List information that must be on all health care records (6 points).

   a. _____

   b. _____

   c. _____

   d. _____

   e. _____

   f. _____

5. Correct the following (5 points):

  a. How do you correct illegible writing? _____

  b. There is an error in charting. It says, "Sent to P.A." It should read, "Sent to P.T." Show how to correct this. _____

  c. "Then I took Mary to the dining room. She enjoyed her friends and ate all of her dinner." _____

  d. "Mr. M. came in for physical therapy today at noon. He needed a diathermy treatment, so I set him up. Mr. M. complained of a lot of pain in his left foot."

  e. Signature on progress note reads, "Mrs. S. Jones." Mrs. Jones is an EKG tech. Show how the signature should be written. _____

  f. What is a graphic chart used to record? _____

There are 25 possible points in this worksheet.

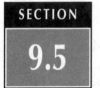

SECTION

9.5   Scheduling and Filing

● **OBJECTIVES**

When you have completed this section, you will be able to do the following:

- Match key terms with their correct meanings.
- List the guidelines for scheduling clients/patients for appointments.
- Describe a tickler file.
- List five filing systems.
- List two kinds of registration forms.
- Demonstrate how to schedule appointments.
- Demonstrate how to schedule a new client/patient: first time visit.
- Demonstrate how to schedule an outpatient diagnostic test.

● **DIRECTIONS**

1. Complete Worksheets 1 and 2 as directed by your teacher.

2. Complete Worksheet/Activity 3.

3. Complete Worksheets 4 and 5.

4. Practice all procedures.

5. Prepare responses to each item listed in Chapter Review.

6. When you are confident that you can meet each objective listed, ask your teacher for the section evaluation.

• EVALUATION METHODS

- Worksheets/Activities
- Class participation
- Written evaluation

• WORKSHEET 1

Match each definition in column B with the correct vocabulary word in column A (8 points).

Column A

_____ **1.** Geographic

_____ **2.** Numerical

_____ **3.** Alphabetical

_____ **4.** Color coding

_____ **5.** Chronological

_____ **6.** Sorting

_____ **7.** Coding

_____ **8.** Indexing

Column B

a. Assigning a color.

b. Order of occurrence.

c. Order by location.

d. In number order.

e. Using the alphabet.

f. Items belonging in a category.

g. Placement according to some system.

h. Order in which items are filed.

There are 8 possible points in this worksheet.

• WORKSHEET 2

1. List five guidelines to follow when scheduling an appointment, and explain why each is important (10 points).

a. _____

b. _____

c. _____

d. _____

e. _____

2. List the six questions you will ask a new client when scheduling an appointment (6 points).

a. _____

b. _____

c. _____

d. _____

e. _____

f. _____

3. List the information you will give a new client when scheduling an appointment (5 points).

a. _____

b. _____

c. _____

d. _____

e. _____

There are 21 possible points in this worksheet.

• WORKSHEET/ACTIVITY 3

Select a procedure (e.g., IVP, UGI, BE) that may be scheduled on an outpatient basis. Call a radiology center to get the answers to the following questions.

1. How long does the procedure take? _____

2. What does the client need to do prior to the procedure? _____

3. What time does the client need to arrive at the hospital? _____

4. Where is the x-ray department located? _____

5. What admitting information does the client need to bring? _____

6. When will the procedure report be sent to the provider? _____

7. What information do you need to give the hospital about the client? _____

There are 70 possible points in this worksheet.

• WORKSHEET 4

1. What does the client information form ask for (3 points)?

2. What is the purpose of the medical history form (2 points)?

3. List the information required on the client information form (5 points).

a. _____

b. _____

c. _____

d. _____

e. _____

4. Call a medical facility or office and ask the following questions (10 points):

a. How often is registration information updated? _____

b. Why are registration forms routinely updated? _____

There are 20 possible points in this worksheet.

• WORKSHEET 5

1. List the five different types of filing systems (5 points)

   a. _____

   b. _____

   c. _____

   d. _____

   e. _____

2. Place the numbers in column A in the correct numerical order in column B (10 points).

Column A	Column B
236	_____
443	_____
198	_____
245	_____
822	_____
323	_____
543	_____
189	_____
637	_____
935	_____

3. Place the names in column A in correct alphabetical order in column B (10 points).

Column A	Column B
Carter	_____
Doors	_____
Spencer	_____
Goulle	_____
Dwight	_____
Mitchell	_____
Salanger	_____
Bradley	_____
Christensen	_____
Lobb	_____

4. Place the names in column A in the correct alphabetical order in column B (12 points).

Column A	Column B
Alec Monroe Goldman	_____
Todd C. Sherman	_____
Kellie Bell-White	_____
Timothy Gallagher O'Bannon	_____
Carlos A. DeLeon	_____
Saint Edward	_____
Father Gerald	_____
Queen Erin	_____
Princess Monica	_____
DeeAnn Sherman, M.D.	_____
Kiley Marie Goldman	_____
Steven Edward Gustov	_____

5. Place the numbers in column A in the correct numerical order in column B (10 points).

Column A	Column B
0535.60	_____
0935.90	_____
0931.60	_____
0933.80	_____
0932.90	_____
0536.80	_____
0935.60	_____
0937.80	_____
432.80	_____
879.90	_____

6. Using the chronological filing system, place the dates in column A in the correct order in column B (6 points).

Column A	Column B
April 8, 1973: Pablo Picasso, one of the greatest artists of the twentieth century, dies.	_____
April 4, 1983: The Challenger space shuttle makes its first flight.	_____
January 25, 1971: The U.S. Supreme Court bars discrimination.	_____
August 9, 1974: Richard Nixon resigns as President of the United States.	_____
December 2, 1982: Barney Clark undergoes the first artificial heart surgery.	_____
December 22, 1970: The U.S. Supreme Court rules that 18-yearolds can vote.	_____

There are 61 possible points in this worksheet.

CHECK-OFF SHEET:
9-1 Scheduling Office Visits

Name _____ Date _____

Directions: Practice this procedure, following each step. When you are ready to have your performance evaluated, give this sheet to your instructor. Review the detailed procedure in your textbook.

Procedure	Pass	Redo	Date Competency Met	Instructor Initials
Student must use Standard Precautions.	☐	☐	_____	_____

Preprocedure

1. Assemble materials.

a. Pen or pencil	☐	☐	_____	_____
b. Appointment book	☐	☐	_____	_____
c. Appointment reminder cards for tickler file	☐	☐	_____	_____
d. Appointment cards	☐	☐	_____	_____
e. Calendar	☐	☐	_____	_____
f. Procedure list with approximate time allotments for each procedure	☐	☐	_____	_____
g. Written instructions for patient/client preparation prior to visit	☐	☐	_____	_____
2. Prepare provider schedules for at least three months.	☐	☐	_____	_____
a. Mark out vacation or holiday times	☐	☐	_____	_____
b. Schedule monthly, weekly, or daily meetings	☐	☐	_____	_____
c. Mark schedule to identify hours for patient/client appointments	☐	☐	_____	_____
3. Follow the correct procedure for the type of appointment system in your office.	☐	☐	_____	_____
4. Write clearly and neatly so that names and procedures are easy to read.	☐	☐	_____	_____

Procedure

5. Schedule appointments.

a. By phone:

(1) Clarify reason for appointment	☐	☐	_____	_____
(2) Discuss most convenient time for client/patient (e.g., a.m., p.m.)	☐	☐	_____	_____
(3) Offer various times	☐	☐	_____	_____
(4) Ask for proper spelling of first and last names once a time is chosen	☐	☐	_____	_____

Procedure	Pass	Redo	Date Competency Met	Instructor Initials
(5) Ask for information, such as birthday or Social Security number, if name is common (e.g., Smith, Jones)	☐	☐	_____	_____
(6) Write patient's/client's telephone number and where he or she can be reached during the day of appointment	☐	☐	_____	_____
(7) Allocate sufficient time for the visit when scheduling a procedure	☐	☐	_____	_____
b. In person:				
(1) Follow steps 1 to 5 of procedure above	☐	☐	_____	_____
(2) Give patient/client an appointment card with date and time of appointment	☐	☐	_____	_____
c. For appointments more than three months in the future:				
(1) Ask patient/client to address an appointment reminder card	☐	☐	_____	_____
(2) Fill in month patient is to return	☐	☐	_____	_____
(3) Instruct patient/client that a card will be sent as a reminder to call and make an appointment	☐	☐	_____	_____
d. Place appointment reminder card in tickler file so that it is sent at the correct time	☐	☐	_____	_____

CHECK-OFF SHEET:

9-2 Scheduling a New Patient/Client: First-Time Visit

Name _____ Date _____

Directions: Practice this procedure, following each step. When you are ready to have your performance evaluated, give this sheet to your instructor. Review the detailed procedure in your textbook.

Procedure	Pass	Redo	Date Competency Met	Instructor Initials
Student must use Standard Precautions.	☐	☐	_____	_____
Preprocedure				
1. Assemble materials.				
a. Appointment book	☐	☐	_____	_____
b. Scheduling guidelines	☐	☐	_____	_____
c. Telephone	☐	☐	_____	_____
d. Pencil	☐	☐	_____	_____
Procedure				
2. Ask patient/client for the following:				
a. First, last, and middle names	☐	☐	_____	_____
b. Birth date	☐	☐	_____	_____
c. Home address	☐	☐	_____	_____
d. Telephone number	☐	☐	_____	_____
3. Ask patient/client if this is a referral. If yes:	☐	☐	_____	_____
a. Determine information you need from the referring provider.	☐	☐	_____	_____
b. Add this information to the medical chart. (Your provider needs to send a consultation report to the referring provider.)	☐	☐	_____	_____
4. Ask what the chief complaint is and when it started.	☐	☐	_____	_____
5. Find the first appointment that allows the appropriate amount of time.	☐	☐	_____	_____
6. Offer a choice of days and times.	☐	☐	_____	_____
7. Enter the following:				
a. Patient's/client's name NP next to name indicating new patient)	☐	☐	_____	_____
b. Time and date of appointment	☐	☐	_____	_____
c. Patient's/Client's day telephone number	☐	☐	_____	_____

Procedure	Pass	Redo	Date Competency Met	Instructor Initials
8. Explain payment procedure (e.g., patient/client must pay for visit, your office will bill).	☐	☐	_____	_____
9. Give directions to the office.	☐	☐	_____	_____
10. Explain parking arrangements.	☐	☐	_____	_____

Postprocedure

11. Repeat day, date, and time the appointment is scheduled.	☐	☐	_____	_____

CHECK-OFF SHEET:
9-3 Scheduling Outpatient Diagnostic Tests

Name _____ **Date** _____

Directions: Practice this procedure, following each step. When you are ready to have your performance evaluated, give this sheet to your instructor. Review the detailed procedure in your textbook.

Procedure	Pass	Redo	Date Competency Met	Instructor Initials
Student must use Standard Precautions.	☐	☐	_____	_____
Preprocedure				
1. Assemble materials.				
a. Written order from provider	☐	☐	_____	_____
b. Patient's chart	☐	☐	_____	_____
c. Test preparation instructions for client/patient	☐	☐	_____	_____
d. Name, address, and phone number of laboratory	☐	☐	_____	_____
e. Telephone	☐	☐	_____	_____
Procedure				
2. Read provider's order.	☐	☐	_____	_____
3. Ask patient/client when he or she is available.	☐	☐	_____	_____
4. Call test lab.	☐	☐	_____	_____
5. Order test	☐	☐	_____	_____
a. Set up time and date	☐	☐	_____	_____
b. Give name, age, address, and telephone number of patient/client	☐	☐	_____	_____
c. Ask if there are special instructions for patient/client prior to the test	☐	☐	_____	_____
6. Provide patient/client with the following:				
a. Name, address, and telephone number of laboratory	☐	☐	_____	_____
b. Date and time	☐	☐	_____	_____
c. Instructions (in writing) for preparation prior to test				
7. Verify instructions with patient/client.	☐	☐	_____	_____
8. Record test time in patient's/client's chart.	☐	☐	_____	_____
Postprocedure				
9. Put a reminder in the tickler file or on a calendar to check for results.	☐	☐	_____	_____

Chapter 10 Medical Terminology

Pronunciation, Word Elements, and Terms

- ## OBJECTIVES

    When you have completed this section, you will be able to do the following:

    - Match key terms with their correct meanings.

    - Define roots, prefixes, and suffixes.

    - Define the word elements listed.

    - Match medical terms with their correct meanings.

    - Divide medical terms into elements.

    - Combine word elements to form medical terms.

- ## DIRECTIONS

    1. Complete Worksheet/Activity 1 as assigned.

    2. Complete Worksheet 2 and Worksheet/Activity 3 as assigned.

    3. Complete Worksheet 4.

    4. When you are confident that you can meet each objective listed above, ask your teacher for the section evaluation.

- ## EVALUATION METHODS

    - Worksheets/activities

    - Class participation

    - Written evaluation

WORKSHEET/ACTIVITY 1

Use index cards to make flash cards to help you learn the prefixes, roots, and suffixes listed in the text. Write each word element on one side of a card, and write its meaning on the other side. Review the cards whenever you have a minute (such as when standing in line or waiting for a ride). Work with your classmates, quizzing each other until you know all of the word elements and their meanings. Learn 12 elements each day. Before going to bed each night, quiz yourself on the 12 elements that you learned that day (1 point for each card).

WORKSHEET 2

1. Fill in the blanks with the appropriate answer (6 points).

   a. ch sounds like _____.

   b. ps sounds like _____.

   c. pn sounds like _____.

   d. c sounds like _____ when it comes before e, i, and y.

   e. g sounds like _____ when it comes before e, i, and y.

   f. i sounds like _____ when added to the end of the word to form a plural.

2. How are medical terms formed (1 point)? _____

3. List three types of word elements (3 points).

   a. _____

   b. _____

   c. _____

4. The element at the beginning of a medical term is known as a _____
   _____ (1 point).

5. The element that is the subject of a medical term is known as a _____
   _____ (1 point).

6. The element found at the end of a medical term is called a _____
   _____ (1 point).

7. Combined vowels are used to help make medical terms easier to _____
   _____ (1 point).

8. Commonly used combined vowels are (a) _____ and (b)
   _____ and sometimes (c) _____ and (d)
   _____ (4 points).

9. Learning word elements gives you the tools necessary to create hundreds of
   _____ (1 point).

10. Use the text to help you put the correct word elements together to form medical terms for the following (10 points).

   _____ a. Slow heart condition

   _____ b. Pertaining to between the ribs

   _____ c. Paralysis of half the body

   _____ d. Condition of hardening of the arteries

_____ e. Cancerous tumor

_____ f. Inflammation of the stomach

_____ g. Condition of the kidney

_____ h. Enlarged extremities

_____ i. Surgical removal of the uterus

_____ j. Incision of the trachea

11. Write the meaning next to the following medical terms (10 points).

a. Epigastric _____

b. Esophagitis _____

c. Melanoma _____

d. Laparotomy _____

e. Postpartum _____

f. Thoracentesis _____

g. Rhinoplasty _____

h. Dermocyanosis _____

i. Craniotomy _____

j. Hepatitis _____

12. Divide the following medical terms into elements (10 points).

a. Acromegaly

b. Antifebrile

c. Bradycardia

d. Carcinoma

e. Dentalgia

f. Gastroenteritis

g. Hemiplegia

h. Intracostal

i. Osteoarthritis

j. Pericarditis

There are 49 possible points in this worksheet.

WORKSHEET/ACTIVITY 3

Go onto the Internet and look at the various free resources that could help you with medical terminology. You may use search engines or go to various health care publishers' Web sites. Look at the textbooks you use for Web addresses as a beginning.

Look up the same terms on different sites and compare what they say. Print out some examples and be ready to tell your classmates which are the best resources and why.

There are 100 possible points in this worksheet.

• WORKSHEET 4

1. Change the following words from singular to plural. Define each word.

Singular	Plural	Definition
a. Stratum	_____	_____
b. Retinoblastoma	_____	_____
c. Decubitus	_____	_____
d. Disease	_____	_____
e. Vena cava	_____	_____
f. Allergy	_____	_____
g. Metastasis	_____	_____

There are 14 possible points in this worksheet.

SECTION

10.2   Abbreviations

• OBJECTIVES

When you have completed this section, you will be able to do the following:

- Match key terms with their correct meanings.
- Replace terms with abbreviations.
- Recognize and define abbreviations that are commonly used by health care workers.

• DIRECTIONS

1. Complete Worksheet/Activity 1 as assigned.
2. Complete Worksheets 2 through 4.
3. Prepare responses to each item listed in Chapter Review.
4. When you are confident that you can meet each objective listed above, ask your teacher for the section evaluation.

• EVALUATION METHODS

- Worksheets/activities
- Class participation
- Written evaluation

• WORKSHEET/ACTIVITY 1

Using index cards, make flash cards to help you learn the abbreviations listed in the text. Write each abbreviation on one side of a card, and write its meaning on the other side. Review the cards whenever you have a minute (such as when standing in line or waiting for a ride). Work with your classmates, quizzing each other until you know all of the abbreviations and their meanings. Learn 12 abbreviations each day. Before going to bed each night, quiz yourself on the 12 elements you learned that day (1 point for each card).

● WORKSHEET 2

Fill in the correct medical term for each of the following abbreviations (50 points).

1. cath.	_____	26. NPO	_____
2. am, AM	_____	27. B/P	_____
3. bid, BID	_____	28. fx	_____
4. hs	_____	29. IV	_____
5. lab	_____	30. spec.	_____
6. hyper	_____	31. ROM	_____
7. CPR	_____	32. po	_____
8. w/c	_____	33. pc	_____
9. qhs	_____	34. qid, QID	_____
10. q	_____	35. Pt, pt	_____
11. amt.	_____	36. q_2h	_____
12. I & O	_____	37. dc, d/c	_____
13. qod, QOD	_____	38. post	_____
14. CA	_____	39. ss	_____
15. c	_____	40. OPD	_____
16. prn	_____	41. postop, ostOp	_____
17. bm, BM	_____	42. BR, br	_____
18. O_2	_____	43. CBC	_____
19. ax	_____	44. stat	_____
20. s	_____	45. c/o	_____
21. wt	_____	46. dx	_____
22. ht	_____	47. cc	_____
23. amb	_____	48. liq.	_____
24. BRP	_____	49. H_2O	_____
25. OOB, oob	_____	50. noct, noc.	_____

There are 50 possible points in this worksheet.

98

● WORKSHEET 3

Fill in the correct medical term for each of the following abbreviations (10 points).

1. adm   _____
2. amb   _____
3. cath.   _____
4. lab   _____
5. CPR   _____
6. B/P   _____
7. ROM   _____
8. NPO   _____
9. prn   _____
10. I & O   _____

There are 10 possible points in this worksheet.

● WORKSHEET 4

Fill in the correct medical abbreviation for each of the following terms (10 points).

1. red blood cell   _____
2. date of birth   _____
3. normal saline   _____
4. licensed practical nurse   _____
5. clear liquids   _____
6. three times a day   _____
7. both ears   _____
8. every 2 hours   _____
9. at once, immediately   _____
10. one thousand   _____

There are 10 possible points in this worksheet.

Chapter **11** Medical Math

SECTION 11.1 Math Review

● OBJECTIVES

When you have completed this section, you will be able to do the following:

- Match key terms with their correct meaning.
- Add and subtract whole numbers, decimals, and percentages.
- Multiply and divide whole numbers, fractions, mixed numbers, decimals, and percentages.
- Convert decimals to percentages and percentages to decimals.

● DIRECTIONS

1. Complete Worksheet 1, Pretest.
2. Read "Introduction to the Math Review" and complete Worksheet 2.
3. Read the information following the Addition and Subtraction headings.
4. Complete Worksheet 3.
5. Read the information following the Multiplication heading.
6. Complete Worksheet/Activity 4.
7. Read the information under the Division heading.
8. Complete Worksheet 5.
9. Read the information following Decimals, Percentages, and Fractions headings.
10. Complete Worksheet 6.

11. When you are confident that you can meet each objective for this section, ask your teacher for the section evaluation.

● EVALUATION METHODS

- Pretest
- Worksheets/Activities
- Class participation
- Written evaluation

● WORKSHEET 1, PRETEST (100 POINTS)

Write the following numbers using commas and decimals in the correct places (5 points).

NUMBER	YOUR ANSWER
1. 9345	
2. 10345	
3. 100345	
4. 9345 $^{40}\!/_{100}$	
5. 123456	

Add commas and decimals to the following numbers. Then write their description as you would describe them to another person.

6. 9345

7. 10345

8. 100345

9. 9345 $^5\!/_{100}$

10. 19345 $^5\!/_{100}$

Calculate the following (show your work).

Addition	Subtraction
11. $3 + 9 =$	**21.** $9 - 3 =$
12. $8 + 4 =$	**22.** $8 - 4 =$
13. $4 + 5 =$	**23.** $5 - 4 =$
14. $12 + 27 =$	**24.** $27 - 12 =$
15. $54 + 72 =$	**25.** $62 - 5 =$
16. $62 + 5 =$	**26.** $15 - 15 =$
17. $15 + 15 =$	**27.** $204 - 186 =$
18. $186 + 204 =$	**28.** $549 - 222 =$
19. $549 + 222 =$	**29.** $89,345 - 1,008 =$
20. $1,008 + 89,345 =$	**30.** $100,000 - 84,694 =$

Multiplication	Division
31. 8 × 4 =	**41.** 6 ÷ 2 =
32. 3 × 3 =	**42.** 12 ÷ 3 =
33. 12 × 6 =	**43.** 42 ÷ 7 =
34. 27 × 9 =	**44.** 25 ÷ 5 =
35. 58 × 18 =	**45.** 72 ÷ 9 =
36. 165 × 10 =	**46.** 240 ÷ 10 =
37. 2,222 × 93 =	**47.** 3,232 ÷ 32 =
38. 624 × 1,000 =	**48.** 960 ÷ 60 =
39. 5,524 × 320 =	**49.** 8,250 ÷ 150 =
40. 8,350 × 600 =	**50.** 5,200 ÷ 16 =

Percentages

Band-aids are packaged in 100 per box. You had four full boxes when you started work yesterday. At the end of the day, you had two full boxes left.

51. What percentage of them were used yesterday? _____

52. What percentage is still left? _____

There are 100 sample bottles of cough medicine in the cupboard.

53. If you give 25 bottles away, how many will you have left? _____

54. What percentage is left in the cupboard? _____

55. What percentage was given away? _____

56–100. _____ Fill in the blank spaces on the following multiplication table.

	1	2	3	4	5	6	7	8	9	10
1										
2										
3										
4										
5										
6										
7										
8										
9										
10										

There are 100 possible points in this worksheet/pretest.

● WORKSHEET 2

Write the place values for each of the digits in the number below. One answer has been completed for you (2,222.22) (20 points).

	2	,	2		2		2	.	2		2

1. _____   2. _____   3. _____   4. _____   5. <u>tenths</u>   6. _____

Write the following numbers using commas and decimals in the correct places.

NUMBER	ANSWER	NUMBER	ANSWER
7. 8492		**11.** 2536	
8. 654 ³⁄₁₀		**12.** 5558555	
9. 92184		**13.** 2645	
10. 108627		**14.** 32323	

15. Describe a whole number._____

16. Describe a non-whole number. _____

17. Describe a mixed number._____

18. Describe a percentage. _____

19. Write a percentage sign. _____

20. Describe the value of a zero in front of a whole number. _____

There are 20 possible points in this worksheet.

● WORKSHEET 3

Add the following numbers (show your work).

1. $8 + 7 =$

2. $9 + 6 + 2 =$

3. $23 + 35 =$

4. $36 + 72 + 18 =$

5. $555 + 398 + 421 =$

6. $746 + 843 + 341 =$

7. $9,742 + 23 + 1,008 + 6,842 =$

8. $43 + 5,432 + 987 + 8,764 =$

9. $8,765 + 964 + 1,053 + 3,338 =$

10. $10,079 + 365 + 5,432 + 89,935 =$

Subtract the numbers in the following problems (show your work for each).

11. $9 - 6 =$

12. $8 - 3 =$

13. $12 - 3 =$

14. $24 - 13 =$

15. $555 - 72 =$

16. $693 - 545 =$

17. $1,003 - 946 =$

18. $1,233 - 895 =$

19. $9,843 - 6,979 =$

20. $6,321 - 93 =$

Show your work as you subtract, and check your answers, in the following:

21. $145 - 68 =$

22. $913 - 43 =$

23. $26 - 10 =$

24. $960 - 96 =$

25. $872 - 154 =$

26. $1,000 - 347 =$

There are 26 possible points in this worksheet.

● WORKSHEET/ACTIVITY 4

Learn the multiplication table from your text, and then fill in the following table by multiplying the top row of numbers against the numbers in the column at the left. Place the correct answer in the square that intersects with the numbers being multiplied. See example below (100 points)

	1	2	3	4	5	6
1						
2						
3						
4						
5					25	
6						

Example: five times five:

	1	2	3	4	5	6	7	8	9	10
1										
2										
3										
4										
5										
6										
7										
8										
9										
10										

Make flash cards by putting each problem represented in the multiplication table on the front side of a card and the answer on the back of the card. Use the cards to review multiplication. Ask a classmate to quiz you using the cards.

There are 150 possible points in this worksheet/activity.

• WORKSHEET 5

Calculate the following (15 points).

1. $225 \div 5 =$

2. $486 \div 3 =$

3. $240 \div 8 =$

4. $8,289 \div 9 =$

5. $1,060 \div 5 =$

6. $3,826 \div 8 =$

7. $4,832 \div 8 =$

8. $2,222 \div 4 =$

9. $6,324 \div 3 =$

10. $7,248 \div 8 =$

11. $963.54 \div 9 =$

12. $339.28 \div 4 =$

13. $637.42 \div 7 =$

14. $2,967.40 \div 5 =$

15. $8,954.73 \div 9 =$

There are 15 possible points in this worksheet.

• WORKSHEET 6

Convert the following decimals to percentages (24 points).

1. $0.33 =$ _____%

2. $0.46 =$ _____%

3. $0.75 =$ _____%

4. $0.13 =$ _____%

5. $0.50 =$ _____%

6. $0.96 =$ _____%

Convert the following percentages to decimals.

7. $100\% =$ _____

8. $20\% =$ _____

9. $64\% =$ _____

10. $85\% =$ _____

Convert the following percentages into fractions.

11. $33\% =$

12. $13\% =$

13. $3\% =$

14. $8\% =$

15. $833\% =$

16. $1,025\% =$

Calculate percentages of the following.

17. 20% of $100 =$

18. 25% of $100 =$

19. 30% of $50 =$

20. 3% of $65 =$

21. 28% of $1,000 =$

22. 15% of $25,000 =$

23. 65% of $90 =$

24. 7.25% of $8 =$

There are 24 possible points in this worksheet.

SECTION

11.2 The Metric System

• OBJECTIVES

When you have completed this section, you will be able to do the following:

- Match key terms with their correct meanings.

- State the metric unit of measure used to determine length, distance, weight, and volume.

- Use metric terms to express 100 and 1,000 units of measure.

- Use metric terms to express 0.1, 0.01, and 0.001 units of measure.

- List four basic rules to follow when using the metric system.

- Identify metric measures of length and volume.

- Convert ounces to cubic centimeters/milliliters, pounds to kilograms, and ounces to grams.

• DIRECTIONS

1. Complete Worksheet 1.

2. Complete Worksheet/Activity 2

3. Complete Worksheets 3 and 4.

4. Ask your teacher for directions to complete Worksheet/Activity 5.

5. When you are confident that you can meet each objective for this section, ask your teacher the section evaluation.

• EVALUATION METHODS

- Worksheets/Activities

- Class participation

- Written evaluation

• WORKSHEET 1

Match each definition or abbreviation in column B to the correct word in column A (12 points). One answer is used more than once.

Column A	Column B
1. Abbreviation	**a.** International System of Units
2. Convert	**b.** A shortened form of a word
3. Decimal	**c.** A number containing a decimal point
4. Metric system	**d.** To transform; to change into another form
5. Meter	**e.** L

6. Gram   **f.** m

7. Liter   **g.** d

8. Kilo   **h.** g

9. Hecto   **i.** c

10. Deci   **j.** k

11. Centi   **k.** h

12. Milli

There are 12 possible points in this worksheet.

• WORKSHEET/ACTIVITY 2

1. Ask your teachers for containers and rulers marked in standard and metric units to help you visualize these measures.

2. What is the metric measure for:

a. Length _____   c. Distance _____

b. Weight _____   d. Volume _____

There are 5 points in this worksheet/activity.

• WORKSHEET 3

1. Write each item below in the space next to the correct measure (8 points).

length and distance   weight   0.01 of a unit

100 units   1,000 units   0.1 of a unit

volume   0.001 of a unit

_____ a. Meter

_____ b. Gram

_____ c. Liter

_____ d. Kilo

_____ e. Hecto

_____ f. Deci

_____ g. Centi

_____ h. Milli

2. Use metric terms to express the following (5 points):

1,000 units _____

100 units _____

1/10 or 0.1 of a unit _____

1/100 or 0.01 of a unit _____

1/1,000 or 0.001 of a unit _____

3. List four basic rules for using the metric system (4 points).

    a. _____

    b. _____

    c. _____

    d. _____

There are 17 possible points in this worksheet.

● WORKSHEET 4

1. There are _____ ml/cc in 1 ounce.

2. To determine the number of ml/ccs in a container marked with ounces, multiply _____.

3. 8 oz. of water = _____ ml/cc.

4. 6 oz. of soup = _____ ml/cc.

5. 16 oz. of juice = _____ ml/cc.

6. 1 lb = _____ kg.

7. 1 kg = _____ lb.

8. To convert pounds to kilograms, multiply the number of pounds by_____.

9. To convert kilograms to pounds, multiply the number of kilograms by ____.

10. Convert 110 lbs. to kilograms. 110 _ _____ = _____ (1 point).

11. Convert 50 k to pounds. 50 _ _____ = _____ (1 point).

12. Convert the following (4 points):

    a. 300 lbs. to kilograms _____

    b. 150 lbs. to kilograms _____

    c. 20 kg to pounds _____

    d. 85 kg to pounds _____

13. To convert ounces to grams, multiply ___ 3 the number of ounces (1 point).

14. To convert grams into ounces, divide 30 into the _____ (1 point).

15. Convert the following (4 points):

    a. 8 oz. to grams_____

    b. 16 oz. to grams_____

    c. 30 g to ounces _____

    d. 120 g to ounces _____

There are 21 possible points in this worksheet.

• WORKSHEET/ACTIVITY 5

Practice weighing your classmates and convert their weight from pounds to kilograms. Practice measuring your classmates and convert from feet to inches and feet to meters. Practice measuring water in centimeters and liters. Convert to cc's.

There are 30 points in this worksheet/activity.

SECTION

11.3 The 24-Hour Clock/Military Time

• OBJECTIVES

When you have completed this section, you will be able to do the following:

- Match vocabulary words with their correct meanings.
- Recognize time on a 24-hour clock.
- Express 24-hour time/military time verbally and in writing.
- Convert Greenwich time to 24-hour time.

• DIRECTIONS

1. Read this section.
2. Complete Worksheet 1.
3. Complete Worksheet/Activity 2.
4. When you are confident that you can meet each objective listed above, ask your instructor for the section evaluation.

• EVALUATION METHODS

- Worksheet
- Class participation
- Written evaluation

• WORKSHEET 1

1. Define *Greenwich time* (1 point). _____

2. Define *24-hour time/military time* (1 point). _____

3. Military time is always expressed in how many digits (1 point)? _____

4. To determine how 5:00 P.M. is expressed in military time, add _____ to 0500 (1 point).

5. Write the correct military time for each of the following Greenwich times (6 points).

   a. 3:00 A.M. _____

   b. 9:00 A.M. _____

   c. 12:00 noon _____

   d. 6:00 P.M. _____

   e. 12:00 midnight_____

   f. 12:30 A.M. _____

6. Write the Greenwich time for each of the following military times (6 points).

   a. 0130 _____

   b. 0500 _____

   c. 1700 _____

   d. 1430 _____

   e. 0045 _____

   f. 0000 _____

There are 16 possible points in this worksheet.

• WORKSHEET/ACTIVITY 2

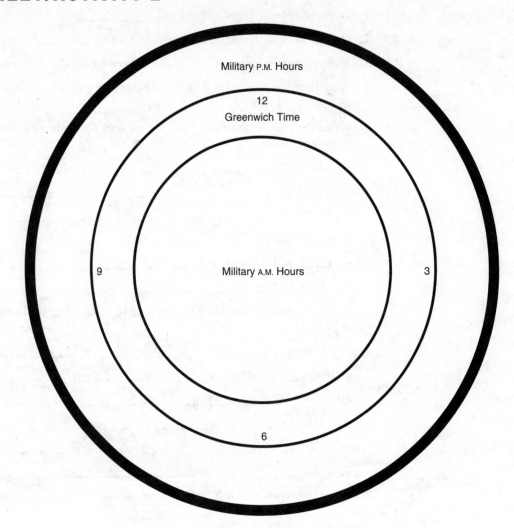

Directions: Fill in the clock diagram with the correct Greenwich and military times. The 3:00, 6:00, 9:00, and 12:00 are reference times in the Greenwich circle to help guide you.

There are 20 points in this worksheet/activity.

Chapter **12** Measurement and the Scientific Process

SECTION
12.1 The Scientific Process

● **OBJECTIVES**

When you have completed this section, you will be able to do the following:

- Match key terms with their correct meanings.
- List eight basic steps of scientific methods.
- Describe a controlled experiment.
- Explain the importance of communication in scientific methods.

● **DIRECTIONS**

1. Complete Worksheet 1.
2. Read the section.
3. Complete Worksheet 2 and Worksheet/Activity 3 as assigned.
4. Complete Worksheet 4.
5. When you are confident that you can meet each objective listed above, ask your teacher for the section evaluation.

● **EVALUATION METHODS**

- Worksheets/Activities
- Class participation
- Written evaluation

● **WORKSHEET 1**

    1. What are scientific methods?_____

    2. Define a hypothesis. _____

    3. What is a controlled experiment? _____

There are 6 possible points in this worksheet.

● **WORKSHEET 2**

    1. List eight basic steps of scientific methods (8 points).

      a. _____

      b. _____

      c. _____

      d. _____

      e. _____

      f. _____

      g. _____

      h. _____

    2. How are observations related to scientific methods? Give an example. (2 points)

    3. What makes a scientific question different from other types of questions? (2 points)

    4. How is a hypothesis related to a scientific question? (2 points)

    5. Why isn't it necessarily a bad thing if a hypothesis is not supported by an investigation? (2 points)

There are 16 possible points in this worksheet.

● **WORKSHEET/ACTIVITY 3**

Placebos are often used in controlled experiments. Conduct research to find out what a placebo is and why it is used. Find an example of an experiment in which a placebo was used. Present your findings in an oral report. Be sure to relate placebos to the variables of a controlled experiment.

There are 25 possible points in this worksheet.

● **WORKSHEET 4**

    1. How do scientists communicate the results of their experiments? (5 points)

    _____

    _____

    2. Why is it important for scientists to communicate the results of their experiments? (5 points)_____

    _____

There are 10 possible points in this worksheet.

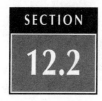

12.2 Measurements

● OBJECTIVES

When you have completed this section, you will be able to do the following:

- Match the key terms with their correct meanings

- Identify tools used to measure length, time, temperature, volume, and mass/weight.

- Identify units used to measure length, time, temperature, volume, and mass/weight.

- Describe the process of estimating.

- Round various numbers.

- Relate accuracy and precision to the validity of results.

- Explain how estimating may affect accuracy and precision.

● DIRECTIONS

1. Complete Worksheet 1 as assigned.

2. Complete Worksheet 2 and Worksheet/Activity 3 as assigned.

3. Complete Worksheets 4 and 5.

4. When you are confident that you can meet each objective listed above, ask your teacher for the section evaluation.

● EVALUATION METHODS

- Worksheets/Activities

- Class participation

- Written evaluation

● WORKSHEET 1

Use the following terms to complete each sentence.

accuracy	mass	volume
estimate	precision	weight

1. If you measure the amount of space an object takes up, you are measuring the object's _____.

2. You can find a(n) _____ when you need only an approximate value.

3. Your _____ is a measure of the force of gravity on your body.

4. The _____ of an object is the amount of matter in it.

5. Several measures show _____ if they are all close to each other.

6. The _____ of a measurement describes how close it is to the actual value.

There are 12 possible points in this worksheet.

• WORKSHEET 2

Name a tool that can be used to take each of the following measurements.

1. Length of a desk _____

2. Temperature of air _____

3. Time taken to run 5 meters _____

4. Volume of water _____

5. Mass of medicine bottle _____

6. Weight of person _____

7. Height of a door _____

8. Temperature of bath water_____

9. Volume of a solid cube _____

10. Mass of a food sample _____

Tell what quantity can be measured by the following units.

11. Kilometer_____

12. Degrees Celsius_____

13. Milliliter_____

14. Gram_____

15. Meter_____

16. Liter_____

17. Pound_____

18. Tablespoon_____

19. Degrees Fahrenheit_____

20. Inch_____

There are 20 possible points in this worksheet.

• WORKSHEET/ACTIVITY 3

Make measurements throughout a day. Your teacher will provide you with examples, such as the length of your desk, the volume of a number cube, and the temperature of a mound of clay. Create a chart in which to record your measurements. Compare with other students. Repeat measurements to eliminate possible errors.

There are 20 possible points in this worksheet/activity.

- ## WORKSHEET 4

Round each of the following numbers to the tenths place.

1. 15.63 _____
2. 126.895_____
3. 8.24_____
4. 57.01_____
5. 100.77_____

Round each of the following numbers to the ones place.

6. 78.20_____
7. 258.6_____
8. 92.4_____
9. 491.10_____
10. 60.8_____

Round each of the following numbers to the tens place.

11. 569_____
12. 2,136_____
13. 742_____
14. 963_____
15. 12,893_____

Round each of the following numbers to the hundreds place.

16. 7,865_____
17. 2,354_____
18. 6,378_____
19. 16,549_____
20. 22,853_____

Round each of the following numbers to the thousands place.

21. 48,111_____
22. 72,621_____
23. 124,263_____
24. 547,309_____
25. 803,563_____

There are 25 possible points in this worksheet.

- ## WORKSHEET 5

Accuracy and precision are often likened to a dart board. The darts represent measurements. Describe each of the following as accurate, precise, or both.

a. Dartboard with all of the darts close together on the edge of the board

b. Dartboard with all of the darts close together in the center of the board

c. Dartboard with all of the darts spread apart all over the board

There are 15 possible points in this worksheet.

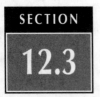
SECTION

12.3 Tables, Graphs, and Charts

- ## OBJECTIVES

  - Match key terms with their correct meanings.

  - Describe three types of graphs.

  - Explain what kind of data is represented by tables and each type of graph.

  - Draw three types of graphs.

- ## DIRECTIONS

  1. Complete Worksheet 1 as assigned.

  2. Complete Worksheet/Activity 2 as assigned.

  3. Complete Worksheets/Activities 3 and 4.

  4. Prepare responses to each item listed in Chapter Review.

  5. When you are confident that you can meet each objective listed above, ask your teacher for the section evaluation.

- ## EVALUATION METHODS

  - Worksheets/Activities

  - Class participation

  - Written evaluation

● WORKSHEET 1

Match each term in Column A to its definition in Column B

Column A	Column B
_____ Data	a. A factor that can change.
_____ Variable	b. Part of a whole.
_____ Proportion	c. A reference line that marks the border of a graph.
_____ Axis	d. Information.
_____ Circle graph	e. Graph in which plotted points are connected.
_____ Line graph	f. Graph in which the height of a column represents data.
_____ Bar graph	g. Graph divided into sections that add to 100%.

There are 7 possible points in this worksheet.

● WORKSHEET/ACTIVITY 2

In a well-developed paragraph, compare line graphs, bar graphs, and circle graphs. Tell what each type of graph looks like and what information is best represented on it. Be sure to type your paragraph using double spacing. Check your spelling and grammar

There are 20 possible points in this worksheet/activity.

● WORKSHEET/ACTIVITY 3

Look through newspapers and magazines to find examples of graphs. Identify an example of a line graph, a bar graph, and a circle graph. Highlight the title of the graph and the information presented on the axes. Note what units the measurements are in. Explain the information represented by the graph as well as any changes or trends that are indicated.

There are 25 possible points in this worksheet/activity.

● WORKSHEET/ACTIVITY 4

Conduct a survey to gather information from your friends, family, or classmates. You might ask about their favorite classes, types of movies, number of siblings, or heights. Record your results in a data table. Then decide which type of graph would be best to represent your results. For example, you might represent favorite types of movies on a circle graph, but heights on a bar graph. Create a graph to represent your data.

There are 25 possible points in this worksheet/activity.

Chapter **13** Your Body and How It Functions

SECTION 13.1 Overview of the Body

● **OBJECTIVES**

When you have completed this section, you will be able to do the following:

- Match key terms with their correct meanings.
- List seven cell functions.
- Identify three main parts of the cell and explain their functions.
- Describe the relationship between cells, tissues, organs, and systems of the body.
- Identify terms relating to the body.
- Label a diagram of the body cavities.
- Explain why health care workers must have a basic knowledge of body structures and how they function.

● **DIRECTIONS**

1. Complete Worksheets 1 and 2.
2. Ask your teacher for directions to complete Worksheet/Activity 3.
3. Complete Worksheets 4 through 6.
4. When you are confident that you can meet each objective for this section, ask your teacher for the section evaluation.

● EVALUATION METHODS

- ■ Worksheets/Activities
- ■ Class participation
- ■ Written evaluation
- ■ Spelling bee preparation

● WORKSHEET 1

Match each definition in column B with the correct vocabulary word in column A.

Column A

_____ **1.** Cell
_____ **2.** Cell membrane
_____ **3.** Composed
_____ **4.** Connective tissue
_____ **5.** Cytoplasm
_____ **6.** Epithelial
_____ **7.** Function
_____ **8.** Microscopic
_____ **9.** Nucleus
_____ **10.** Nutrients
_____ **11.** Reproduction
_____ **12.** Sacral region
_____ **13.** Structure
_____ **14.** Tissue

Column B

a. The form in which the body is made.

b. A thin, soft layer of tissue that surrounds the cell and holds it together.

c. The action or work of tissues, organs, or body parts.

d The smallest structural unit in the body that is capable of independent functioning.

e. Formed by putting many parts together.

f. Jellylike liquid that carries on the activities of the cell.

g. Tissue specialized to bind together and support other tissues.

h. A group of cells of the same type that act together to perform a specific function.

i. Too small to be seen by the eye but large enough to be seen through a microscope.

j. The area where the sacrum is located.

k. The part of a cell that is vital for its growth, metabolism, reproduction, and transmitted characteristics.

l. Food.

m. The process that takes place in animals to create offspring.

n. Pertaining to the covering of the internal and external organs of the body.

There are 14 possible points in this worksheet.

● WORKSHEET 2

1. Label the three main parts of a basic cell (3 points).

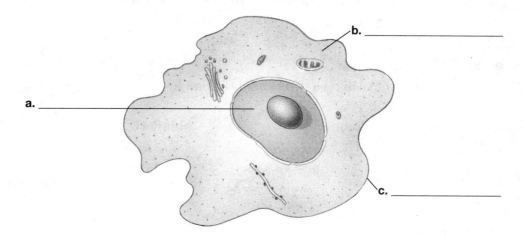

a. _____

b. _____

c. _____

2. Name the three main parts of a cell, and explain the function of each (6 points).

Cell Part   **Function**

a. _____   _____

b. _____   _____

c. _____   _____

3. Explain how cells, tissues, organs, and systems form a body (5 points).

_____

_____

_____

4. List the five primary kinds of tissues found in the body (5 points).

a. _____

b. _____

c. _____

d. _____

e. _____

5. Name the eleven body systems that will be discussed in this chapter (11 points).

a. _____   g. _____

b. _____   h. _____

c. _____   i. _____

d. _____   j. _____

e. _____   k. _____

f. _____

There are 30 possible points in this worksheet.

● WORKSHEET/ACTIVITY 3

Study the new terms in Section 13.1. Prepare to participate in a spelling bee by learning to spell and define the new terms in this unit.

There are 50 possible points for this worksheet/activity.

● WORKSHEET 4

Match each statement in column B with the correct word in column A (15 points).

Column A

_____ **1.** Superior
_____ **2.** Inferior
_____ **3.** Ventral or anterior
_____ **4.** Dorsal or posterior
_____ **5.** Cranial
_____ **6.** Caudal
_____ **7.** Medial
_____ **8.** Lateral
_____ **9.** Proximal
_____ **10.** Distal
_____ **11.** Cranial cavity
_____ **12.** Spinal cavity
_____ **13.** Thoracic cavity
_____ **14.** Abdominal cavity
_____ **15.** Pelvic cavity

Column B

a. Contains the heart, lungs, and large blood vessels.

b. Near the surface or front of the body.

c. Below or lower.

d. Near the head.

e. Near the center or midline of the body.

f. Above or in a higher position.

g. Nearest the point of attachment.

h. Away from the midline.

i. Near the back of the body.

j. Farthest from the point of attachment.

k. Encloses the spinal cord.

l. Tail end or sacral region.

m. Contains the stomach, most of the intestines, the kidneys, liver, gallbladder, pancreas, and spleen.

n. Houses the brain.

o. Contains urinary bladder, rectum, and parts of the reproductive system.

There are 15 possible points in this worksheet.

● WORKSHEET 5

Label the cavities of the body on the following diagram. Then indicate which are the ventral cavities and which are the dorsal cavities by writing *V* or *D* in spaces 6 and 7.

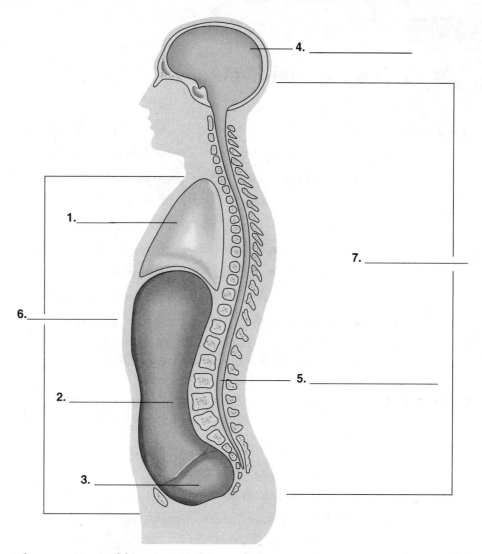

4. _____

1. _____

7. _____

6. _____

5. _____

2. _____

3. _____

There are 7 possible points in this worksheet.

• WORKSHEET 6

Select one career from each health service area, and explain why a worker in that service must have a basic knowledge of body structures and how they function (8 points).

1. a. Diagnostic services career title: _____

   b. Explanation: _____

2. a. Therapeutic services career title: _____

   b. Explanation: _____

3. a. Environmental services career title: _____

   b. Explanation: _____

4. a. Informational services career title: _____

   b. Explanation: _____

There are 8 possible points in this worksheet.

SECTION
13.2

The Skeletal System

- ## OBJECTIVES

When you have completed this section, you will be able to do the following:

- Match key terms with their correct meanings.
- Label a diagram of major bones in the body.
- Select from a list the functions of bones.
- Name the long, short, flat, and irregular bones of the body.
- Identify immovable, slightly movable, and freely movable joints of the body.
- Identify common disorders of the skeletal system.
- Label a diagram of four types of bone fractures.
- Explain why a health care worker must have a basic knowledge of the skeletal system and how it functions.

- ## DIRECTIONS

1. Complete Worksheet 1 before beginning the reading.
2. Read this section.
3. Complete Worksheets 2 through 5 as assigned.
4. Complete Worksheet 6.
5. Ask your teacher for directions to complete Worksheets/Activities 7 and 8.
6. When you are confident that you can meet each objective for this section, ask your teacher for the section evaluation.

- ## EVALUATION METHODS

- Worksheets/Activities
- Class participation
- Written evaluation

- ## WORKSHEET 1

Match each definition in column B with the correct vocabulary word in column A (15 points).

Column A	Column B
_____ 1. Appendicular	a. Parts or elements of a whole.
_____ 2. Axial	b. Living human being during the first eight weeks of development in the uterus
_____ 3. Brittle	c. Pertaining to the central structures of the body.
_____ 4. Calcify	d. Pertaining to any body part added to the axis.
_____ 5. Cartilage	e. To harden by forming calcium deposits.
_____ 6. Components	f. Bonelike.
_____ 7. Concave	

Column A

_____ **8.** Conception

_____ **9.** Embryo

_____ **10.** Flexible

_____ **11.** Lateral

_____ **12.** Osseous

_____ **13.** Penetrates

_____ **14.** Porous

_____ **15.** Spontaneous

Column B

g. Fragile, easy to break.

h. Enters or passes through.

i. Occurs when the male sperm fertilizes the female ovum and a new organism begins to develop.

j. Tough connective tissue.

k. Able to bend easily.

l. Relating to the sides or side of.

m. Filled with tiny holes.

n. Curved inward; depressed; dented.

o. Occurring naturally without apparent cause.

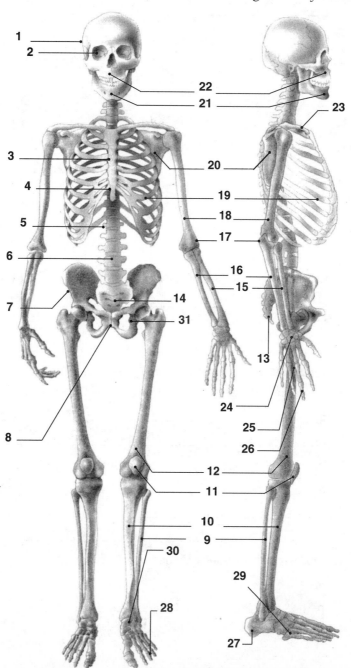

There are 15 possible points in this worksheet.

- ## WORKSHEET 2

Label the bones of the skeletal system shown on the diagram (31 points).

1. _____   17. _____
2. _____   18. _____
3. _____   19. _____
4. _____   20. _____
5. _____   21. _____
6. _____   22. _____
7. _____   23. _____
8. _____   24. _____
9. _____   25. _____
10. _____   26. _____
11. _____   27. _____
12. _____   28. _____
13. _____   29. _____
14. _____   30. _____
15. _____   31. _____
16. _____

There are 31 possible points in this worksheet.

- ## WORKSHEET 3

1. List the four functions of bones (4 points).

   a. _____
   b. _____
   c. _____
   d. _____

2. Name the long bones of the body (6 points).

   a. _____
   b. _____
   c. _____
   d. _____
   e. _____
   f. _____

3. Name the short bones of the body (2 points).

   a. _____
   b. _____

4. Name the flat bones of the body (4 points).

   a. _____
   b. _____

c. _____

d. _____

5. Name the irregular bones of the body (3 points).

a. _____

b. _____

c. _____

6. Define joint (1 point). _____

7. Name three types of joints (3 points).

a. _____

b. _____

c. _____

There are 23 possible points in this worksheet.

• WORKSHEET 4

Complete the table identifying common bone disorders.

Condition	Disorder	Symptoms
Arthritis	_____	Pain and swelling in the joints
Osteoarthritis	Inflammation of the membrane of the joint.	_____
_____	Abnormal outward curvature of the thoracic vertebrae (hunchback).	Bent appearance and sometimes pain
Lordosis	_____	Curved appearance

Condition	Disorder	Symptoms
_____	The bones do not calcify	Aches and pains in the lumbar (lower back) region and thighs, spreading later to the arms and ribs.
Osteomyelitis	_____	_____
_____	The bone becomes porous, causing it to break easily.	Pain, especially in the lower back.
Rickets	_____	Bowlegs and knock-knees enlarged.
_____	An autoimmune disease that causes chronic inflammation of the joints	Fatigue, lack of appetite, low grade fever, muscle and joint aches, and stiffness.
_____	A lateral curvature	Congenital malformation of spine.

There are 11 possible points in this worksheet.

• WORKSHEET 5

Label the fractures shown on the following diagram (4 points).

a. _____

b. _____

c. _____

d. _____

There are 4 possible points in this worksheet.

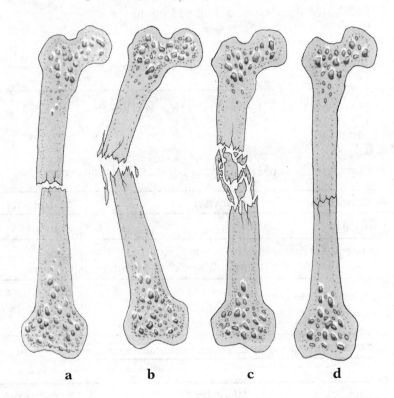

a   b   c   d

• WORKSHEET 6

Select two careers from different health services areas, and explain why a worker in that service must have a basic knowledge of the skeletal system and how it functions (6 points).

1. a. Name of health care service: _____

   b. Career title: _____

   c. Explanation: _____

2. a. Name of health care service: _____

   b. Career title: _____

   c. Explanation: _____

There are 6 possible points in this worksheet.

- **WORKSHEET/ACTIVITY 7**

    Study the new terms in Section 13.2 and memorize the bones of the body and their locations. Be prepared to label the bones of the body on a skeleton.

    There are 10 possible points in this worksheet/activity.

- **WORKSHEET/ACTIVITY 8**

    Learn the joints of the body, their locations, and their functions. Be prepared to identify, label, and explain the movement of each joint of the body.

    There are 10 possible points in this worksheet/activity.

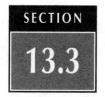

SECTION 13.3 The Muscular System

- **OBJECTIVES**

    When you have completed this section, you will be able to do the following:

    - Match key terms with their correct meanings.
    - Explain the difference between muscle and bone functions.
    - List three major functions of the muscles.
    - Match common disorders of the muscular system with their descriptions.
    - Match basic muscle movements to their correct names.
    - Label a diagram of the muscular system.
    - Describe how muscles provide support and movement.
    - Explain why the health care worker's understanding of the muscular system is important.

- **DIRECTIONS**

    1. Complete Worksheet 1.
    2. Complete Worksheets 2 through 5 as assigned.
    3. When you are confident that you can meet each objective for this section, ask your teacher for the section evaluation.

- **EVALUATION METHODS**

    - Worksheets
    - Class participation
    - Written evaluation

• WORKSHEET 1

Match each definition statement in column B with the correct vocabulary word in column A (8 points).

Column A	Column B
_____ 1. Axis	a. To break down.
_____ 2. Contract (v.)	b. Not under control.
_____ 3. Deteriorate	c. Damage to the body caused by an injury, wound, or shock.
_____ 4. Digestion	d. Under the control of the person.
_____ 5. Elastic	e. A center point.
_____ 6. Involuntary	f. Easily stretched.
_____ 7. Trauma	g. To shorten; to draw together.
_____ 8. Voluntary	h. Process of breaking down food mechanically and chemically.

There are 8 possible points in this worksheet.

• WORKSHEET 2

1. List the three main functions of muscles (3 points).

   a. _____

   b. _____

   c. _____

2. Write each word listed below in the space next to the statement that best defines it (6 points).

   adduct   flex   rotate

   abduct   extended   sphincter

   _____ a. To move a body part away from the midline.

   _____ b. Circular muscle that controls an opening.

   _____ c. To move a body part toward the midline.

   _____ d. To turn a body part on its axis.

   _____ e. To straighten a body part by moving it away from the body.

   _____ f. To bend a body part toward the body.

3. Write the name of the correct muscular system disorder beside each of the definitions below (4 points).

   a. Disease that progressively deteriorates muscle tissue _____

   b. Trauma to the muscle, usually caused by a violent contraction _____

   c. Muscle pain _____

   d. Tear of the muscle tissue _____

There are 13 possible points in this worksheet.

● WORKSHEET 3

Label the parts of the muscular system on the following diagram (19 points).

1._____ 8._____ 14._____

2._____ 9._____ 15._____

3._____ 10._____ 16._____

4._____ 11._____ 17._____

5._____ 12._____ 18._____

6._____ 13._____ 19._____

7._____

There are 19 possible points in this worksheet.

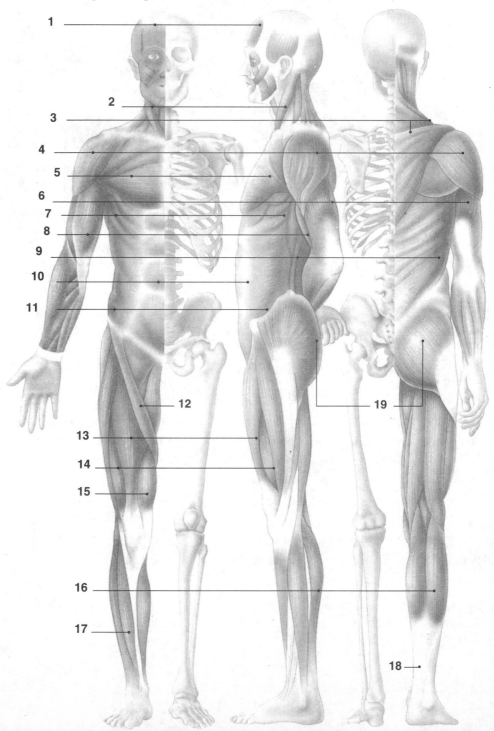

● **WORKSHEET 4**

Fill in the crossword puzzle using the common disorders and terminology list from Section 13.3 in your text.

[ ] Indicates a space between two words.

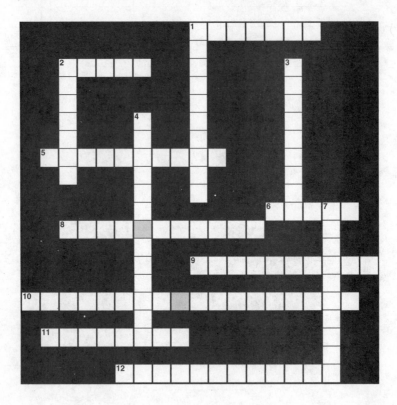

Clues

Across

1. Muscular protrusion (bulge) through a muscle.
2. Resembling muscle.
5. Inflammation of connective tissue.
6. Tumor containing muscle tissue.
8. Tear of the muscle tissue.

9. Weakness or partial paralysis of a muscle.
10. Disease that progressively deteriorates muscle tissue.
11. Beginning in the muscle.
12. Pain of the abdominal muscle.

Down

1. Heart muscle or cardiac muscle.
2. Muscle pain.
3. Record of muscle contractions.

4. Trauma to the muscle, usually caused by a violent contraction.
7. Muscle weakness.

There are 12 possible points in this worksheet.

● WORKSHEET 5

1. Describe how muscles provide support for the body (5 points). _____

_____

_____

_____

_____

2. Describe how muscles allow movement (5 points). _____

_____

_____

_____

_____

3. Select two careers from different health service areas, and explain why a worker in that service must have a basic knowledge of the muscular system and how it functions (6 points).

   a. Name of health care service: _____

   b. Career title: _____

   c. Explanation: _____

   _____

   _____

   _____

   d. Name of health care service: _____

   e. Career title: _____

   f. Explanation: _____

   _____

   _____

   _____

There are 16 possible points in this worksheet.

SECTION 13.4 The Circulatory System

• OBJECTIVES

When you have completed this section, you will be able to do the following:

- Match key terms with their correct meanings.
- Name the major organs of the circulatory system.
- Label a diagram of the heart and blood vessels.
- Recognize functions of the circulatory system.
- Identify the common disorders of the circulatory system.
- List the parts of the circulatory system through which blood flows.
- Describe how the circulatory system supports life.
- Explain why the health care worker's understanding of the circulatory system is important.

• DIRECTIONS

1. Complete Worksheet 1.
2. Complete Worksheets 2 through 6 as assigned.
3. When you are confident that you can meet each objective for this section, ask your teacher for the section evaluation.

• EVALUATION METHODS

- Worksheets
- Class participation
- Written evaluation

● WORKSHEET 1

Fill in the crossword puzzle using the vocabulary words from Section 13.4 in your text.

Indicates a space between two words.

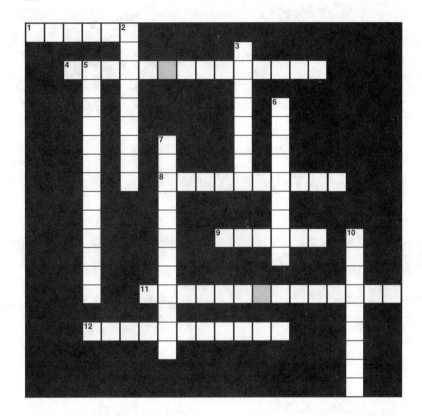

Clues

Across

1. Element in the atmosphere that is essential for maintaining life.
4. Elements that are unfit for the body's use and are eliminated from the body.
8. Containing oxygen.

Down

2. Food substances that supply the body with necessary elements for good health.
3. Enough, sufficient.
5. Things that are not usual, that differ from the standard.

There are 12 possible points in this worksheet.

9. Defective or imperfect.
11. A gas, heavier than air; a waste product from the body.
12. Arms, legs, hands, and feet.

6. For the most part; chiefly.
7. Lacking oxygen.
10. Pertaining to old age; over 65 years.

● WORKSHEET 2

Label the parts of the circulatory system on the following diagram.

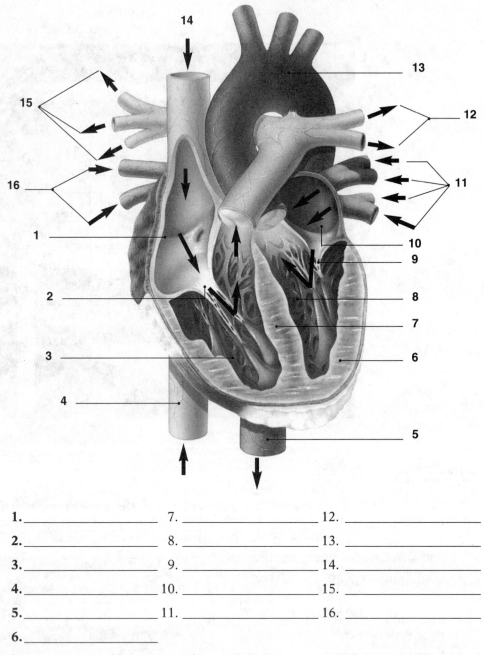

1._____	7. _____	12. _____
2._____	8. _____	13. _____
3._____	9. _____	14. _____
4._____	10. _____	15. _____
5._____	11. _____	16. _____
6._____		

There are 16 possible points in this worksheet.

● WORKSHEET 3

Label the following diagram, indicating the names of vessels and showing the movement of oxygen (O_2) and carbon dioxide (CO_2) in the cells of body organs.

1. _____

2. _____

3. _____

4. _____

5. _____

There are 5 possible points in this worksheet.

• WORKSHEET 4

List the parts of the circulatory system through which blood flows. Begin at the right atrium and return to the right atrium.

1. Right atrium _____ **11.** _____

2. _____ **12.** _____

3. _____ **13.** _____

4. _____ **14.** _____

5. _____ **15.** _____

6. _____ **16.** _____

7. _____ **17.** _____

8. _____ **18.** _____

9. _____ **19.** _____

10. _____ **20.** _____

There are 20 possible points in this worksheet.

• WORKSHEET 5

1. Describe how the circulatory system supports life (1 point.) _____

_____

_____

_____

_____

_____

2. Explain why your understanding of the circulatory system is important (1 point). _____

_____

_____

_____

_____

_____

_____

There are 2 possible points in this worksheet.

● WORKSHEET 6

Briefly describe the disorder associated with each of the following conditions.

a. Aneurysm _____

b. Arteriosclerosis _____

c. Endocarditis _____

d. Heart murmur _____

e. Hypertension _____

f. Myocardial infarction (MI) _____

g. Myocarditis _____

h. Pericarditis _____

i. Varicose veins _____

There are 18 possible points in this worksheet.

SECTION

13.5 The Lymphatic System

● OBJECTIVES

When you have completed this section, you will be able to do the following:

- Match key terms with their correct meanings.
- Describe the general functions of the lymphatic system.
- Describe what lymph is.
- Match lymph vessels and organs to their function.
- Explain the difference between an antigen and an antibody.
- Identify common disorders of the lymphatic system.
- Describe how the lymphatic system helps provide immunity.

• DIRECTIONS

1. Complete Worksheet 1.

2. Complete Worksheets 2 through 4 as assigned.

3. When you are confident that you can meet each objective for this section, ask your teacher for the section evaluation.

• EVALUATION METHODS

- Worksheets
- Class participation
- Written evaluation

• WORKSHEET 1

Fill in the crossword puzzle using the vocabulary words and terminology list from Section 13.5 in your text.

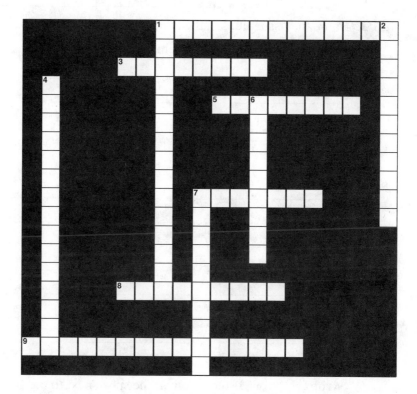

Clues

Across

1. Abnormally high number of lymphocytes in the blood.

3. Tumor made up of lymphatic tissue.

5. Absence of a spleen.

7. Foreign matter that causes the body to produce antibodies.

8. Cell that surrounds, eats, and digests microorganisms.

9. Surgical removal of the lymph nodes.

Down

1. Abnormally low number of lymphocytes in the blood.
2. Surgical removal of the spleen.
4. Enlargement of the lymph nodes.

There are 11 possible points in this worksheet.

6. Pertaining to an organism that lives in or on another organism, taking nourishment from it.
7. Substances made by the body to produce immunity to an antigen.

● WORKSHEET 2

1. What other system does the lymphatic system work closely with (1 point)?

   _____

2. What are the main functions of the lymphatic system (4 points)?

   a. _____

   b. _____

   c. _____

   d. _____

3. Name the tissue fluid in the lymphatic system (1 point). _____

4. What does the lymphatic system protect the body against (1 point)? _____

   _____

   _____

5. List the parts of the lymphatic system (10 points).

   a. _____

   b. _____

   c. _____

   d. _____

   e. _____

   f. _____

   g. _____

   h. _____

   i. _____

   j. _____

6. Write each word listed below in the space next to the statement that best describes it (8 points).

lymph	capillaries	lymph	tonsils
thymus	lymphocytes	lymph nodes	
lymph	vessels	spleen	

   _____ a. Help the body defend itself.

   _____ b. Lie along the lymph vessels.

   _____ c. Tubes that reach into the interstitial spaces of most body tissues.

_____ d. Filters microorganisms and waste products from the blood.

_____ e. Have valves to help move the lymph from the tissues.

_____ f. Tissue fluid that is in a capillary.

_____ g. Stores lymphocytes that work with the lymphatic system to defend the body.

_____ h. Filter tissue fluid, not lymph.

There are 25 possible points in this worksheet.

• WORKSHEET 3

1. Describe the difference between an antigen and an antibody (1 point).

_____

_____

_____

2. Explain how the lymphatic system helps provide immunity (1 point).

_____

_____

_____

_____

_____

3. Describe how you would have to live if your immune system did not protect you from bacteria (1 point).

_____

_____

_____

_____

There are 3 possible points in this worksheet.

• WORKSHEET 4

1. What are allergies?

2. How is anaphylactic shock related to, but different from, common allergies?

3. In what way is elephantiasis related to the lymphatic system?

4. Describe lymphadenitis.

There are 4 possible points in this worksheet.

13.6 The Respiratory System

● OBJECTIVES

When you have completed this section, you will be able to do the following:

- Match key terms with their correct meanings.
- Label major organs of the respiratory system on a diagram.
- Describe the flow of oxygen through the body.
- Identify common disorders of the respiratory system.
- Describe how the respiratory system supports life.
- Explain why the health care worker's understanding of the respiratory system is important.

● DIRECTIONS

1. Complete Worksheet 1 after reading the section.
2. Complete Worksheets 2 through 5 as assigned.
3. When you are confident that you can meet each objective for this section, ask your teacher for the section evaluation.

● EVALUATION METHODS

- Worksheets
- Class participation
- Written evaluation

● WORKSHEET 1

Fill in the crossword puzzle using the vocabulary words and terminology list from Section 13.6 in your text.

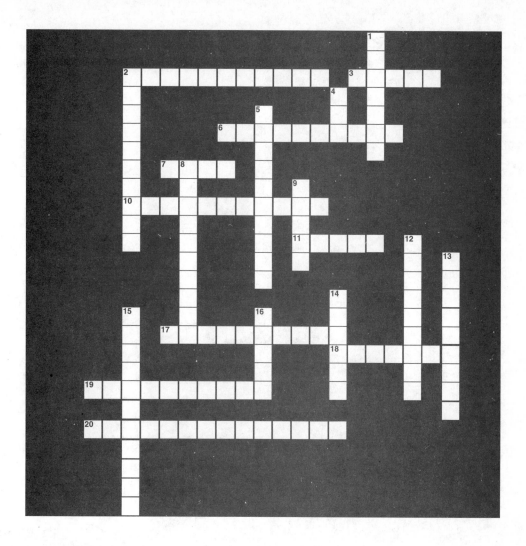

Clues

Across

2. Getting rid of.
3. Cessation of breathing.
6. Inflammation of the bronchial tubes.
7. Abbreviation for "eye, ear, nose, throat."
10. Process of breathing in air during respiration (see also 18).

11. Hairlike projections that move rhythmically on the inside lining of the bronchial tubes.
17. Process of breathing in air during respiration (see also 11).
18. Difficult or painful breathing.
19. Inflammation of the larynx.
20. Dilation of the bronchi.

Down

1. Lack of oxygen.
2. Process of forcing air out of the body during respiration (see also 8).
4. Abbreviation for "upper respiratory infection."
5. Things that contaminate the air.
8. Process of forcing air out of the body during respiration (see also 2).

9. Small bag or sac.
12. Rapid breathing.
13. Nosebleed.
14. To cause to be or become.
15. Between the ribs.
16. Nostrils.

There are 21 possible points in this worksheet.

● WORKSHEET 2

1. Label the parts of the respiratory system on the following diagram (10 points).

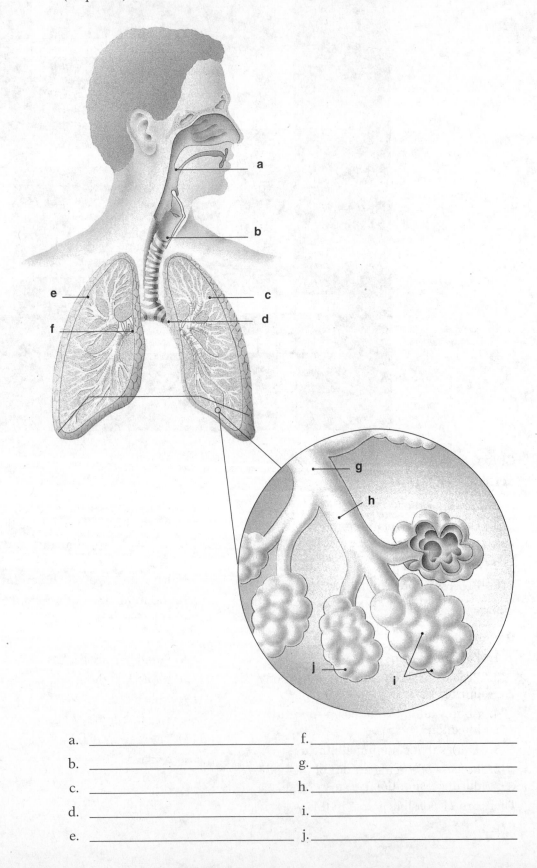

a. _____   f. _____

b. _____   g. _____

c. _____   h. _____

d. _____   i. _____

e. _____   j. _____

2. Describe the flow of oxygen through the body, starting with the nose or mouth and ending at the cell (10 points).

a. nose or mouth_____   f._____

b. _____   g._____

c. _____   h._____

d. _____   i._____

e. _____   j._____

There are 20 possible points in this worksheet.

• WORKSHEET 3

Write the appropriate word for each of the following definitions.

_____   **1.** Condition in which the alveoli become stretched and unable to force carbon dioxide out of the lungs.

_____   **2.** Essential life-giving element.

_____   **3.** Process of forcing air out of the body during respiration.

_____   **4.** Condition in which the walls of the bronchial tubes become narrow and less air passes through.

_____   **5.** Gaseous waste product of the cell.

_____   **6.** Inflammation of the lungs.

_____   **7.** Things that contaminate the air.

_____   **8.** Breathing.

_____   **9.** Infectious disease caused by the tubercle bacillus.

_____   **10.** Process of breathing in air during respiration.

There are 10 possible points in this worksheet.

• WORKSHEET 4

1. Describe how the respiratory system supports life (1 point). _____

_____

_____

_____

2. Explain why your understanding of the respiratory system is important (1 point). _____

_____

_____

_____

There are 2 possible points in this worksheet.

● WORKSHEET 5

Write the name of each condition described.

_____ **1.** Progressive disease can result in disability, and in severe cases, heart or respiratory failure and death. Symptoms include anxiety, shortness of breath, difficulty breathing, cough, cyanosis, and rapid heartbeat.

_____ **2.** Infectious disease caused by the tubercle bacillus. Symptoms include listlessness, vague chest pain, decreased appetite, fever, night sweats, and weight loss.

_____ **3.** A condition in which the bronchial tube walls spasm, narrowing the passageways. This makes it difficult to exhale and creates a suffocating feeling.

_____ **4.** A contagious illness that can be caused by a number of different types of viruses. May cause a person to feel tired along with having nasal stuffiness, sore throat, hoarseness, cough and sometimes fever and headache.

_____ **5.** Inflammation of the lungs, usually caused by bacteria, viruses, or an irritation by chemicals. Symptoms include chills, fever, chest pain headache, and cough.

There are 10 possible points in this worksheet.

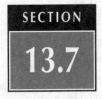

SECTION 13.7 The Digestive System

● OBJECTIVES

When you have completed this section, you will be able to do the following:

- Match key terms with their correct meanings.

- Label a diagram of the digestive system and its accessory organs.

- Explain the functions of the digestive system.

- Recognize the function of organs associated with the digestive system.

- Match common disorders of the digestive system with their descriptions.

- Describe how the digestive system absorbs nutrients.

- Explain why the health care worker's understanding of the digestive system is important.

● DIRECTIONS

1. Complete Worksheets 1 through 5 as assigned.

2. When you are confident that you can meet each objective for this section, ask your teacher for the section evaluation.

• EVALUATION METHODS

- Worksheets
- Class participation
- Written evaluation

• WORKSHEET 1

Match each definition in column B with the correct vocabulary word in column A (9 points).

Column A	Column B
_____ **1.** Absorption	a. Outlet from which the body expels solid
_____ **2.** Alimentary canal waste.	b. Creamy semifluid mixture of food and digestive juices.
_____ **3.** Antibodies	c. Passage of watery stool at frequent intervals.
_____ **4.** Anus	d. Pertaining to the area over the pit of the stomach.
_____ **5.** Chyme	e. The digestive tube from the mouth to the anus.
_____ **6.** Defecation	f. Process of breaking down food mechanically and chemically.
_____ **7.** Diarrhea	g. Process of taking in, absorbing.
_____ **8.** Digestion	h. The pushing of solid material from the bowel.
_____ **9.** Epigastric	i. Substances produced by the body to destroy disease-causing organisms and foreign matter that attacks the body.

Write each word listed below in the space next to the statement that best defines it (8 points).

liver	evacuated	insulin
minute (adj.)	feces	sphincter
peristalsis	secrete	

_____ **10.** Emptied out.

_____ **11.** Solid waste that is evacuated from the body.

_____ **12.** Largest gland in the body.

_____ **13.** Hormone secreted by the pancreas that is essential for maintaining the correct blood sugar level.

_____ **14.** Exceptionally small.

_____ **15.** Progressive, wavelike motion that occurs involuntarily in hollow tubes of the body.

_____ **16.** To discharge a substance.

_____ **17.** Circular muscle that allows the opening and closing of a body part.

There are 17 possible points in this worksheet.

● WORKSHEET 2

Label the parts of the digestive system on the following diagram.

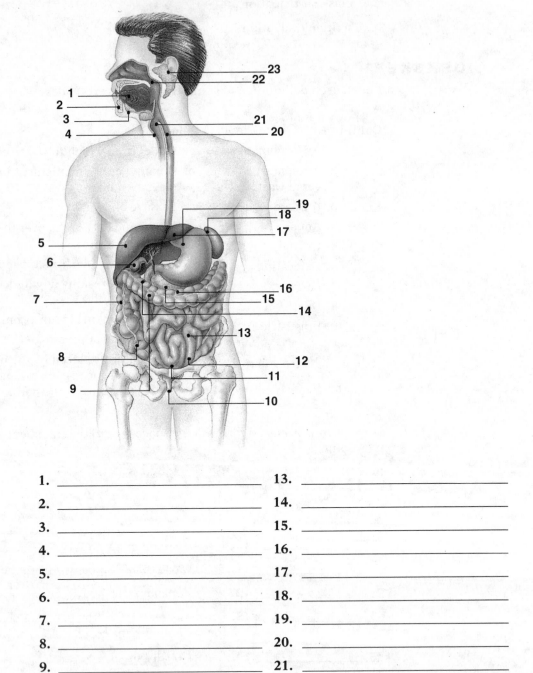

1. _____   13. _____

2. _____   14. _____

3. _____   15. _____

4. _____   16. _____

5. _____   17. _____

6. _____   18. _____

7. _____   19. _____

8. _____   20. _____

9. _____   21. _____

10. _____   22. _____

11. _____   23. _____

12. _____

There are 23 possible points in this worksheet.

• WORKSHEET 3

Write the appropriate word next to each of the following statements.

_____ **1.** Process of changing food into a usable substance by the body.

_____ **2.** A passageway for food located at the back of the oral cavity.

_____ **3.** Rhythmic wavelike motion.

_____ **4.** Produces secretions that dissolve food and coat food with mucus.

_____ **5.** Long muscular tube that begins at the mouth and ends at the anus.

_____ **6.** Creamy semifluid mixture of food and digestive juices.

_____ **7.** Flap that covers the trachea.

_____ **8.** Where food enters the body.

_____ **9.** First 10 to 12 inches of the small intestine.

_____ **10.** Last 6 to 8 inches of the alimentary canal.

_____ **11.** Receives food and water from the pharynx.

_____ **12.** Minute projections that line the small intestine.

_____ **13.** Is attached to the small intestine and absorbs water.

_____ **14.** Ringlike muscle found at the far end of the stomach.

_____ **15.** Receives food and water from the esophagus.

_____ **16.** Portion of the alimentary canal where most absorption takes place.

_____ **17.** End of the alimentary canal.

_____ **18.** Produces pancreatic juices.

_____ **19.** Produces bile, heparin, and antibodies.

_____ **20.** Sac that stores bile.

_____ **21.** Condition that occurs when the cells of the liver become damaged.

_____ **22.** Inflammation of the pancreas.

_____ **23.** Inflammation of the liver.

_____ **24.** Presence of a stone in the gallbladder.

There are 24 possible points in this worksheet.

• WORKSHEET 4

1. Describe how the digestive system absorbs nutrients (1 point). _____

_____

_____

_____

_____

_____

_____

2. Explain why your understanding of the digestive system is important (1 point). _____

_____

_____

_____

_____

_____

There are 2 possible points in this worksheet.

• WORKSHEET 5

Fill in the crossword puzzle using the terminology list from Section 13.7 in your text.

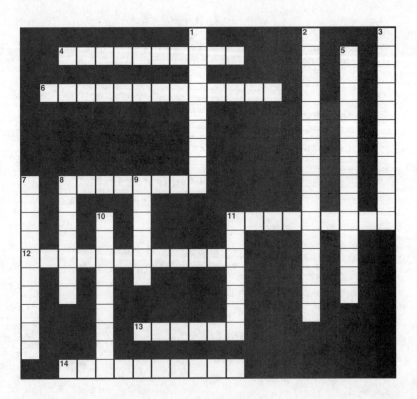

Clues

Across

4. Cyst of the intestinal wall.
6. Pertaining to the intestines and the liver.
8. Lack of appetite.
11. Opening into the colon.

Down

1. Difficult or painful swallowing.
2. Pertaining to the stomach and intestines.
3. Any disease of the liver.
5. Incision for the removal of a gall-stone.
7. Process by which food is changed into energy for the body's use.

12. Pertaining to the cheek and tongue.
13. Vomiting.
14. Hernia involving the intestine.

8. Without acid.
9. Substance that induces vomiting.
10. Gallbladder.
11. Inflammation of the colon.

There are 16 possible points in this worksheet.

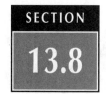

SECTION 13.8

The Urinary System

● OBJECTIVES

When you have completed this section, you will be able to do the following:

- Match key terms with their correct meanings.
- Label a diagram of the urinary system.
- Identify the function of organs in the urinary system.
- Match common disorders of the urinary system with their descriptions.
- Describe how the urinary system removes liquid waste and eliminates it from the body.
- Explain why the health care worker's understanding of the urinary system is important.

● DIRECTIONS

1. Complete Worksheet 1 before beginning the reading.
2. Read this section.
3. Complete Worksheets 2 through 4 as assigned.
4. When you are confident that you can meet each objective for this section, ask your teacher for the section evaluation.

● EVALUATION METHODS

- Worksheets
- Class participation
- Written evaluation

• WORKSHEET 1

1. Define the following vocabulary words. Look in a medical dictionary for words that are not in your glossary (7 points).

    a. Nephron _____

    b. Hemodialysis _____

    c. Micturition _____

    d. Urination _____

    e. Peritoneal cavity _____

    f. Excrete _____

    g. Mechanism _____

2. Write each word listed below in the space next to the statement that best defines it. Look in a medical dictionary (7 points).

waste product   dialysis   obstruction   edema

elimination   symptom   infuses

_____ a. Any change in the body or its functions that indicates a disease.

_____ b. Flows into the body by gravity.

_____ c. Process of removing waste from body fluids.

_____ d. Process of getting rid of something.

_____ e. Blockage or clogging.

_____ f. Material that is unfit for the body's use and is eliminated from the body.

_____ g. Abnormal or excessive collection of fluid in the tissues.

There are 14 possible points in this worksheet.

• WORKSHEET 2

Label the parts of the urinary system on the following diagram.

1. _____   7. _____

2. _____   8. _____

3. _____   9. _____

4. _____   10. _____

5. _____   11. _____

6. _____   12. _____

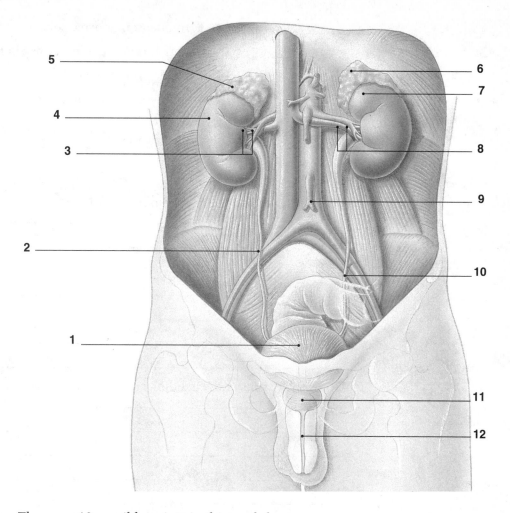

There are 12 possible points in this worksheet.

● WORKSHEET 3

Write the appropriate word next to each of the following statements.

_____ **1.** Liquid waste product of the body.

_____ **2.** Inner part of the kidney.

_____ **3.** Inflammation of the kidney.

_____ **4.** Kidney stones.

_____ **5.** Sac surrounding the kidney.

_____ **6.** Abnormal or excessive collection of fluid in the tissue.

_____ **7.** Inflammation of the urethra.

_____ **8.** Chief filtering mechanism of the kidney.

_____ **9.** Cuplike capsule.

_____ **10.** Inflammation of the urinary bladder.

_____ **11.** Tiny twisted tube of the nephron.

_____ **12.** Accumulation of urine substances in the blood.

_____ **13.** Common treatment for kidney failure.

_____ **14.** Expanded renal pelvis.

_____ **15.** Condition in which the nephron of the kidney is unable to filter waste.

There are 15 possible points for this worksheet.

● WORKSHEET 4

1. Describe how the urinary system removes liquid waste and eliminates it from the body (1 point). _____

_____

_____

_____

_____

_____

2. Explain why your understanding of the urinary system is important (1 point). _____

_____

_____

_____

_____

_____

There are 2 possible points in this worksheet.

SECTION

13.9 The Endocrine Systems

● OBJECTIVES

When you have completed this section, you will be able to do the following:

- Match key terms with their correct meanings.
- Label endocrine glands on a diagram.
- Identify functions of the endocrine glands.
- Identify common disorders of the endocrine glands.
- Explain the difference between the endocrine and exocrine glands.

■ Describe the effects of the endocrine glands on the body.

■ Explain why the health care worker's understanding of the glandular systems is important.

● DIRECTIONS

1. Complete Worksheets 1 through 4 as assigned.

2. When you are confident that you can meet each objective for this section, ask your teacher for the section evaluation.

● EVALUATION METHOD

■ Worksheets

■ Class participation

■ Written evaluation

● WORKSHEET 1

Match each definition in column B to the correct vocabulary word in column A (6 points).

Column A

_____ **1.** Duct

_____ **2.** Hormone

_____ **3.** Lacrimal

_____ **4.** Sebaceous

_____ **5.** Excrete

_____ **6.** Metabolism

Column B

a. Narrow, round tube that carries secretions from a gland.

b. Throw off or eliminate as waste product.

c. Body's process of using food to make energy and use nutrients.

d. Pertaining to tears.

e. Protein substance secreted by an endocrine gland directly into the blood.

f. Pertaining to fatty secretions.

There are 6 possible points in this worksheet.

● WORKSHEET 2

Label the parts of the glandular system on the following diagram.

1. _____

2. _____

3. _____

4. _____

5. _____

6. _____

7. _____

8. _____

9. _____

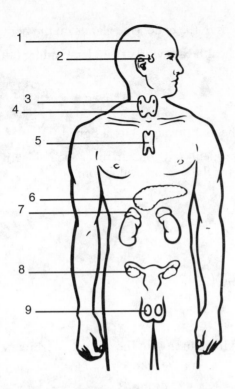

There are 9 possible points in this worksheet.

● WORKSHEET 3

Write the appropriate word next to each of the following statements.

_____ **1.** Fluids that are carried to a nearby organ or to the outside of the body.

_____ **2.** Glands that have ducts.

_____ **3.** Gland that produces thyroxin.

_____ **4.** Hormones that are carried to all parts of the body through the blood and lymph systems.

_____ **5.** Gland that produces adrenalin.

_____ **6.** Glands without ducts.

_____ **7.** Gland that produces parathyroid hormones.

_____ **8.** Gland that produces TSH, ACTH, FSH, LH, oxytocin, prolactin, and somatotropic hormones.

_____ **9.** Gland that produces insulin.

_____ **10.** Glands that produce estrogen and progesterone.

_____ **11.** Gland that produces corticoids.

_____ **12.** Glands that produce testosterone.

_____ **13.** Deficiency of sugar in the blood.

_____ **14.** Decreased production of the thyroid secretion.

_____ **15.** Insufficient amount of hormones from the adrenal glands.

_____ **16.** Overabundance of sugar in the blood.

_____ **17.** Increased production of the thyroid secretion.

There are 17 possible points in this worksheet.

• WORKSHEET 4

1. Describe ways the glandular systems help regulate body processes (7 points). _____

_____

_____

_____

_____

2. Explain why your understanding of the glandular systems is important (1 point)._____

_____

_____

_____

_____

3. Explain how endocrine glands are different from exocrine glands. (3 points)._____

_____

_____

_____

_____

There are 11 possible points in this worksheet.

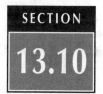

SECTION

13.10 The Nervous System

• OBJECTIVES

When you have completed this section, you will be able to do the following:

- Match key terms with their correct meanings.

- Match and select the functions of various parts of the nervous system.

- Label diagrams of the eye and ear.

- Match common disorders of the nervous system with their correct names.

- Describe the influence of the nervous system on the body.

- Explain why the health care worker's understanding of the nervous system is important.

158

• DIRECTIONS

1. Complete Worksheets 1 through 6 as assigned.

2. When you are confident that you can meet each objective for this section, ask your teacher for the section evaluation.

• EVALUATION METHODS

- Worksheets
- Class participation
- Written evaluation

• WORKSHEET 1

Write the appropriate word next to each of the following statements (5 points).

_____ 1. To increase or elevate a sound.

_____ 2. State of balance.

_____ 3. Three small bones in the middle ear that amplify sound.

_____ 4. Nerve; includes the cell and the long fiber coming from the cell.

_____ 5. Elements in the external or internal environment that are strong enough to set up a nervous impulse.

Match each definition in column B with the correct vocabulary word in column A (9 points).

Column A

_____ 6. Cerebrum
_____ 7. Peripheral
_____ 8. CNS
_____ 9. Ganglia
_____10. Pigmented
_____11. Receptor
_____12. Response
_____13. Scattering
_____14. Translate

Column B

a. Colored

b. Nerve that responds to stimuli.

c. Spreading in many directions; dispersing.

d. Action or movement due to a stimulus.

e. Portion of the brain that controls voluntary movements.

f. Mass of nerve tissue composed of nerve cell bodies.

g. Situated away from a central structure.

h. Central nervous system.

i. To make understandable.

There are 14 possible points in this worksheet.

• WORKSHEET 2

Complete the following sentences.

1. The central nervous system includes the (a) _____ and the (b) _____ (2 points).

2. The peripheral nervous system includes the (a) _____ and (b) _____ outside the brain and spinal cord (2 points).

3. The nervous system is a system of nerve cells linked together to

(a) _____ stimuli and (b) _____ to stimuli (2 points).

4. The nervous system works together in _____ messages to the brain (1 point).

5. Each specialized neuron leads into a passage that delivers the message or stimuli to the areas in the brain that can (a) _____ and cause a (b) _____ (2 points).

There are 9 possible points in this worksheet.

• WORKSHEET 3

1. Label the parts of the eye on the following diagram (10 points).

a. _____   f. _____

b. _____   g. _____

c. _____   h. _____

d. _____   i. _____

e. _____   j. _____

2. List three things that protect the eye (3 points).

a. _____

b. _____

c. _____

3. The white of the eye is the _____ (1 point).

4. The heavily pigmented second coating of the eye is
the_____ (1 point).

5. The clear front portion of the sclera is the _____ (1 point).

6. The innermost coating of the eye, which senses vision, is
the_____ (1 point).

7. The nerve that receives a picture and sends it to the brain for interpretation
is the _____ (1 point).

There are 18 possible points in this worksheet.

• WORKSHEET 4

1. Label the parts of the ear on the following diagram (11 points).

a. _____   g._____

b. _____   h._____

c. _____   i._____

d. _____   j._____

e. _____   k._____

f. _____

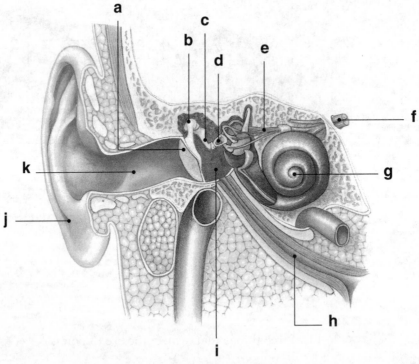

2. Name the three main parts of the ear (3 points).

a. _____

b. _____

c. _____

3. The middle ear contains (a) _____ [number] bones called
   (b) _____ (2 points).

4. The semicircular canals of the inner ear (a) _____ sound
   waves to the (b) _____ that allow us to (c)
   _____ sound (3 points).

There are 19 possible points in this worksheet.

● WORKSHEET 5

1. Taste is sensed by receptors called _____ (1 point).

2. Name the four main tastes (4 points).

   a. _____   c. _____

   b. _____   d. _____

3. The receptor that receives smells is called the _____ (1
   point).

4. Our special senses of sight, hearing, taste, and smell are limited to certain
   areas of the body. List the four general senses that are found throughout
   the body (4 points).

   a. _____   c. _____

   b. _____   d. _____

5. Write the appropriate word for each of the following definitions (6 points).

   _____ a. Clouding of the lens of the eye.

   _____ b. Condition in which blisters appear on the nerves
   and cause a great deal of pain.

   _____ c. Condition that causes deafness because the bones
   in the ear change.

   _____ d. Inflammation of a nerve.

   _____ e. Inflammation of the eyelid lining.

   _____ f. Condition that can cause deterioration of the optic
   nerve.

There are 16 possible points in this worksheet.

● WORKSHEET 6

1. Describe the influence of the nervous system on the body (7 points). _____

   _____

   _____

   _____

   _____

   _____

   _____

2. Explain why your understanding of the nervous system is important (1 point). _____

_____

_____

_____

_____

There are 8 possible points in this worksheet.

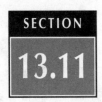

SECTION

13.11

The Reproductive System

• OBJECTIVES

When you have completed this section, you will be able to do the following:

- Match key terms with their correct meanings.

- Label a diagram of the male and female reproductive systems.

- Match the various organs in the reproductive systems with their functions.

- Match common disorders of the reproductive system with their descriptions.

- Describe how the reproductive system affects the body.

- Explain why the health care worker's understanding of the reproductive system is important.

• DIRECTIONS

1. Complete Worksheets 1 through 5 as assigned.

2. When you are confident that you can meet each objective for this section, ask your teacher for the section evaluation.

• EVALUATION METHODS

- Worksheets
- Class participation
- Written evaluation

• WORKSHEET 1

Match each definition in column B with the correct vocabulary word in column A (7 points).

Column A

_____ **1.** Cilia

_____ **2.** Fetus

_____ **3.** Ova

_____ **4.** Semen

_____ **5.** Menstruation

_____ **6.** Peristalsis

_____ **7.** Endometrium

Column B

a. Female reproductive cells that, when fertilized by the male, develop into a new organism.

b. Cyclic deterioration of the endometrium.

c. Infant developing in the uterus after the first three months until birth.

d. Interlining of the uterus.

e. Hairlike projections that move rhythmically.

f. Fluid from the testes, seminal vesicles, prostate gland, and bulbourethral glands that contains water, mucin, proteins, salts, and sperm.

g. Progressive, wavelike movement that occurs involuntarily in hollow tubes of the body.

Define the following words (6 points).

8. Estrogen _____

9. Mature _____

10. Sex cell _____

11. Testosterone _____

12. Spermatozoa _____

13. Projections _____

There are 13 possible points in this worksheet.

• WORKSHEET 2

1. Label the parts of the female reproductive system on the following diagram (10 points).

a. _____ f. _____

b. _____ g. _____

c. _____ h. _____

d. _____ i. _____

e. _____ j. _____

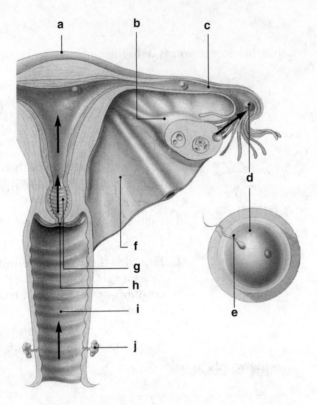

2. Write each organ listed below in the space next to the statement that best defines its function (5 points).

ovaries   fallopian tubes   fimbriae

uterus   vagina

_____ a. Houses and nourishes the fertilized ovum.

_____ b. Houses the neck of the uterus and is known as the birth canal.

_____ c. Produce ova and estrogen.

_____ d. Function as passageways through which ova travel into the uterus.

_____ e. Create a current that sweeps the ovum into the fallopian tube.

There are 15 possible points in this worksheet.

● WORKSHEET 3

1. Label the parts of the male reproductive system on the following diagram (14 points).

a. _____

b. _____

c. _____

d. _____

e. _____

f. _____

g. _____

h. _____

i. _____

j. _____

k. _____

l. _____

m. _____

n. _____

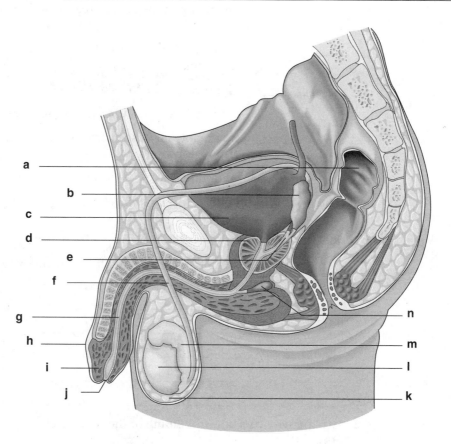

2. Write each organ listed below in the space next to the statement that best defines its function (6 points).

testes   epididymis   vas deferens

seminal   vesicles   prostate gland   urethra

_____ a. Produce a thick yellow secretion that adds to the volume of semen and nourishes the sperm.

_____ b. Functions as a passageway for sperm.

_____ c. Produces a secretion that maintains the mobility of sperm.

_____ d. Serves as a passageway for sperm and urine.

_____ e. Stores sperm until they mature.

_____ f. Produce spermatozoa and testosterone.

There are 20 possible points in this worksheet.

● WORKSHEET 4

Write the appropriate disorder next to each of the following descriptions (8 points).

_____ 1. Contagious disease characterized by a discharge of pus from the urethra.

_____ 2. Hidden testes.

_____ 3. Contagious disease characterized by recurrent lesions appearing in the genital region and the mucosa of the mouth.

_____ 4. Nonbloody vaginal discharge usually caused by an infection.

_____ 5. Tightness of the foreskin.

_____ 6. Tumors in women that are usually benign.

_____ 7. Contagious disease characterized by lesions that may not appear for months.

_____ 8. Inflammation of the testes.

There are 8 possible points in this worksheet.

● WORKSHEET 5

1. Describe how the reproductive system affects the body (3 points).

_____

_____

_____

_____

_____

2. Explain why your understanding of the reproductive system is important (1 point).

_____

_____

_____

_____

_____

There are 4 possible points in this worksheet.

13.12 The Integumentary System

- ## OBJECTIVES

  When you have completed this section, you will be able to do the following:

  - Match key terms with their correct meanings.
  - Label a diagram of a cross section of skin.
  - List the five main functions of skin.
  - Identify three main layers of the skin.
  - Match common disorders of the integumentary system with their descriptions.
  - Describe how the integumentary system protects the body.
  - Explain why the health care worker's understanding of the integumentary system is important.

- ## DIRECTIONS

  1. Read this section.
  2. Complete Worksheets 1 and 2 as assigned.
  3. When you are confident that you can meet each objective for this section, ask your teacher for the section evaluation.

- ## EVALUATION METHODS

  - Worksheets
  - Class participation
  - Written evaluation

- ## WORKSHEET 1

  1. Write each word listed below in the space next to the statement that best defines it (3 points).

     epidermis   sloughed   subcutaneous

     _____ a. Under the skin.

     _____ b. Outer layer of skin.

     _____ c. Discarded; separated from.

2. Label the parts of the cross section of skin on the following diagram (14 points).

a. _____

b. _____

c. _____

d. _____

e. _____

f. _____

g. _____

h. _____

i. _____

j. _____

k. _____

l. _____

m. _____

n. _____

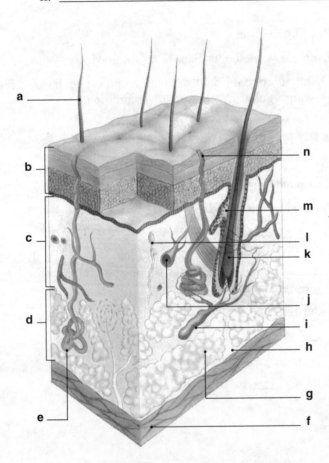

There are 17 possible points in this worksheet.

• WORKSHEET 2

1. Name the two kinds of glands that are present in the skin (2 points).

a. _____

b. _____

2. Name the kinds of tissues found in the skin (3 points).

a. _____

b. _____

c. _____

3. List the five main functions of the skin (5 points).

a. _____

b. _____

c. _____

d. _____

e. _____

4. List the three main layers of tissue (3 points).

a. _____

b. _____

c. _____

5. Write the appropriate word next to each of the following statements (10 points).

_____ a. Caused by a fungus; usually involves the toes and soles of the feet.

_____ b. Refers to any skin condition.

_____ c. Caused by bacteria entering the hair follicles or sebaceous glands.

_____ d. Appears as itchy, reddened areas on the surface of the skin.

_____ e. Waxlike in appearance.

_____ f. Inflammation of the sebaceous gland.

_____ g. Scaly skin.

_____ h. Baldness.

_____ i. Hives.

_____ j. Hardened, thickened skin.

There are 23 possible points in this worksheet.

SECTION 13.13 Genetics

- ## OBJECTIVES

  When you have completed this section, you will be able to do the following:

  - Match key terms with their correct meanings.

  - Describe the structure of DNA.

  - Describe the role of DNA in human heredity.

  - Match common genetic disorders with their descriptions.

  - Explain why the health care worker's understanding of genetics is important.

- ## DIRECTIONS

  1. Complete Worksheet 1.

  2. Complete Worksheet/Activity 2 as assigned.

  3. Complete Worksheet 3 and 4.

  4. When you are confident that you can meet each objective for this section, ask your teacher for the section evaluation.

- ## EVALUATION METHODS

  - Worksheets/Activities

  - Class participation

  - Written evaluation

• WORKSHEET 1

Match each definition in column B with the correct vocabulary word in column A.

Column A

_____ **1.** chromosomes

_____ **2.** dominant

_____ **3.** gene

_____ **4.** trait

_____ **5.** genome

_____ **6.** deoxyribonucleic acid

_____ **7.** alleles

_____ **8.** recessive

_____ **9.** nucleotides

Column B

a. A genetically determined characteristic or condition

b. The complete set of a body's DNA

c. Description of a trait that shows influence or control.

d. Forms of a gene that influence a trait or set of traits.

e. Subunits of DNA that each contain a phosphate, sugar, and base.

f. Structures that contain coiled and condensed portions of the cell's DNA.

g. A molecule found in all living cells that contains information for building proteins and influencing traits.

h. A portion of DNA that contains instructions for a trait.

i. Description of a trait that is passive or hidden.

There are 9 possible points in this worksheet.

• WORKSHEET/ACTIVITY 2

Gather household items from which you can make a model of DNA. Consider simple items such as straws, toothpicks, candies, or coins. Construct your model. Prepare a key to explain what each item represents. For example, a red gumdrop might represent adenine. Present your model to the class.

There are 25 possible points in this worksheet.

• WORKSHEET 3

1. What is the role of DNA in human heredity (2 points)? _____

_____

_____

_____

_____

2. Why might it be important for a health care worker to understand genetics (2 points)? _____

_____

_____

_____

_____

There are 4 possible points in this worksheet.

● WORKSHEET 4

Write the name of the genetic disorder that matches each description below.

Cystic Fibrosis

Down Syndrome

Duchene's Muscular Dystrophy

Sickle Cell Anemia

_____ **1.** A genetic disorder linked to genes on the X-chromosome that causes muscle weakness and degeneration.

_____ **2.** A blood disorder that creates deformed red blood cells that have trouble carrying oxygen.

_____ **3.** An illness causing serious lung problems that occurs when offspring inherit two recessive alleles for the disease.

_____ **4.** Delayed development and mental retardation caused by an extra copy of chromosome 21.

There are 4 possible points in this worksheet.

Chapter **14** Human Growth and Development

Development and Behavior

- **OBJECTIVES**

    When you have completed this section, you will be able to do the following:

    - Match key terms with their correct meanings.
    - Identify three stages of development between conception and birth.
    - List four common developments of growth in the first year of life and the age at which they usually occur.
    - Define and describe characteristics of adolescent development.
    - Interview a person between the ages of 50 and 80.
    - Compare your life experiences to each stage described in this chapter.
    - Design a bulletin board representing one stage of growth and development, including age-specific communication requirements.

- **DIRECTIONS**

    1. Complete Worksheets 1 and 2.
    2. Follow your teacher's directions to complete Worksheets/Activities 3 through 6.
    3. When you are confident that you can meet each objective for this section, ask your teacher for the section evaluation.

174

● EVALUATION METHODS

- ■ Worksheets/Activities
- ■ Class participation
- ■ Written evaluation

● WORKSHEET 1

Match each definition in column B with the correct vocabulary word in column A.

Column A

_____ **1.** Adolescent

_____ **2.** Continuum

_____ **3.** Coordination

_____ **4.** Decade

_____ **5.** Embryo

_____ **6.** Fetus

_____ **7.** Menstruation

_____ **8.** Prone

_____ **9.** Supine

_____ **10.** Viable

_____ **11.** Zygote three months until birth.

Column B

a. Lying on the stomach.

b. Living human being during the first eight weeks of development in the uterus.

c. Pertaining to the period of life between childhood and maturity.

d. Capable of living.

e. Progression from start (birth) to finish (death).

f. Period of 10 years.

g. Infant developing in the uterus after the first.

h. Lying on the back.

i. Cyclic deterioration of the endometrium.

j. Any cell formed by the coming together of two reproductive (sex) cells.

k. State of harmonized action.

There are 11 possible points in this worksheet.

● WORKSHEET 2

1. Identify the three stages of development between conception and birth (3 points).

   a. _____

   b. _____

   c. _____

2. List four common developments of growth in the first year of life and the age at which they usually occur (8 points).

Developments of Growth	Age
a.	
b.	
c.	
d.	

3. List three characteristics of adolescent development (3 points).

a. _____

b. _____

c. _____

There are 14 possible points in this worksheet.

• WORKSHEET/ACTIVITY 3

Design a bulletin board representing one of the growth and development stages listed below (e.g., a collage of infants doing different activities, paired with their age, or photos of various ages depicting each developmental stage). Include age-specific communication requirements.

- Infant
- Toddler stage (18 months to 3 years)
- Preschool and elementary age (3 to 8 years)
- Preteen years or preadolescent years (8 to 13 years)
- Adolescent or teenage years (13 to 18 years)
- Young adult (18 to 20 years)
- Adulthood (20 and older)

There are 100 possible points in this worksheet/activity.

• WORKSHEET/ACTIVITY 4

Interview an individual between the ages of 50 and 80. Ask the following question, plus at least four more of your own (100 points).

Interviewee's name _____ Birth year _____

1. What was your daily life like, including family roles (mother's role, father's role, and children's role)?

Use the following worksheet as a guide for your interviews.

	Mother's Role	Father's Role	Children's Role
a. Before you were 20 years old?	_____	_____	_____
b. Between 20 and 40 years of age?	_____	_____	_____
c. Between 40 and 60 years of age?	_____	_____	_____

2. What were the clothing fads when you were in your teens?

a. Shoes _____

b. Hats _____

c. Coats_____

d. Length of women's skirts_____

e. Bathing suits _____

3. What were you doing the day . . .

    a. Sputnik was launched? _____

    b. Iran took hostages at the U.S. embassy? _____

    c. The Challenger exploded? _____

    d. President Kennedy was assassinated? _____

    e. The Vietnam War ended? _____

4. What gave or gives you the most enjoyment . . .

    a. As a teenager? _____

    b. In middle school? _____

    c. Now? _____

5. When did you first . . .

    a. Own a car? _____

    b. Fly in an airplane? _____

    c. Own a television set? _____

6. Can you tell me what an Edsel is? _____

    _____

    _____

7. What type of music was popular when you were in your teens? _____

    _____

    _____

8. What was a common weekend like when you were a child? _____

    _____

    _____

9. What was your favorite activity, hobby, sport, and so on? _____

    _____

    _____

10. What was your first job? How old were you when you started? What was your starting salary? _____

    _____

    _____

There are 100 possible points in this worksheet/activity.

● WORKSHEET/ACTIVITY 5

Compare and contrast your life experience and that of the subject of your interview.

Age	My Experience	Interviewee's Experience
Example:		
16	I got my first job after school at a fast-food restaurant.	He worked on the farm after school, beginning in elementary school.

There are 500 possible points in this worksheet/activity.

● WORKSHEET/ACTIVITY 6

Using Worksheet 4 and additional research, develop a two- to five-minute skit or report depicting the 10-year time period assigned by your instructor. All group members must actively participate in the presentation. The presentation must give a picture of:

- The time period
- Common leisure activities of the time
- Popular clothing styles (through pictures or wearing or describing the clothes of the time)
- Popular music or songs
- Comedians of the era
- News events
- Modes of transportation

There are 100 possible points in this worksheet/activity.

SECTION 14.2 Aging and Role Change

● OBJECTIVES

When you have completed this section, you will be able to do the following:

■ Match key terms with their correct meanings.

■ Identify six body systems and the common physical changes that occur with aging.

■ Identify basic human needs that are met through work, environment, socialization, and family relationships.

■ Write an "action plan" to assist another person cope with changes caused by aging.

● DIRECTIONS

1. Complete Worksheet/Activity 1.

2. Complete Worksheet 2 as assigned.

3. Follow your teacher's directions to complete Worksheets 3 through 5.

4. When you are confident that you can meet each objective for this section, ask your teacher for the section evaluation.

● EVALUATION METHODS

■ Worksheets

■ Class participation

■ Written evaluation

● WORKSHEET/ACTIVITY 1

Select four or five individuals from among family, friends, and neighbors. Be sure to have a wide range of ages from children to the elderly. Interview them about their favorite pastimes, such as sports, music, dancing, gardening, and reading.

Think how aging and role changes have changed these activities and prepare a brief report for your classmates to identify any trends you have observed.

There are 50 possible points in this worksheet/activity.

● WORKSHEET 2

Fill in the crossword puzzle using the vocabulary words from Section 14.2.

Indicates a space between two words.

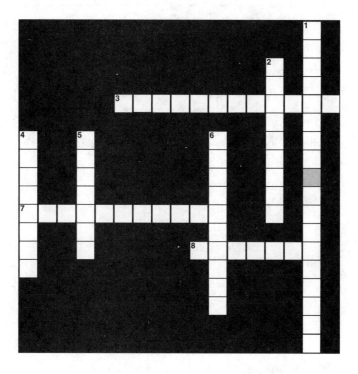

Clues

Across

3. Infrequent or difficult emptying of the bowel.

7. Surroundings we live in.

Down

1. Air sacs in the lungs.

2. Keeping elements within the body that are normally eliminated.

8. Elements in the environment that are strong enough to set up a nervous impulse.

4. Involuntary actions that occur when a nerve is stimulated.

5. Body's strength or energy.

6. Adjustment.

There are 8 possible points in this worksheet.

● WORKSHEET 3

1. List three changes that may occur in the nervous system with aging (3 points).

a. _____

b. _____

c. _____

2. List three disorders of the musculoskeletal system that are found in the elderly (3 points).

   a. _____

   b. _____

   c. _____

3. The lungs become less (a) _____ and the (b) _____ membrane thickens; this makes (c) _____ more difficult (3 points).

4. Arteries may become (a) _____ and (b) _____ (2 points).

5. Bladder _____ may occur from retention of urine in the bladder (1 point).

There are 12 possible points in this worksheet.

● WORKSHEET 4

1. List four role changes that may occur in the elderly (4 points).

   a. _____

   b. _____

   c. _____

   d. _____

2. Give two ways an individual can adapt to the loss of family relationships (2 points).

   a. _____

   b. _____

3. What are two losses experienced when the work role is changed (2 points)?

   a. _____

   b. _____

4. Give two possible effects of change in environment (2 points).

   a. _____

   b. _____

There are 10 possible points in this worksheet.

● WORKSHEET 5

Complete the following action plan.

1. Name a person you know who is coping with the changes caused by aging.

2. List the changes you see in this person's daily life.

3. List things that might help this person cope with the changes you listed above.

4. Write a plan that could help this person cope with these changes.

Note: Always determine the other person's desire for assistance before trying to help him or her.

There are 25 possible points in this worksheet.

Disabilities and Role Changes

● OBJECTIVES

When you have completed this section, you will be able to do the following:

- Match key terms with their correct meanings.
- Define *health*.
- List three examples of activities of daily living (ADL).
- Define assistive/adaptive devices.
- Identify ways to encourage independence.
- List eight birth defects.
- List ten debilitating illnesses.
- Identify seven common changes that occur following the loss of body functions.
- State the goal of rehabilitation.
- Select a disability and summarize your feelings and expectations concerning:
  - What you think it would be like to live with that disability
  - The type of care you would expect
  - The way others respond to the disability

● DIRECTIONS

1. Complete Worksheet 1.

2. Complete Worksheet/Activity 2 as assigned.

3. Complete Worksheet 3 as assigned.

4. Complete Worksheet/Activity 4 as assigned.

5. When you are confident that you can meet each objective for this section, ask your teacher for the section evaluation.

● EVALUATION METHODS

- Worksheets/Activities
- Class participation
- Written report
- Written evaluation

• WORKSHEET 1

Match each definition in column B with the correct vocabulary word in column A.

Column A

_____ 1. Passed from parent to child.

_____ 2. Impaired or abnormal functioning.

_____ 2. Deep sleep; unconscious state for a long period of time.

_____ 4. A number of symptoms occurring together.

_____ 5. Removal of a body part.

_____ 6. State of poisoning or becoming poisoned.

_____ 7. Shortage.

_____ 8. Moving forward, following steps toward an end product.

_____ 9. Causing weakness or impairment.

_____ 10. State of being confused about time, place, and identity of persons and objects.

_____ 11. Pertaining to the embryo.

_____ 12. Substance that causes a change to occur in other substances.

_____ 13. Events in a series.

_____ 14. Defect present at birth.

_____ 15. State of being weakened or deteriorated.

_____ 16. Pertaining to the nervous system.

_____ 17. To change, to become suitable.

_____ 18. Unsound or unhealthy state of being.

_____ 19. Condition of hardening of the arteries.

_____ 20. Fat.

_____ 21. Infections that occur when the immune system is weakened.

_____ 22. Belief in oneself.

There are 22 possible points in this worksheet.

Column B

a. Adapt
b. Amputation
c. Arteriosclerosis
d. Birth defect
e. Coma
f. Debilitating
g. Deficiency
h. Dysfunction
i. Embryonic
j. Hereditary
k. Impairment
l. Infirmity
m. Intoxication
n. Neurological
o. Opportunistic infections
p. Progressive
q. Self-esteem
r. Lipid
s. Syndrome
t. Episodes
u. Enzyme
v. Disorientation

• WORKSHEET/ACTIVITY 2

Work with your group to develop a verbal report on the disability assigned by your instructor.

1. Explain how daily life changes for those with your assigned disability.

_____

_____

_____

_____

_____

2. List the types of jobs a person with this disability could do that would promote independence.

_____

_____

_____

_____

_____

3. List the types of leisure activities a person with this disability could participate in.

_____

_____

_____

_____

4. List common attitudes about this disability.

_____

_____

_____

_____

5. Decide which part of the above information each person in the group will present to the class.

Student Name	**Report Responsibility**
_____	_____
_____	_____
_____	_____
_____	_____
_____	_____

There are 50 possible points in this worksheet/activity.

● WORKSHEET 3

1. List eight birth defects (8 points).

a. _____

b. _____

c. _____

d. _____

e. _____

f. _____

g. _____

h. _____

2. List 11 debilitating illnesses (11 points).

a. _____

b. _____

c. _____

d. _____

e. _____

f. _____

g. _____

h. _____

i. _____

j. _____

k. _____

3. What is the goal of rehabilitation (1 point)?_____

_____

4. Mark an X in the space next to the seven common changes that occur following the loss of body function (7 points).

_____ a. Family

_____ b. Eating habits

_____ c. Animals

_____ d. Elimination of waste

_____ e. Ability to move

_____ f. Communication skills

_____ g. Sensory awareness

_____ h. Ability to think and comprehend

_____ i. Sexual activity

5. List three examples of activities of daily living (ADL) (3 points).

a. _____

b. _____

c. _____

6. What are assistive or adaptive devices (1 point)? _____

_____

7. Mark an X in the space next to the ways that you can encourage independence in your patients (3 points).

_____ a. Allow patients to help choose their clothing.

_____ b. Always brush your patients' teeth for them.

_____ c. Let patients do as many ADLs as possible.

_____ d. Comb your patients' hair for them.

_____ e. Do everything you can for your patients.

_____ f. Help patients comb their hair.

8. Mrs. Wong is trying to comb her hair. She had a stroke two months ago and is still very slow. You have several more residents to care for and barely enough time to finish. What will you do, and why (2 points)?

_____

_____

_____

9. Jaime Garcia is a young athlete. He was badly injured during a football game. He is very frustrated because he cannot move his right arm. He is trying to learn how to eat with his left hand. During breakfast, he throws the cereal across the room. What will you do, and why (2 points)?

_____

_____

_____

There are 38 possible points in this worksheet.

● WORKSHEET/ACTIVITY 4

Select a disability, and summarize your feelings and expectations about the disability in a one-page paper.

- What do you think it would be like to live with the disability?

- What type of care would you expect if you had the disability?

- How would others respond to the disability?

Follow these guidelines when preparing your paper:

- Use 8.5-by-11-inch paper.

- Type, word-process, or write neatly in ink.

- Use correct spelling and grammar.

There are 10 possible points in this worksheet/activity.

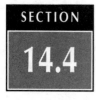

SECTION

14.4 End-of-Life Issues

● OBJECTIVES

When you have completed this section, you will be able to do the following:

- Match key terms with their correct meanings.

- Match the psychological stages of a long terminal illness with their names.

- Identify and discuss your feelings about terminal illness.

- Explain the philosophy of hospice care.

• DIRECTIONS

1. Complete Worksheet 1.

2. Complete Worksheet 2.

3. Follow your instructor's directions to complete Worksheet/Activity 3.

4. Prepare responses to each item listed in Chapter Review.

5. When you are confident that you can meet each objective for this section, ask your teacher for the section evaluation.

• EVALUATION METHODS

- Worksheets/Activities
- Class participation
- Written evaluation
- Written report

• WORKSHEET 1

Fill in the crossword puzzle using the vocabulary words from Section 14.4 in your text.

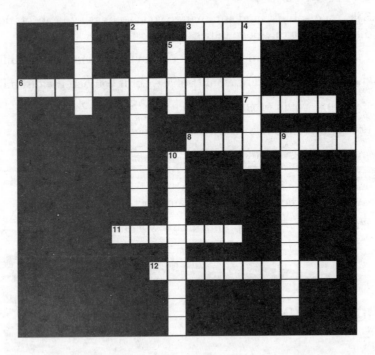

Clues

Across

3. Psychological stage one: unable to believe they are really going to die.

6. Pertaining to the mind.

7. Psychological stage two: mad because they are going to die.

8. About to happen.

11. Facility that helps the terminally ill live each day to the fullest.

12. Psychological stage three: admit they are dying but say they must live for a certain time or event.

Down

1. Psychological stage one: experience disbelief and amazement ("Not me!").

2. Theory; a general principle used for a specific purpose.

4. Limited in contact with others.

5. Psychological stage two: experience uncontrolled anger.

9. Psychological stage four: feel sadness, grief, and loss.

10. Psychological stage five: acknowledge that they are going to die.

There are 12 possible points in this worksheet.

● WORKSHEET 2

1. List the five psychological stages often experienced by the terminally ill, in the order in which they usually occur (5 points).

   a. _____

   b. _____

   c. _____

   d. _____

   e. _____

2. Explain the philosophy of hospice (1 point). _____

   _____

3. Mrs. Nygun has a terminal illness. Until recently, she had been able to care for herself and was fairly independent. You have become friends over several months. Recently she became ill with pneumonia and unable to care for herself. She tells you to get away from her and calls you names. Why do you think she is so angry? Explain how you will respond to her and why (2 points). _____

   _____

4. You are assigned Mr. Hong. He is near death. When you care for him, you notice that his breathing is very difficult. He feels cold to the touch, and he is losing control of body functions. How will you treat him? What do you think you might feel while caring for him (2 points)? _____

   _____

   _____

There are 10 possible points in this worksheet.

● WORKSHEET/ACTIVITY 3

Describe your experience with someone who is or was terminally ill. If you have no previous experience, describe what you think you might feel when you first learn of a terminal illness.

Follow these guidelines when preparing your paper:

- Use 8.5-by-11-inch paper.

- Type, word-process, or write neatly in ink.

- Use correct spelling and grammar.

There are 10 possible points in this worksheet/activity.

Chapter **15** Mental Health

Mental Illness

- **OBJECTIVES**

    When you have completed this section, you will be able to do the following:

    - Define mental illness.
    - Identify seven types of mental illnesses.
    - Identify three types of risk factors for mental illness.
    - Describe four anxiety disorders.
    - Describe two mood disorders.
    - List three symptoms of attention deficit hyperactivity disorder.
    - Describe two eating disorders.
    - Relate substance abuse to mental illness.
    - Describe Alzheimer's disease.

- **DIRECTIONS**

    1. Complete Worksheets 1 and 2 as assigned.
    2. Complete Worksheets 3 through 6 as assigned.
    3. When you are confident that you can meet each objective for this section, ask your teacher for the section evaluation.

- **EVALUATION METHODS**
  - Worksheets
  - Class participation
  - Written evaluation

- **WORKSHEET 1**

    1. Define mental illness (1 point). _____

    _____

    2. Identify seven types of mental illnesses (7 points). _____

    _____

    _____

    _____

    _____

    _____

    _____

    _____

    3. Identify three types of risk factors for mental illness (3 points). _____

    _____

    _____

    _____

    There are 11 possible points in this worksheet.

- **WORKSHEET 2**

    1. What is anxiety (1 point)? _____

    _____

    2. How is an anxiety disorder different from everyday anxiety (1 point)? _____

    _____

    _____

    3. Describe four anxiety disorders (8 points).

    a. _____

    _____

    b. _____

    _____

    c. _____

    _____

    d. _____

    _____

    There are 10 possible points in this worksheet.

● WORKSHEET 3

    1. What is a mood disorder (2 points)? _____

_____

_____

    2. How is person affected by bipolar disorder (5 points)? _____

_____

_____

_____

    3. How is person affected by depression (5 points)? _____

_____

_____

_____

    4. List nine possible characteristics of depression (9 points). _____

_____

_____

_____

_____

_____

_____

_____

_____

_____

    There are 21 possible points in this worksheet.

● WORKSHEET 4

    1. What does ADHD stand for (1 point)? _____

_____

    2. Describe three characteristics of ADHD (6 points)? _____

_____

_____

_____

    3. What are three general groups of people with ADHD (3 points)?

        a. _____

        b. _____

        c. _____

    There are 10 possible points in this worksheet.

192

- **WORKSHEET 5**

  1. What is anorexia nervosa (2 points)? _____
  _____

  2. What is bulimia nervosa (2 points)? _____
  _____

  3. How are eating disorders related to other mental illnesses (2 points)? _____
  _____

  _____

  4. How are mental illnesses related to substance abuse (2 points)? _____
  _____

  _____

  There are 8 possible points in this worksheet.

- **WORKSHEET 6**

  1. What is Alzheimer's disease (2 points)? _____

  _____

  _____

  _____

  2. What are two primary risk factors for Alzheimer's disease (2 points)?
  a. _____
  b. _____

  3. How does Alzheimer's disease affect brain cells (4 points)? _____
  _____

  _____

  4. List and describe the three main stages of Alzheimer's disease (6 points).
  a. _____

  _____
  b. _____
  c. _____

  _____

  There are 14 possible points in this worksheet.

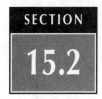

SECTION

15.2 **Techniques for Treating Mental Illness**

● **OBJECTIVES**

When you have completed this section, you will be able to do the following:

- List three ways to treat mental illness.
- List consequences of not treating mental illness.
- Explain why mental illness patients may stop taking medications.
- Define *psychotherapy*.
- List four benefits of psychotherapy.
- Explain why treatment for drug abuse involves hospitalization.
- Describe why the treatment for Alzheimer's disease differs from the treatment for most other mental illnesses.

● **DIRECTIONS**

1. Complete Worksheet 1 as assigned.
2. Complete Worksheet/Activity 2 as assigned.
3. Prepare responses to reach item listed in Chapter Review.
4. When you are confident that you can meet each objective for this section, ask your teacher for the section evaluation.

● **EVALUATION METHODS**

- Worksheets
- Class participation
- Written evaluation
- Interview

● **WORKSHEET 1**

1. List three ways to treat mental illness (3 points).

_____

_____

_____

2. Describe consequences of not treating mental illness (2 points).

_____

_____

_____

3. What is a common reason why mental illness patients may stop taking medications (2 points)?

_____

_____

4. What is psychotherapy (1 point)?

_____

_____

5. List four benefits of psychotherapy (4 points).

a. _____

b. _____

c. _____

d. _____

6. Explain why treatment for drug abuse involves hospitalization (3 points).

_____

_____

_____

There are 15 possible points in this worksheet.

● WORKSHEET/ACTIVITY 2

Prepare interview questions for a health care provider who cares for patients suffering from Alzheimer's disease. Consider the following ideas:

- How is caring for Alzheimer's patients different from caring for other patients?

- What do you consider the most difficult challenges of caring for these patients?

- How is your work rewarding to you?

- What personality traits do you have that enable you to perform this role?

Have your questions approved by your instructor. Then set up an interview at a local facility. Conduct the interview in person or by telephone. Present your findings to the class.

There are 50 possible points in this worksheet.

CHECK-OFF SHEET:
15-1 Activities with Alzheimer's Patients

Name _____ Date _____

Directions: Practice this procedure, following each step. When you are ready to have your performance evaluated, give this sheet to your instructor. Review the detailed procedure in your textbook.

Procedure	Pass	Redo	Date Competency Met	Instructor Initials
Student must use Standard Precautions.	☐	☐	_____	_____
Preprocedure				
1. Wash hands.	☐	☐	_____	_____
2. Identify the patient and the activity in which he or she will be participating. Pay attention to	☐	☐	_____	_____
a. the patient's skills and abilities	☐	☐	_____	_____
b. what the patient enjoys	☐	☐	_____	_____
c. physical problems	☐	☐	_____	_____
d. the physician's recommendations	☐	☐	_____	_____
3. Gather equipment for the activity (if needed).	☐	☐	_____	_____
4. Break the activity into small, measurable steps.	☐	☐	_____	_____
Procedure				
5. Greet the patient, and tell him or her what you are going to do today.	☐	☐	_____	_____
6. Help the patient get started with the activity.	☐	☐	_____	_____
7. Explain each step of the activity using simple terms. It may be necessary to repeat the explanation or to clarify in terms the patient understands.	☐	☐	_____	_____
8. Help the patient through difficult steps or if he or she appears frustrated. As much as possible, let the patient do most of the activity on his or her own.	☐	☐	_____	_____
9. Do not criticize or correct the patient.	☐	☐	_____	_____
Postprocedure				
10. Put away equipment.	☐	☐	_____	_____
11. Wash hands.	☐	☐	_____	_____
12. Record the patient's response to the activity.	☐	☐	_____	_____

CHECK-OFF SHEET:
15-2 Music Therapy

Name _____ Date _____

Directions: Practice this procedure, following each step. When you are ready to have your performance evaluated, give this sheet to your instructor. Review the detailed procedure in your textbook.

Procedure	Pass	Redo	Date Competency Met	Instructor Initials
Student must use Standard Precautions.	☐	☐	_____	_____
Preprocedure				
1. Identify the patient.	☐	☐	_____	_____
2. Identify the type of music that the patient enjoys.	☐	☐	_____	_____
3. Provide a comfortable space in which the patient can listen to the music.	☐	☐	_____	_____
4. Gather and set up equipment. Choose music, something to play it on, pictures that mean something to the patient to help them recall memories.	☐	☐	_____	_____
5. Block other sources of sound. Close windows and doors, turn off televisions and other radios, and reduce background noise as much as possible.	☐	☐	_____	_____
Procedure				
6. Start the music.	☐	☐	_____	_____
7. Encourage the patient to clap or sing along with the music. When appropriate, encourage the patient to dance or move with the music.	☐	☐	_____	_____
8. While playing the music, show the patient pictures to help with memories.	☐	☐	_____	_____
Postprocedure				
9. Put away equipment.	☐	☐	_____	_____
10. Record the patient's response to the activity.	☐	☐	_____	_____

CHECK-OFF SHEET:
15-3 Art Therapy

Name _____ Date _____

Directions: Practice this procedure, following each step. When you are ready to have your performance evaluated, give this sheet to your instructor. Review the detailed procedure in your textbook.

Procedure	Pass	Redo	Date Competency Met	Instructor Initials
Student must use Standard Precautions.	☐	☐	_____	_____
Preprocedure				
1. Identify the patient.	☐	☐	_____	_____
2. Assemble materials. Avoid potentially harmful materials, such as sharp blades and tools. Materials may include the following:	☐	☐	_____	_____
a. nontoxic acrylic paints or watercolor paints	☐	☐	_____	_____
b. brushes and canvases or watercolor paper	☐	☐	_____	_____
c. clay	☐	☐	_____	_____
3. Prepare a work area for the patient. Neatly arrange materials and cover surfaces to protect them from spillage.	☐	☐	_____	_____
Procedure				
4. Help the patient start the project.	☐	☐	_____	_____
5. Encourage the patient to talk about what he or she is doing. Ask the patient to remember events related to the project or to tell a story about the project.	☐	☐	_____	_____
6. Help the patient through difficult steps or if he or she appears frustrated. As much as possible, let the patient do most of the project on his or her own.	☐	☐	_____	_____
7. Do not criticize or correct the patient.	☐	☐	_____	_____
8. When the patient is finished with the project, help him or her clean up.	☐	☐	_____	_____
Postprocedure				
9. Put away equipment.	☐	☐	_____	_____
10. Clean work space.	☐	☐	_____	_____
11. Record the patient's response to the activity.	☐	☐	_____	_____

Chapter 16 Nutrition

16.1 Basic Nutrition

- ● **OBJECTIVES**

   When you have completed this section, you will be able to do the following:

   - Match key terms with their correct meanings.

   - Name the four functions of food.

   - Name the five basic nutrients and explain how they maintain body function.

   - List five problems associated with obesity.

   - Perform basic volume conversions.

   - Explain the USDA food pyramid.

   - Compare your diet with the recommendations in the USDA food pyramid.

- ● **DIRECTIONS**

   1. Complete Worksheet 1.

   2. Complete Worksheet/Activity 2.

   3. Complete Worksheets 3 through 5 after your teacher discusses this chapter in class.

   4. Complete Worksheets/Activities 6 and 7.

   5. Complete Worksheet 8.

   6. When you are confident that you can meet each objective for this section, ask your teacher for the section evaluation.

- ## EVALUATION METHODS
  - Worksheets/Activities
  - Class participation
  - Written evaluation

- ## WORKSHEET 1

  Write each word listed below in the space next to the statement that best defines it.

vitality	nutrients	resistance
regulate	absorbed	protein
vitamins	minerals	essential
metabolism	stamina	hemoglobin
fecal	obesity	calories

  _____ **1.** Ability of the body to protect itself from disease.

  _____ **2.** Group of substances necessary for normal metabolism, growth, and body function.

  _____ **3.** Ability of an organism to go on living.

  _____ **4.** The body's process of using food to make energy and nutrients.

  _____ **5.** Substances that nourish the body.

  _____ **6.** Body's strength or energy.

  _____ **7.** To control or adjust.

  _____ **8.** Necessary.

  _____ **9.** Complex chemical in the blood; carries oxygen and carbon dioxide.

  _____ **10.** Extreme fatness; abnormal amount of fat on the body.

  _____ **11.** Taken up or received.

  _____ **12.** Inorganic elements that occur in nature; essential to every cell.

  _____ **13.** Complex compound found in plant and animal tissues; essential for heat, energy, and growth.

  _____ **14.** Units of measurement of the fuel value of food.

  _____ **15.** Pertaining to feces, a solid waste product.

  There are 15 possible points in this worksheet.

- ## WORKSHEET/ACTIVITY 2

  Make a poster identifying foods that supply different nutrients such as vitamins and their sources. Food pictures can be found in magazines or on the Internet, or you may draw them.

  There are 50 possible points in this worksheet.

- ## WORKSHEET 3

   1. Name the four functions of food (4 points).

      a. _____ c._____

      b. _____ d._____

   2. Name the five basic nutrients, and explain how they maintain body function (10 points).

Basic Nutrients	**How They Maintain Body Function**
a. _____	_____
b. _____	_____
c. _____	_____
d. _____	_____
e. _____	_____

   3. Describe the food pyramid, and explain why it is important (2 points).

      _____

      _____

      _____

   There are 16 possible points in this worksheet.

- ## WORKSHEET 4

   1. Following the example in this first question, keep a record of what you eat for two full days. At the end of each day, determine whether you had a balanced diet. If not, how could you have balanced it?

      Example:

MEAL	FOOD EATEN	FOOD GROUP/SERVING AMOUNT
Breakfast	1 banana 1 slice toast with jelly ½ cup milk coffee	2 servings fruit 1 serving bread and cereal ½ serving dairy zero

Lunch	fast-food hamburger:
	    3 oz. meat patty
	    bun
	    lettuce and tomato
	20 French Fries
	8 oz. soda
		1 serving meat
		2 servings bread and cereal
		½ serving fruit and vegetable
		2 servings vegetable
		zero

Snack	apple	1 serving fruit

Dinner	spaghetti with tomato sauce:
	    ⅔ cup spaghetti
	    ½ cup tomato sauce
	Lettuce salad
	1 cup milk
		1 serving bread and cereal
		1 serving fruit and vegetable
		1 serving vegetable
		1 serving dairy

Snack	candy bar	zero

2. Total the number of servings from each food group in the food pyramid on your daily menu. Show how it is balanced, or what you could add to balance your diet.

If you are an adult, you might add cheese and a glass of milk to lunch. A teen might add cheese to lunch and ice cream for an evening snack.

Day 1

MEAL	FOOD EATEN	FOOD GROUP/ SERVING AMOUNT	FOODS NEEDED TO BALANCE DIET
Breakfast Lunch Dinner Snack			

Total _____

To balance diet add: _____

Day 2

MEAL	FOOD EATEN	FOOD GROUP/ SERVING AMOUNT	FOODS NEEDED TO BALANCE DIET
Breakfast Lunch Dinner Snack			

Total _____

To balance diet add: _____

There are 50 possible points in this worksheet.

● **WORKSHEET 5**

1. Summarize what you learned from Worksheet 4 in the space below.

I Need to Eat More: **I Need to Eat Less:**

_____   _____

_____   _____

_____   _____

_____   _____

2. Write a realistic action plan to help you follow the food pyramid guidelines.

_____
_____
_____
_____
_____
_____
_____
_____
_____
_____
_____

There are 25 possible points in this worksheet.

● WORKSHEET/ACTIVITY 6

Prepare a one-week menu for your family. Total the food group servings for each day and demonstrate whether the daily intake is balanced according to the food pyramid.

There are 100 possible points in this worksheet/activity.

● WORKSHEET/ACTIVITY 7

Your teacher will divide the class into groups and ask each group to identify food preferences of a specific ethnic group. Plan a two-day balanced menu which includes some of each group's ethnic food preferences.

There are 100 possible points in this worksheet/activity.

● WORKSHEET 8

Complete each of the following conversions (10 points).

1. 6 teaspoons = _____ ml

2. 4 tablespoons = _____ cc

3. 8 tablespoons = _____ cup (s)

4. 2 pints = _____ fluid ounces

5. 250 ml = _____ cc

6. 12 teaspoons = _____ tablespoons

7. 4 tablespoons = _____ teaspoons

8. 10 fluid ounces = _____ ml

9. 3 pints = _____ cc

10. 2 cups = _____ ml

Solve the following problems (3 points).

1. A dose of medicine is 1 tablespoon. How many doses does a 12-ounce bottle contain?_____

2. A container holds 10 pints of water. How many milliliters are needed to fill the container? _____

3. A patient receives 720 cc of blood. How many pints of blood did the patient receive? _____

There are 13 possible points in this worksheet/activity.

SECTION 16.2 Therapeutic Diets

• OBJECTIVES

When you have completed this section, you will be able to do the following:

- Match key terms with their correct meaning.
- List three factors that influence food habits.
- Select a correct therapeutic diet for physical disorders.
- Discuss characteristics and treatment of common eating disorders
- List four commonly abused substances and their negative impacts on the human body.

• DIRECTIONS

1. Complete Worksheet 1.
2. Complete Worksheet 2 as assigned.
3. Complete Worksheet/Activity 3.
4. Complete Worksheets 4 and 5.
5. Prepare responses to each item listed in Chapter Review.
6. When you are confident that you can meet each objective for this section, ask your teacher for the section evaluation.

• EVALUATION METHODS

- Worksheets/Activities
- Class participation
- Written evaluation

• WORKSHEET 1

Write each word listed below in the space next to the statement that best defines it.

therapeutic	preferences	metabolic
edema	gastrointestinal	deficient
colitis	ileitis	diabetes mellitus
soluble	atherosclerosis	anorexia nervosa
hypertension	lactation	

_____ **1.** Pertaining to all of the physical and chemical changes that take place in living organisms and cells.

_____ **2.** Lacking something.

_____ **3.** Pertaining to the treatment of disease or injury.

_____ **4.** Able to break down or dissolve in liquid.

_____ **5.** Priorities; first choices.

_____ **6.** Condition of hardening of the arteries due to fat deposits that narrow the space through which blood flows.

_____ **7.** Body's process of producing milk to feed newborns.

_____ **8.** Swelling; abnormal or excessive collection of fluid in the tissues.

_____ **9.** Inflammation of the ileum.

_____ **10.** Pertaining to the stomach and intestine.

_____ **11.** Inflammation of the colon.

_____ **12.** Condition that develops when the body cannot change sugar into energy.

_____ **13.** Loss of appetite with serious weight loss; considered a mental disorder.

_____ **14.** High blood pressure.

There are 14 possible points in this worksheet.

• WORKSHEET 2

1. List three factors that influence food habits (3 points).

a. _____

b. _____

c. _____

2. Name the therapeutic diet for each of the following (8 points).

    a. For a patient having trouble chewing or swallowing: _____

    b. To soothe the gastrointestinal system: _____

    c. For a patient with anorexia nervosa: _____

    d. To regulate the cholesterol in the blood: _____

    e. To reduce salt intake: _____

    f. To replace fluids lost by vomiting: _____

    g. For a patient with diabetes mellitus: _____

    h. For a patient with gallbladder and liver disease:_____

There are 11 possible points in this worksheet.

● WORKSHEET/ACTIVITY 3

Choose a therapeutic diet and make a poster depicting the foods in the diet. Tell why the diet is necessary.

There are 100 possible points in this worksheet/activity.

● WORKSHEET 4

Compare and contrast anorexia nervosa with bulimia nervosa. Include a description of the disorders and their treatments.

_____

_____

_____

_____

_____

_____

_____

_____

_____

There are 25 possible points in this worksheet/activity.

● WORKSHEET 5

List four commonly abused substances and their impacts on the body.

    1. Substance:_____

    Impact:_____

    _____

    2. Substance:_____

    Impact:_____

    _____

3. Substance:_____

    Impact:_____

    _____

4. Substance:_____

    Impact:_____

    _____

There are 8 possible points in this worksheet/activity.

Chapter 17 Controlling Infection

The Nature of Microorganisms

- **OBJECTIVES**

   When you have completed this section, you will be able to do the following:

   - Match key terms with their correct meanings.
   - Define pathogenic and nonpathogenic.
   - List conditions affecting the growth of bacteria.
   - List ways that microorganisms and viruses cause illness.
   - List ways that microorganisms and viruses spread.
   - List five ways to prevent the spread of microorganisms and viruses.
   - Describe generalized and localized infections.
   - Explain the difference in signs and symptoms of generalized and localized infections.

- **DIRECTIONS**

   1. Complete Worksheet 1.
   2. Complete Worksheet 2 as assigned.
   3. Ask your teacher for directions to complete Worksheets/Activities 3 and 4.
   4. When you are confident that you can meet each objective for this section, ask your teacher for the section evaluation.

212

• EVALUATION METHODS

- Worksheets/Activities
- Class participation
- Return demonstration
- Written evaluation

• WORKSHEET 1

Match each definition in column *B* with the correct vocabulary word in column *A*.

Column A

_____ 1. Aerobic
_____ 2. Generalized
_____ 3. Anaerobic
_____ 4. Contaminated
_____ 5. Localized
_____ 6. Decompose
_____ 7. Enterotoxin
_____ 8. Feces
_____ 9. Host
_____10. Inhabit
_____11. Nonpathogenic
_____12. Pathogenic
_____13. Toxin
_____14. Susceptible
_____15. Spirochetes
_____16. Microorganisms

Column B

a. Affecting all of the body.
b. Poisonous substance that is produced in, or originates in, the contents of the intestine.
c. Able to grow and function without air or oxygen.
d. Organism from which microorganism takes nourishment.
e. Not causing disease.
f. Soiled, unclean; not suitable for use.
g. Poisonous substance.
h. Slender, coil-shaped organisms.
i. Requiring oxygen.
j. Causing disease.
k. To decay; to break down.
l. To dwell; to live.
m. Solid waste evacuated from the body through the anus.
n. Organisms so small that they can be seen only through a microscope.
o. Capable of being affected or infected.
p. Affecting one area of the body.

There are 16 possible points in this worksheet.

• WORKSHEET 2

1. Write each word listed below in the space next to the statement that best defines it (4 points).

bacteria   viruses   protozoa   fungi

_____ a. Are smaller than bacteria.
_____ b. Cause amebic dysentery.
_____ c. Are a very low form of plant life.
_____ d. Causes strep throat.

2. List three ways that microorganisms affect the body and cause illness (3 points).

    a. _____

    b. _____

    c. _____

3. List six conditions that affect the growth of bacteria (6 points).

    a. _____

    b. _____

    c. _____

    d. _____

    e. _____

    f. _____

4. Define *pathogen* and *nonpathogen* (2 points).

_____

_____

5. List two ways that microorganisms are spread, and give three examples of each (8 points).

Ways Microorganisms Spread   **Examples**

    a. _____   _____

    b. _____   _____

6. What two organisms always inhabit health care environments (2 points)?

    a. _____

    b. _____

7. List five ways the health care worker can prevent the spread of microorganisms (5 points).

    a. _____

    b. _____

    c. _____

    d. _____

    e. _____

8. Explain the difference in signs and symptoms of generalized and localized infection (4 points).

_____

_____

_____

9. Explain why understanding microorganisms is important to health care workers (5 points).

_____

_____

_____

There are 39 possible points in this worksheet.

• WORKSHEET/ACTIVITY 3

Read about microorganisms in a reference book from the classroom or the library. Choose one microorganism, and write a two-to-three-page, double-spaced paper about it. Include the following in your paper:

- The microorganism's shape and size
- Its pattern of growth
- Whether it is aerobic or anaerobic
- How it affects the body (e.g., toxins, cell invasion, and so on)
- The symptoms it causes

Follow these guidelines when preparing your report:

- Use 8.5-by-11-inch paper.
- Type, word-process, or write neatly in ink.
- Use correct spelling and grammar.

There are 100 possible points in this worksheet/activity.

20 points—format: introduction, body, summary

40 points—topic development

20 points—grammar

20 points—appearance, professional look

• WORKSHEET/ACTIVITY 4

Find a partner to work with. Take a sheet of paper each and divide the paper into three columns. List the infections that you have had in the first column and the signs and symptoms of those infections in the second column.

Switch papers and fill in the final column, which is a list of the possible causes of the infection.

When you are finished, switch back to your original paper and talk with your classmate about passing along infection. See if the known ways of getting an infection match with your recollection of how you may have gotten infected.

There are 10 possible points each in this worksheet/activity.

SECTION

17.2 | Asepsis and Standard Precautions

- **OBJECTIVES**

  When you have completed this section, you will be able to do the following:

  - Match key terms with their meanings.
  - Define medical asepsis.
  - Match terms related to medical asepsis with their correct meanings.
  - List five aseptic techniques.
  - List some of the Standard Precaution guidelines concerning the use of protective equipment.
  - Demonstrate appropriate handwashing techniques.
  - Explain the difference between bactericidal and bacteriostatic.
  - List reasons why asepsis is important.

- **DIRECTIONS**

  1. Complete Worksheet 1.
  2. Complete Worksheet 2.
  3. Complete Worksheet/Activity 3 as assigned.
  4. When you are confident that you can meet each objective for this section, ask your teacher for the section evaluation.

- **EVALUATION METHODS**

  - Worksheets
  - Class participation
  - Return demonstration
  - Written evaluation

• WORKSHEET 1

Match each definition in column B with the correct vocabulary word in column A.

Column A

_____ 1. Asepsis

_____ 2. Exposed

_____ 3. Aseptic technique

_____ 4. Autoclaves

_____ 5. Isolation

_____ 6. Protective

_____ 7. Disinfection

_____ 8. Dysfunction

_____ 9. Sterilized

_____10. Standard precautions

Column B

a. Methods used to make the environment, the worker, and the patient as germ-free as possible.

b. Abnormal functioning.

c. Standard procedures that protect patients, health care workers, and visitors from pathogens.

d. Process of freeing from microorganisms by physical or chemical means.

e. Sterilizers that use steam under pressure to kill all forms of bacteria on fomites.

f. Made free from all living microorganisms.

g. Sterile condition; free from all germs.

h. Guarding another from danger; providing a safe environment.

i. Condition of having limited contact with others.

j. Left unprotected.

There are 10 possible points in this worksheet.

WORKSHEET 2

1. What is medical asepsis (1 point)? _____

   _____

2. What is a solution that slows the growth of microorganisms called (1 point)?_____

3. What is a solution that kills microorganisms called (1 point)? _____

   _____

4. Mark each of the following statements *T* for true or *F* for false (6 points).

   _____ a. Skin and hair can be sterilized.

   _____ b. Spores are killed when exposed to steam sterilization and high temperature.

   _____ c. Disinfection is a method of controlling the spread of infection.

   _____ d. There is only one kind of sterilization.

   _____ e. Proper handwashing helps control the spread of infection.

   _____ f. Handwashing is one of the most important controls of infection.

5. What does aseptic technique include (6 points)?

a. _____ d. _____

b. _____ e. _____

c. _____ f. _____

6. Explain why Standard Precautions are important (6 points). _____

_____

7. What is a common household cleaner that is effective against microorganisms (1 point)? _____

_____

_____

8. What dilution do you use when preparing this cleaner for disinfecting (1 point)?_____

_____

9. What method of sterilization destroys spore-forming bacteria (1 point)?

_____

10. There are three types of sterilization. What are they (3 points)?

a. _____

b. _____

c. _____

11. List four major factors in the control of microorganisms (4 points).

a. _____

b. _____

c. _____

d. _____

12. You are carrying supplies down the hall. You notice you've dropped a towel. When you pick it up, it looks clean. What will you do, and why (2 points)?

_____

_____

_____

There are 33 possible points in this worksheet.

WORKSHEET/ACTIVITY 3

Many people do not wash their hands properly. They either rush through the activity too quickly or do not wash thoroughly. Demonstrate proper the proper technique for handwashing for a partner. Allow your partner to critique your demonstration so you can make improvements. Then do the same for your partner.

There are 15 possible points in this worksheet/activity.

17.3 Standard Precautions

OBJECTIVES

When you have completed this section, you will be able to do the following:

- Match key terms with their meanings.
- Name primary levels of precautions identified in the guidelines developed by the Centers for Disease Control and Prevention (CDC).
- Identify three types of Transmission-Based Precautions.
- Demonstrate the correct procedure for entering and leaving an area where Transmission-Based Precautions are followed.
- Differentiate between Standard Precautions and Transmission-Based Precautions.

DIRECTIONS

1. Complete Worksheet 1.
2. Complete Worksheet/Activity 2.
3. When you are confident that you can meet each objective for this section, ask your teacher for the section evaluation.

EVALUATION METHODS

- Worksheets
- Class participation
- Return demonstration
- Written evaluation

WORKSHEET 1

Match the following statements with the appropriate terms listed at the left (8 points).

Terms

_____ **1.** Standard precautions

_____ **2.** Transmission-based precautions

_____ **3.** Nosocomial

_____ **4.** Droplet precautions

_____ **5.** Airborne precautions

_____ **6.** Micron

_____ **7.** Contact precautions

_____ **8.** HBV

Statements

a. Reduce the spread of pathogens 5 microns or smaller in size.

b. Reduce the risk of pathogen transmission through direct or indirect contact.

c. Hepatitis B Virus.

d. Primary strategy for successfully preventing hospital-acquired infections.

e. Hospital-acquired infection.

f. Reduce the risk of transmission by a particle larger than 5 microns.

g. Care for known or suspected patients infected with pathogens.

h. One-millionth of a meter in size.

9. When should Standard Precautions be followed (1 point)? _____

_____

_____

10. Why are Transmission-based Precautions necessary (1 point)? _____

_____

_____

11. What is the difference between Transmission-based Precautions and Standard Precautions (6 points)? _____

_____

_____

12. Which precautions require the room door to be closed (1 point)? _____

_____

_____

13. When working with a client in Droplet Precautions, when do you put on a mask (1 point)? _____

_____

14. When working with a client in Contact Precautions, when do you take your gloves off (1 point)? _____

_____

15. Which of the three Transmission-based Precautions requires a private room with specific ventilation criteria (1 point)?_____

_____

16. Name the three Transmission-based Precautions (3 points).

a. _____

b. _____

c. _____

17. Name two primary levels of precautions identified in the guidelines developed by the Center for Disease Control (2 points).

a. _____

b. _____

There are 25 possible points in this worksheet.

WORKSHEET/ACTIVITY 2

With a partner, demonstrate the correct procedure for entering and leaving an area where Transmission-Based Precautions are followed. Allow your partner to critique your demonstration. Then do the same for your partner.

There are 15 possible points in this worksheet/activity.

CHECK-OFF SHEET:

17-1 Hand Hygiene (Washing)

Name _____ Date _____

Directions: Practice this procedure, following each step. When you are ready to have your performance evaluated, give this sheet to your instructor. Review the detailed procedure in your textbook.

Procedure	Pass	Redo	Date Competency Met	Instructor Initials
Student must use Standard Precautions.	☐	☐	_____	_____
Preprocedure				
1. Wash your hands between patient contacts.	☐	☐	_____	_____
2. Wash your hands after removing protective gloves.	☐	☐	_____	_____
3. Wash your hands after contact with body fluids, even if gloves have been worn.	☐	☐	_____	_____
Procedure				
4. Stand at sink. Avoid contact of your uniform with the sink. Roll a paper towel out to have ready to use after washing your hands.	☐	☐	_____	_____
5. Turn on water and adjust water temperature.	☐	☐	_____	_____
6. Wet hands and wrist area. Keep hands lower than elbows.	☐	☐	_____	_____
7. Using soap from dispenser, lather thoroughly.	☐	☐	_____	_____
8. Using soap and friction, wash the palms, backs of the hands, fingers, between the fingers, knuckles, wrists and forearms. Clean nails. If no nail brush is available, rub fingernails on palms of hands.	☐	☐	_____	_____
9. Continue washing for at least 15 seconds.	☐	☐	_____	_____
10. Rinse thoroughly with fingertips downward.	☐	☐	_____	_____
11. Dry hands.	☐	☐	_____	_____
12. Use paper towel to turn off faucet and open door, if necessary.	☐	☐	_____	_____
13. Use lotion on hands to prevent chapping, if needed.	☐	☐	_____	_____

CHECK-OFF SHEET:
17-2 Personal Protective Equipment

Name _____ Date _____

Directions: Practice this procedure, following each step. When you are ready to have your performance evaluated, give this sheet to your instructor. Review the detailed procedure in your textbook.

Procedure	Pass	Redo	Date Competency Met	Instructor Initials
Student must use Standard Precautions.	☐	☐	_____	_____

Preprocedure

1. Determine the expected level of exposure.	☐	☐	_____	_____
2. Refer to the CDC guidelines for the use of Personal Protective Equipment to determine the appropriate PPE equipment to use.	☐	☐	_____	_____
3. Always practice safe work practices, which includes:	☐	☐	_____	_____
a. Keep hands away from face.				
b. Work from clean to dirty.				
c. Limit surfaces touched.	☐	☐	_____	_____
d. Change when torn or heavily contaminated.	☐	☐	_____	_____
e. Perform hand hygiene.	☐	☐	_____	_____

Procedure

NOTE: When using Personal Protective Equipment, done in the order the procedures are given. Prior to donning protective equipment:

a. Remove your watch or push it well up your arm.	☐	☐	_____	_____
b. Wash your hands.	☐	☐	_____	_____

Gown

1. Untie the gown's waist strings; then put the gown on and wrap it around the back of your uniform.	☐	☐	_____	_____
2. Tie or snap the gown at the neck and at the waist making sure your uniform is completely covered.	☐	☐	_____	_____

Mask

Surgical type masks are used to cover the nose and mouth and provide protection from contact with large infectious droplets (over 5 mm in size). For protection from inhalation of small particles or droplet nuclei particulate respirators are recommended. The health care worker must be fitted for these masks prior to use in order to maintain appropriate seal and protection. The infection control department staff will do fit testing for the employee during the employees orientation period.

1. Determine the appropriate type of face mask to be used.	☐	☐	_____	_____
2. Place the mask snugly over your nose and mouth. Secure the mask by tying the strings behind your head or placing the loops around your ears.	☐	☐	_____	_____

Procedure	Pass	Redo	Date Competency Met	Instructor Initials
3. If the mask has a metal strip, squeeze it to fit your nose firmly.	☐	☐	_____	_____
4. If you wear eyeglasses, tuck the mask under their lower edge.	☐	☐	_____	_____

Goggles/Face Shield

Goggles or face shield should be worn when there is a risk of contaminating the mucous membranes of the eyes.	☐	☐	_____	_____

Ventilation Devices

Use a ventilation device, which provides protection for the caregiver from oral contact and secretions, as alternative to mouth to mouth resuscitation.	☐	☐	_____	_____

Gloves

Gloves should be worn when there is risk of touching blood or body fluids. Gloves are worn only once and are discarded according to agency policy. Some care activities for an individual patient may require changing gloves more than once. Hands should be thoroughly washed after gloves are removed.	☐	☐	_____	_____
1. Use clean, disposable gloves.	☐	☐	_____	_____
2. Select a glove that provides appropriate fit.	☐	☐	_____	_____
3. Place the gloves on the hands so that they extend to cover the wrist of the isolation gown.	☐	☐	_____	_____

Removing Personal Protective Equipment

Remember that the outside surfaces of your Personal Protective Equipment are contaminated.

1. While wearing gloves, untie the gowns waist strings.	☐	☐	_____	_____
2. With your gloved left hand, remove the right glove by pulling on the cuff, turning the glove inside out as you pull.	☐	☐	_____	_____
3. Remove the left glove by placing two fingers in the glove and pulling it off, turning it inside out as you remove it. Discard. Wash your hands.	☐	☐	_____	_____
4. Untie the neck strings of your gown. Grasp the outside of the gown at the back of the shoulders and pull the gown down over your arms, turning it inside out as you remove it.	☐	☐	_____	_____
5. Holding the gown well away from your uniform, fold it inside out. Discard it in the laundry hamper.	☐	☐	_____	_____

Procedure	Pass	Redo	Date Competency Met	Instructor Initials
6. Wash your hands. Turn off the faucet using a paper towel and discard the towel in trash container.	☐	☐	_____	_____
7. Remove the mask/goggles to avoid contaminating your face or hair in the process. Untie your mask and/or remove your goggles by holding only the strings/strap. Discard.	☐	☐	_____	_____
8. Wash your hands and forearms with soap or antiseptic after leaving the room.	☐	☐	_____	_____

CHECK-OFF SHEET:
17-3 Caring For Soiled Linens
Name _____ **Date** _____

Directions: Practice this procedure, following each step. When you are ready to have your performance evaluated, give this sheet to your instructor. Review the detailed procedure in your textbook.

Procedure	Pass	Redo	Date Competency Met	Instructor Initials
Student must use Standard Precautions.	☐	☐	_____	_____
Preprocedure				
1. Wash hands.	☐	☐	_____	_____
2. Don disposable gloves.	☐	☐	_____	_____
Procedure				
3. Fold the soiled bed linens inward upon themselves when removing them from the bed.	☐	☐	_____	_____
4. Hold the linens away from your uniform when removing from room.				
5. Place in the nearest hamper.	☐	☐	_____	_____
6. Should the outside surface of the linen hamper bag become soiled it should be placed in a clean outer bag prior to pickup by the laundry staff.	☐	☐	_____	_____

CHECK-OFF SHEET:
17-4 Disposing of Sharps

Name _____ Date _____

Directions: Practice this procedure, following each step. When you are ready to have your performance evaluated, give this sheet to your instructor. Review the detailed procedure in your textbook.

Procedure	Pass	Redo	Date Competency Met	Instructor Initials
Student must use Standard Precautions.	☐	☐	_____	_____

Preprocedure

Procedure	Pass	Redo	Date Competency Met	Instructor Initials
1. Select the safest method of using sharps, using a needleless system whenever possible.	☐	☐	_____	_____
2. Wash hands.	☐	☐	_____	_____
3. Don disposable gloves.	☐	☐	_____	_____
4. Locate the closest sharps container to the area you will be working in.	☐	☐	_____	_____

Procedure

Procedure	Pass	Redo	Date Competency Met	Instructor Initials
5. After the use of any needle place the protective sheath before leaving the patient area.	☐	☐	_____	_____
6. If sharps are used during a procedure, carefully separate them from other items on the tray and cover them with the procedure tray cover.	☐	☐	_____	_____
7. Place any disposable sharps items in the closest sharps container.	☐	☐	_____	_____
8. For non-disposable sharps items place them in the designated area of the closest dirty utility room.	☐	☐	_____	_____
9. Remove and discard disposable gloves.	☐	☐	_____	_____
10. Wash hands.	☐	☐	_____	_____ .

CHECK-OFF SHEET:
17-5 Wrap Instruments for Autoclave
Name _____ Date _____

Directions: Practice this procedure, following each step. When you are ready to have your performance evaluated, give this sheet to your instructor. Review the detailed procedure in your textbook.

Procedure	Pass	Redo	Date Competency Met	Instructor Initials
Student must use Standard Precautions.	☐	☐	_____	_____

Preprocedure

Procedure	Pass	Redo	Date Competency Met	Instructor Initials
1. Retrieve/receive instruments and equipment to be decontaminated.	☐	☐	_____	_____
2. Don appropriate attire:	☐	☐	_____	_____
a. Scrub uniform	☐	☐	_____	_____
b. Head cover	☐	☐	_____	_____
c. Cover gown	☐	☐	_____	_____
d. Gloves	☐	☐	_____	_____
e. Goggles and/or face mask	☐	☐	_____	_____

Procedure

Procedure	Pass	Redo	Date Competency Met	Instructor Initials
3. Sort grossly soiled instruments from those less soiled.	☐	☐	_____	_____
4. Soak instruments that have gross soil in approved enzymatic hospital cleaner. If manual scrubbing is necessary, a soft bristled brush will be used below the water line to decrease the possibility of aerosol contamination.	☐	☐	_____	_____
5. Place instruments with moving parts or hard to reach areas in Sonic Cleaner in open position for cycle (see procedure for operating Sonic Cleaner). All large surface instruments, retractors and elevators will be cleaned manually.	☐	☐	_____	_____
6. Rinse all instruments, washed mechanically or manually, in standing tap water, and running tap water.	☐	☐	_____	_____
7. Immerse instruments with moving parts in instrument lubricant for 45 seconds.	☐	☐	_____	_____
8. Wash instrument trays, washbasins, and rubber items in warm water.	☐	☐	_____	_____
9. Rinse items in standing tap water and running tap water, and dry before wrapping.	☐	☐	_____	_____

Procedure	Pass	Redo	Date Competency Met	Instructor Initials
10. Wash glassware, such as syringes, in warm water and appropriate cleaner. Rinse in standing, running tap water, and distilled water.	☐	☐	_____	_____
11. Air-dry syringes before preparing for sterilization.	☐	☐	_____	_____
12. After the cleaning process, move all instruments to the assembly table in the clean processing room.	☐	☐	_____	_____
13. Assemble, using the appropriate item list for each tray. Note any shortages and try to locate any missing instruments.	☐	☐	_____	_____
14. Make note of any sets with missing instruments.	☐	☐	_____	_____
15. Place tray with items onto designated wrapper. Fold each side of the wrapper in towards the middle. Secure the wrapper with autoclave tape.	☐	☐	_____	_____
16. Notify autoclave personnel of trays, items when readied for sterilizing.	☐	☐	_____	_____

Postprocedure

17. Personnel are responsible for maintaining a clean area.	☐	☐	_____	_____
18. Hand washing is mandatory prior to leaving the area.	☐	☐	_____	_____

CHECK-OFF SHEET:
17-6 Putting on Sterile Gloves and Removing Them

Name _____ **Date** _____

Directions: Practice this procedure, following each step. When you are ready to have your performance evaluated, give this sheet to your instructor. Review the detailed procedure in your textbook.

Procedure	Pass	Redo	Date Competency Met	Instructor Initials
Student must use Standard Precautions.	☐	☐	_____	_____
Preprocedure				
1. Assemble equipment.	☐	☐	_____	_____
2. Wash hands.	☐	☐	_____	_____
Procedure				
3. Pick up wrapped gloves.	☐	☐	_____	_____
4. Check to be certain that they are sterile.	☐	☐	_____	_____
a. Package intact	☐	☐	_____	_____
b. Seal of sterility	☐	☐	_____	_____
5. Place on clean, flat surface.	☐	☐	_____	_____
6. Open wrapper by handling only the outside.	☐	☐	_____	_____
7. Maintain sterility of wrap and gloves.	☐	☐	_____	_____
8. Position with cuff end toward self.	☐	☐	_____	_____
9. Use your left hand to pick up the right-handed glove at folded cuff edge, touching only the inside of glove.	☐	☐	_____	_____
10. Grasp inside of glove with thumb and forefinger.	☐	☐	_____	_____
11. Lift glove out and insert other hand.	☐	☐	_____	_____
12. Put on glove while maintaining sterility.	☐	☐	_____	_____
13. Put glove on right hand.	☐	☐	_____	_____
14. Use gloved right hand to pick up left-handed glove.	☐	☐	_____	_____
15. Place finger of gloved right hand under cuff of left-handed glove.	☐	☐	_____	_____
16. Lift glove up and away from wrapper to pull onto left hand.	☐	☐	_____	_____
17. Continue pulling left glove under wrist. (Be certain that gloved right thumb does not touch skin or clothing.)	☐	☐	_____	_____
18. Place fingers under cuff of right glove and pull cuff up over right wrist with gloved left hand.	☐	☐	_____	_____
19. Adjust fingers of gloves as necessary.	☐	☐	_____	_____

Procedure	Pass	Redo	Date Competency Met	Instructor Initials
20. Keep hands in view and above waist one sterile gloves are on.	☐	☐	_____	_____
21. If either glove tears, remove and discard. Begin with new gloves!	☐	☐	_____	_____
Postprocedure				
22. Turn gloves inside out as you remove them.	☐	☐	_____	_____

CHECK-OFF SHEET:

17-7 Transmission-Based Precautions: Applying Personal Protective Equipment

Name _____ Date _____

Directions: Practice this procedure, following each step. When you are ready to have your performance evaluated, give this sheet to your instructor. Review the detailed procedure in your textbook.

Procedure	Pass	Redo	Date Competency Met	Instructor Initials
Student must use Standard Precautions.	☐	☐	_____	_____
Preprocedure				
1. Assemble equipment.	☐	☐	_____	_____
2. Wash hands.	☐	☐	_____	_____
Procedure				
3. Cover all hair on head with a paper cap.	☐	☐	_____	_____
4. Put on a mask by:	☐	☐	_____	_____
a. Unfolding mask if appropriate.	☐	☐	_____	_____
b. Cover mouth and nose with mask.	☐	☐	_____	_____
c. Secure mask by:				
(1) Pulling elastic on each side of mask over ear, or	☐	☐	_____	_____
(2) Tying top string at sides of mask at back of head and tie lower string at back of neck.	☐	☐	_____	_____
5. Put on gown with opening at back. Slip arms into sleeves of gown.	☐	☐	_____	_____
a. Tie bow at back of neck.	☐	☐	_____	_____
b. Overlap gown edges.	☐	☐	_____	_____
c. Tie at waist with bow or fasten with Velcro strip.	☐	☐	_____	_____
d. Make sure that uniform is completely covered.	☐	☐	_____	_____

CHECK-OFF SHEET:
17-8 Transmission-Based Precautions: Removing Personal Protective Equipment

Name _____ Date _____

Directions: Practice this procedure, following each step. When you are ready to have your performance evaluated, give this sheet to your instructor. Review the detailed procedure in your textbook.

Procedure	Pass	Redo	Date Competency Met	Instructor Initials
Student must use Standard Precautions.	☐	☐	_____	_____
Preprocedure				
1. Untie waist tie of gown.	☐	☐	_____	_____
Procedure				
2. Remove gloves by:				
a. With dominant hand, remove other glove by grasping it just below wrist.	☐	☐	_____	_____
b. Pulling the first glove inside out as you remove it from hand.				
c. With first two fingers of ungloved hand, reach inside glove without touching outside of glove— pull glove off hand covering the first glove. (The second glove removed surrounds the first and both are inside out.) Discard.	☐	☐	_____	_____
3. Wash hands.	☐	☐	_____	_____
4. Untie gown at neck.	☐	☐	_____	_____
5. Remove gown by:				
a. Crossing arms and grasping shoulder of gown with each hand.	☐	☐	_____	_____
b. Pull gown forward causing it to fold inside out.	☐	☐	_____	_____
c. Roll gown so that all contaminated portions are inside of roll, and place in dirty hamper marked Toxic Waste or Hazardous Waste inside room.	☐	☐	_____	_____
6. Wash hands.	☐	☐	_____	_____
7. Remove cap and mask, and discard.	☐	☐	_____	_____
Postprocedure				
8. Use paper towel to open door.	☐	☐	_____	_____
9. Discard towel inside room.	☐	☐	_____	_____
10. Wash hands immediately after leaving the room.	☐	☐	_____	_____

CHECK-OFF SHEET:
17-9 Changing a Sterile Dressing

Name _____ Date _____

Directions: Practice this procedure, following each step. When you are ready to have your performance evaluated, give this sheet to your instructor. Review the detailed procedure in your textbook.

Procedure	Pass	Redo	Date Competency Met	Instructor Initials
Student must use Standard Precautions.	☐	☐	_____	_____
Preprocedure				
1. Wash hands.	☐	☐	_____	_____
2. Assemble supplies.	☐	☐	_____	_____
a. Pair of nonsterile examination gloves	☐	☐	_____	_____
b. Pair of sterile examination gloves	☐	☐	_____	_____
c. Sterile dressing material	☐	☐	_____	_____
d. Tape	☐	☐	_____	_____
e. Biohazardous waste container	☐	☐	_____	_____
3. Explain procedure to patient.	☐	☐	_____	_____
4. Position patient.	☐	☐	_____	_____
Procedure				
5. Put on nonsterile gloves.	☐	☐	_____	_____
6. Remove soiled dressing and examination gloves. Note appearance of wound (size, color, drainage).	☐	☐	_____	_____
7. Discard in biohazardous waste container.	☐	☐	_____	_____
8. Wash hands.	☐	☐	_____	_____
9. Designate a site to be used as a sterile field.	☐	☐	_____	_____
a. Place sterile drape on site.	☐	☐	_____	_____
b. Open and place all sterile dressing supplies on sterile field.	☐	☐	_____	_____
c. Pour wound-cleaning solution or antiseptic into sterile container.	☐	☐	_____	_____
10. Put on sterile gloves.	☐	☐	_____	_____
11. Medicate wound as directed by physician.	☐	☐	_____	_____
12. Apply a double layer of gauze to wound or incision.	☐	☐	_____	_____

Procedure	Pass	Redo	Date Competency Met	Instructor Initials
Postprocedure				
13. Remove gloves and place in biohazardous waste container.	☐	☐	_____	_____
14. Wash hands.	☐	☐	_____	_____
15. Secure dressing with tape.	☐	☐	_____	_____
16. Document the following:	☐	☐	_____	_____
a. Date	☐	☐	_____	_____
b. Time	☐	☐	_____	_____
c. Type of dressing applied	☐	☐	_____	_____
d. Appearance of wound	☐	☐	_____	_____
e. Your name and certification	☐	☐	_____	_____

Chapter 18 Measuring Vital Signs and Other Clinical Skills

Temperature, Pulse, and Respiration

● **OBJECTIVES**

When you have completed this section, you will be able to do the following:

- List the vital signs.
- List fourteen factors that influence body temperature.
- Name the sites where temperature can be measured.
- Tell how normal temperature differs depending on the site.
- Describe how to measure oral, rectal, and axillary temperature.
- Describe a common method for measuring a pulse.
- List six factors that influence the pulse rate.
- Demonstrate counting and recording a radial pulse.
- Recognize the two parts of a respiration.
- List eight factors that affect respiration.

● **DIRECTIONS**

1. Complete Worksheets 1 and 2.
2. Complete Worksheets 3, 4, and 5.
3. Complete Worksheet/Activity 6.
4. When you are confident that you can meet each objective for this section, ask your teacher for the section evaluation.

- **EVALUATION METHODS**
  - Worksheets/Activities
  - Class participation
  - Return demonstrations
  - Written evaluation

- **WORKSHEET 1**

  Fill in the crossword puzzle using the vocabulary words from Section 18.1 in your text.

  ▣ Indicates a space between two words.

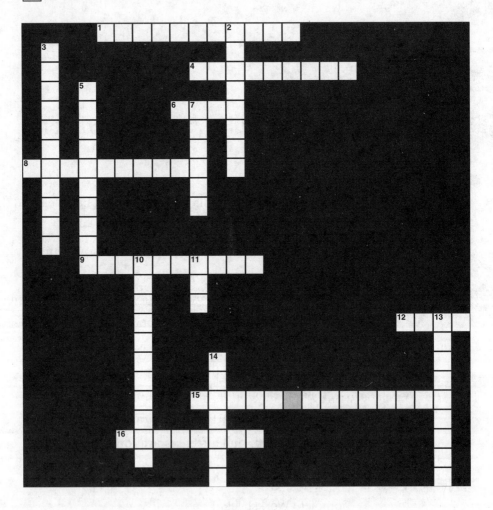

Clues

Across

1. Constant balance within the body.
4. The mixing together of oxygen and another element.
6. Referring to the mouth.
8. Measure of heat; abbreviated F.
9. Process of pushing air out of the lungs during respiration.
12. Pointed end of something.
15. Highest and lowest pressure against the walls of blood vessels.
16. Leaping; strong or forceful.

Down

2. Referring to the armpit.
3. Standard measure.
5. Large amount of bleeding.
7. Referring to the far end of the large intestine just above the anus.

10. Process of breathing in air during respiration.
11. Temperature, pulse, and respiration.
13. Process of eliminating waste material.
14. Measure of heat; abbreviated C.

There are 16 possible points in this worksheet.

● WORKSHEET 2

1. What do homeostatic mechanisms regulate (1 point)? _____
_____

2. List the vital signs (6 points).

a. _____

b. _____

c. _____

d. _____

e. _____

f. _____

3. Which measurements are referred to as TPR (3 points)?

a. _____

b. _____

c. _____

There are 10 possible points in this worksheet.

● WORKSHEET 3

Write each word listed below in the space next to the statement that best defines it (9 points).

afebrile	Celsius	hypothermia
axillary	Fahrenheit	rectal
calibration	febrile	TPR

_____1. Standard measure—e.g., each line on a thermometer or a ruler is a _____.

_____2. Measure of heat: abbreviated F.

_____3. Referring to the far end of the large intestine just above the anus.

_____4. Without fever.

_____5. Condition in which the body temperature is below normal.

_____6. Referring to the armpit.

_____7. Temperature, pulse, and respiration.

_____**8.** Measure of heat; abbreviated C.

_____**9.** Feverish.

Fahrenheit Thermometers

10. Write the correct reading for each of the following thermometers (3 points).

a. _____

b. _____

c. _____

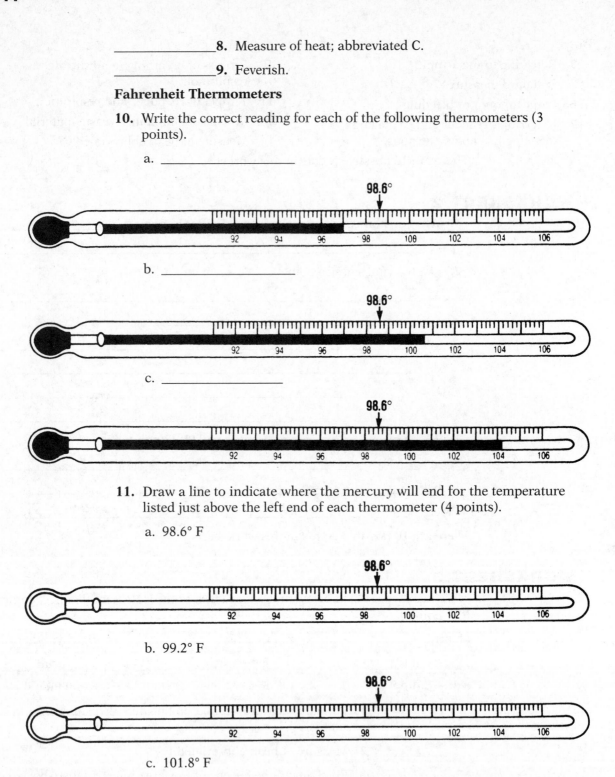

11. Draw a line to indicate where the mercury will end for the temperature listed just above the left end of each thermometer (4 points).

a. 98.6° F

b. 99.2° F

c. 101.8° F

d. 103° F

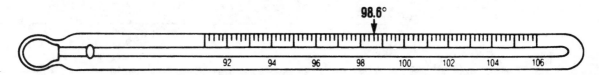

Celsius Thermometers

12. Write the correct reading for each of the following thermometers (2 points).

a. _____

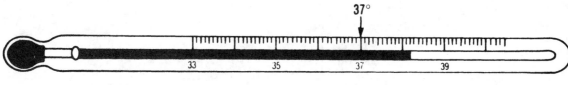

b. _____

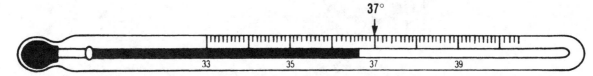

13. Draw a line to indicate where the mercury will end for the temperature listed just above the left end of each thermometer (3 points).

a. 37.2° C

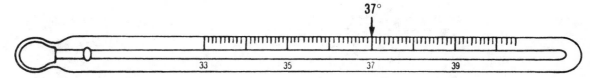

b. 39.4° C

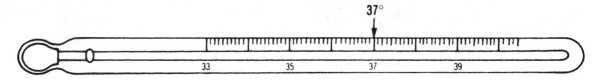

c. 38.6° C

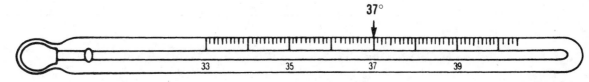

There are 21 possible points in this worksheet.

WORKSHEET 4

1. Define the following words (6 points).

   a. Apex _____

   b. Arrhythmia _____

   c. Bounding_____

   d. Bradycardia _____

   e. Hemorrhage _____

   f. Tachycardia _____

2. Label the pulse points on the following diagram (7 points).

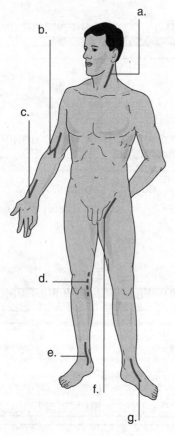

a. _____   e._____

b. _____   f._____

c. _____   g._____

d. _____

3. Mark each of the following statements T for true or F for false (5 points).

_____ a. The pulse rate indicates the number of times the heart beats in one minute.

_____ b. When you take a pulse, you should use your thumb.

_____ c. The apical pulse is the most common pulse that we take.

_____ d. A normal pulse rate for an adult is 130 to 140.

_____ e. A normal pulse rate for an adult is 60 to 80.

4. List six factors that affect the pulse rate (6 points).

a. _____ d. _____

b. _____ e. _____

c. _____ f. _____

5. Define pulse oximetry (1 point). _____

_____

There are 25 possible points in this worksheet.

• WORKSHEET 5

1. Define the following words (6 points).

a. Cheynes-Stokes _____

b. Apnea _____

c. Rales _____

d. Inspiration _____

e. Expiration _____

f. Dyspnea _____

2. List four types of abnormal respirations (4 points).

a. _____

b. _____

c. _____

d. _____

3. List eight factors that affect respiration (8 points).

a. _____ e. _____

b. _____ f. _____

c. _____ g. _____

d. _____ h. _____

There are 18 possible points in this worksheet.

• WORKSHEET/ACTIVITY 6

Ask people of various ages if you can practice counting their pulse and respirations. Complete the chart below with the appropriate information.

	Age	Pulse Rate	Note Characteristics of Pulse	Respiratory Rate	Note Characteristics of Respirations
1					
2					
3					
4					
5					
6					
7					
8					
9					
10					
11					

There are 25 points possible when you record the practice results of 5 people.

There are 50 points possible when you record the practice results of 11 people.

SECTION

18.2 Blood Pressure

• OBJECTIVES

When you have completed this section, you will be able to do the following:

- Match key terms with their correct meanings.
- Define blood pressure.
- Match descriptions of systolic and diastolic blood pressure.
- List four factors that increase blood pressure.
- List four factors that can reduce blood pressure.
- State the normal range of blood pressure.
- Demonstrate how to measure and record a blood pressure accurately.
- Explain how vital signs provide information about the patient's health.

• DIRECTIONS

1. Complete Worksheet 1.
2. Complete Worksheets 2 and 3 as assigned.

3. Practice all procedures using the skills check-off sheets in your workbook.

4. When you are confident that you can meet each objective for this section, ask your teacher for the section evaluation.

● EVALUATION METHODS

- Worksheets

- Class participation

- Written evaluation

- Return demonstration

● WORKSHEET 1

Fill in the crossword puzzle using the vocabulary words from Section 18.2 in your text (14 points).

Indicates a space between two words.

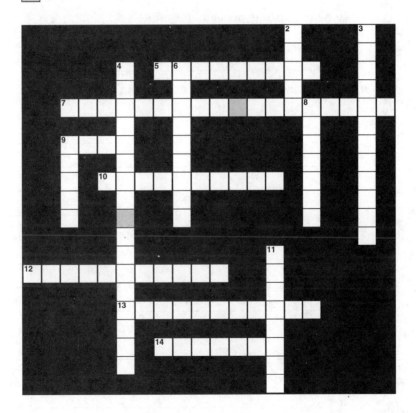

Clues

Across

5. Equipment needed to perform a task.

7. Lowest pressure against the blood vessels of the body.

9. Refers to pressure.

10. Measure of length.

12. Below normal blood pressure range.

13. Instrument used to amplify sound.

14. To swell or fill up with air.

Down

2. Standard scale for measurement.
3. High blood pressure.
4. First heart sound or beat heard when taking a blood pressure.

6. Feeling.
8. Refers to pulse.
9. Refers to measure.
11. Out of date.

There are 14 possible points in this worksheet.

● WORKSHEET 2

1. Define *blood pressure* (1 point).

_____

_____

2. Explain systolic pressure (1 point).

_____

_____

3. Explain diastolic pressure (1 point).

_____

_____

4. List five factors that increase blood pressure (5 points).

a. _____

b. _____

c. _____

d. _____

e. _____

5. List four factors that decrease blood pressure (5 points).

a. _____

b. _____

c. _____

d. _____

e. _____

6. List three types of blood pressure apparatus (3 points).

a. _____

b. _____

c. _____

7. What is the normal range of blood pressure (1 point)? _____

8. Define hypertension (1 point). _____

9. Define hypotension (1 point). _____

There are 19 possible points in this worksheet.

● WORKSHEET 3

Write the pressures indicated on the following diagrams in the spaces provided (6 points).

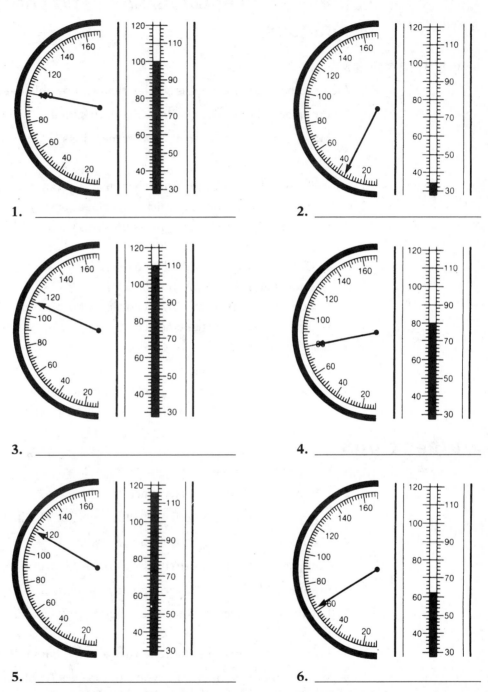

1. _____

2. _____

3. _____

4. _____

5. _____

6. _____

There are 6 possible points in this worksheet.

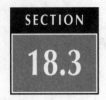

SECTION 18.3

Nursing Skills and Assistive and Therapeutic Techniques

● OBJECTIVES

When you have completed this section, you will be able to do the following:

- Complete all objectives in Part One of this book.

- Match key terms with their correct meanings.

- Identify the following:
  — Responsibilities of the nurse or nurse assistant
  — Four skin conditions requiring special attention
  — Areas on the body where pressure sores usually develop
  — Antipressure aids
  — Occupied bed, closed bed, and open bed
  — Causes and symptoms of dehydration
  — Common types of specimens collected for analysis
  — Six common prosthetic devices

- List the following:
  — Four types of bathing
  — Two body areas requiring special attention during the bathing process
  — Four changes in the skin that may indicate the beginning of a pressure sore

● DIRECTIONS

1. Complete Worksheet 1.

2. Complete Worksheet 2 as assigned.

3. Complete Worksheets/Activities 3 through 5 as directed by your teacher.

4. Complete Worksheets 6 through 8 as assigned.

5. Complete Worksheets/Activities 9 through 11 as directed by your teacher.

6. Complete Worksheets 12 through 15 as assigned.

7. Use the skills check-off sheets to practice and demonstrate all procedures in the chapter.

8. Prepare responses to each item listed in the Chapter Review.

9. When you are confident that you can meet each objective for this section, ask your teacher for the section evaluation.

● EVALUATION METHODS

- Worksheets/Activities

- Class participation

- Written evaluation

- Return demonstrations

● WORKSHEET 1

Fill in the crossword puzzle using the vocabulary words from Chapter 18 in your text.

▢ Indicates a space between two words.

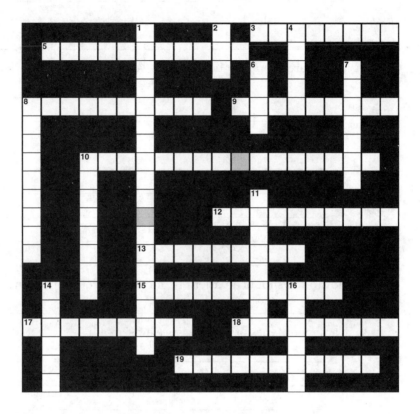

Clues

Across

3. Left over.
5. Severe loss of fluid from tissue and cells.
8. Walking.
9. Fecal material tightly wedged into the bowel.
10. Soft restraints used to protect residents.
12. Removal.

13. To get rid of something.
15. Unable to control the bowel or bladder.
17. Tubes inserted into a body opening or cavity.
18. Holding or keeping.
19. Ability to bend easily.

Down

1. Artificial parts made for the body.
2. Range of motion (abbreviation).
4. Opening.
6. Arm or leg.
7. Involuntary muscle contraction and relaxation.
8. Keeping a resident in proper position is called body _____.

10. Region between the vulva and anus in a female, or between the scrotum and anus in the male.
11. Liquid or pill that causes evacuation of the bowel.
14. Cold and wet.
16. Vomit.

There are 21 possible points in this worksheet.

• WORKSHEET 2

1. What are four skin conditions you should look for when bathing a patient?

a. _____
b. _____
c. _____
d. _____

2. Which areas on the body are very sensitive to pressure?

a. _____
b. _____
c. _____
d. _____
e. _____
f. _____
g. _____
h. _____

3. How often should a patient be moved to prevent pressure sores? _____
_____

4. Name four types of antipressure aids?

a. _____
b. _____
c. _____
d. _____

• WORKSHEET/ACTIVITY 3

Find a partner and talk about how each of you likes to wake up in the morning and go to sleep at night. Be prepared to share your discussion with the class and think about the insights your own preferences give you into helping clients in your care with morning and nighttime routines.

There are 5 possible points in this worksheet/activity.

• WORKSHEET/ACTIVITY 4

Ask your teacher for directions. Bring a toothbrush to class for practice. In teams of three (a resident, nurse assistant, and observer), practice Self-Care Oral Hygiene, Brushing the Resident's Teeth, Oral Hygiene: Ambulatory Resident, Denture Care, and Oral Hygiene for the Unconscious Resident.

The observer is responsible for checking that you carefully follow the procedure.

There are 50 possible points for each check-off sheet you return and demonstrate. There are 200 points in this worksheet/activity. Points for practice and demonstration are assigned according to your participation and ability to return demonstrate the procedure to your teacher.

• WORKSHEET/ACTIVITY 5

Ask your teacher for directions. In teams of three (a resident, nurse assistant, and observer), use the skills check-off list to practice Offering the Bedpan, Offering the Urinal, and Bedside Commode.

Each student will participate as (a) resident, (b) nurse assistant, and (c) observer. The observer is responsible for checking that you carefully follow the procedure.

There are 50 possible points for each check-off sheet you return and demonstrate. There are 150 points in this worksheet/activity. Points for practice and demonstration are assigned according to your participation and ability to return demonstrate the procedure to your teacher.

• WORKSHEET 6

List seven reasons why ambulating the patient is important (7 points).

1. _____
2. _____
3. _____
4. _____
5. _____
6. _____
7. _____

List eight complications of poor body alignment (8 points).

8. _____
9. _____
10. _____
11. _____
12. _____
13. _____
14. _____
15. _____

Match the following position names with their description (6 points).

_____**16.** Supine position   a. Facing down.

_____**17.** Semiprone   b. Sitting position.

_____**18.** Semisupine   c. Lying on side.

_____**19.** Prone position   d. Lying on side, front of body toward the mattress.

_____**20.** Laterial   e. Lying on side with back of body leaning toward mattress.

_____**21.** Fowler's position   f. Flat on back facing upward.

There are 21 possible points in this worksheet.

• WORKSHEET 7

1. List nine steps in preparing the patient for a meal (9 points).

a. _____

b. _____

c. _____

d. _____

e. _____

f. _____

g. _____

h. _____

i. _____

2. Place the letter *E* next to causes of edema. Place the letter D next to causes of dehydration (12 points).

_____ a. diarrhea

_____ b. vomiting

_____ c. high salt intake

_____ d. bleeding

_____ e. infections

_____ f. excessive perspiration

_____ g. injuries, burns

_____ h. certain kidney diseases

_____ i. certain heart diseases

_____ j. poor fluid intake

_____ k. infiltration of IV

_____ l. sitting too long in one position

3. Place the letter E next to the symptoms of edema. Place the letter *D* next to symptoms of dehydration (8 points).

_____ a. decrease in urine output

_____ b. gain in weight

_____ c. fever

_____ d. sometimes shortness of breath

_____ e. concentrated urine

_____ f. weight loss

_____ g. puffiness or swelling

_____ h. increase in urine output

There are 29 possible points in this worksheet.

• WORKSHEET 8

1. From the following list, identify the nine items to be measured when the resident is on I & O. Circle the letter next to the appropriate items (9 points).

a. water

b. cereal

c. gelatin

d. egg salad sandwich

e. juice

f. fruit salad

g. tea

h. apple

i. toast

j. meat

k. milk

l. soup

m. ice cream

n. coffee

o. custard

2. List the items of patient output you will measure when the patient is on I & O (5 points).

   a. _____

   b. _____

   c. _____

   d. _____

   e. _____

3. Ask your teacher for an I & O form. Convert ounces to cubic centimeters (cc) on those of the following food items that would be listed on the I & O sheet. Place the number of cc to the right of the foods you would measure (there are 15). Total the day's fluid intake and record in cc (15 points).

   Breakfast
   4 oz. glass of tomato juice
   2 poached eggs
   11/2 slices toast with butter
   8 oz. cup of tea
   2 oz. water

   Midmorning snack
   2 graham crackers
   4 oz. cup of bouillon
   During bedbath
   1/2 of a 4 oz. glass of water

   Lunch
   3 oz. beef stew
   1 serving green beans
   1 serving fruit salad
   1 slice whole wheat bread with butter
   8 oz. glass of skimmed milk
   6 oz. cup of tea

   Midafternoon snack
   3 oz. dish of custard
   2½ oz. of water
   6 oz. cup of tea

   Dinner
   4 oz. glass of apple juice
   1 cheese sandwich
   1 6 oz. bowl of tomato soup
   3 oz. of a 6 oz. dish of jello

   During PM care
   8 oz. glass of water

   Bedtime
   1/2 of an 8 oz. glass of water

   Total _____cc

4. Compute the patient output from the following list. Record the total in cubic centimeters (5 points).

6:30 A.M.	voided	300cc
8:00 A.M.	emesis	225cc
9:00 A.M.	voided	350cc
12:00 P.M.	voided	300cc
3:45 P.M.	voided	100cc

Total _____

There are 34 possible points in this worksheet.

• WORKSHEET/ACTIVITY 9

Ask your teacher for directions. In teams of three (a *resident*, *nurse assistant*, and *observer*), use the skills check-off sheets in Chapter 18 to practice: Ambulating with a Walking BeltPivot Transfer Wheelchair, Sliding from Bed to Wheelchair and Back, Sliding from Bed to Gurney and Back, Two-Person Lift from Bed to Chair and Back, Lifting with a Mechanical Lift, Moving a Resident on a Gurney, and Moving Resident in a Wheelchair. Each student will participate as (a) resident, (b) nurse assistant, and (c) observer. The observer is responsible for checking that you carefully follow the procedure.

There are 50 possible points in each skills check-off sheet. There are 50 possible points in this worksheet/activity. Points for practice and demonstration are assigned according to your participation and ability to return demonstrate the procedure to your teacher.

• WORKSHEET/ACTIVITY 10

Ask your teacher for directions. In teams of three (a *resident*, *nurse assistant*, and *observer*), use the skills check-off list to practice. Each student will participate as (a) resident, (b) nurse assistant, and (c) observer. The observer is responsible for checking that you carefully follow the procedure. Use the skills check-off sheets provided in your book and by your teacher to practice: Assisting Resident to Sit Up in Bed, Helping the Helpless Resident to Move Up in Bed, Logrolling, Turning Resident Away from You, and Turning Resident Toward You.

There are 50 points in each skills check-off sheet.

There are 250 points in this worksheet/activity.

• WORKSHEET/ACTIVITY 11

You will be required to bring shorts and a tank top or a bathing suit to practice procedures.

Ask your teacher for directions. In teams of three (a resident, nurse assistant, and observer), use the skills check-off list to practice. Each student will participate as (a) resident, (b) nurse assistant, and (c) observer. The observer is responsible for checking that you carefully follow the procedure. Use the skills check-off sheets provided in your book and by your teacher to practice: Resident Gown Change, Giving a Bed Bath, Giving a Partial Bath (Face, Hands,

Axillae, Buttocks, and Genitals), Tub/Shower Bath, Shampooing the Hair in Bed, Shampooing in Shower or Tub, Arranging the Hair, Nail Care, and Shaving the Resident.

There are 50 points in each skills check-off sheet.

There are 450 points in this worksheet/activity.

• WORKSHEET 12

1. List five types of enema (5 points).

   a. _____

   b. _____

   c. _____

   d. _____

   e. _____

2. Why is an ostomy required (1 point)? _____

3. List six causes of urinary incontinence (6 points).

   a. _____

   b. _____

   c. _____

   d. _____

   e. _____

   f. _____

4. Explain what is meant by bladder training (1 point).

   _____

   _____

   _____

5. What are three things you should note about urine (3 points)?

   a. _____

   b. _____

   c. _____

6. What are three things you should note about a bowel movement (3 points)?

   a. _____

   b. _____

   c. _____

7. Explain why a urinary drainage bag is not raised above the resident's hips (1 point).

There are 20 possible points in this worksheet.

• WORKSHEET 13

1. Identify common specimens you will be asked to collect by circling them on the following list (4 points).

sputum   bone marrow   blood

nasal drainage   feces   routine urine

24-hour urine   wound   drainage

2. List 13 symptoms of diabetic coma that can be easily identified (13 points).

a. _____   h. _____

b. _____   i. _____

c. _____   j. _____

d. _____   k. _____

e. _____   l. _____

f. _____   m. _____

g. _____

3. List nine symptoms of insulin shock that can be easily identified (9 points).

a. _____   f. _____

b. _____   g. _____

c. _____   h. _____

d. _____   i. _____

e. _____

4. List oxygen safety rules (5 points).

a. _____

b. _____

c. _____

d. _____

e. _____

5. List four causes of seizures (4 points).

a. _____

b. _____

c. _____

d. _____

There are 35 possible points in this worksheet.

• WORKSHEET 14

1. List four symptoms that may indicate that a patient is about to faint (4 points).

a. _____

b. _____

c. _____

d. _____

2. List five things you must do when you use postural supports on a patient (5 points).

a. _____

b. _____

c. _____

d. _____

e. _____

3. Define soft postural supports (1 point).

_____

_____

4. Preparing a body after death is called _____ (1 point).

There are 11 possible points in this worksheet.

• WORKSHEET 15

1. Mrs. Sherman is 96 years old. She experienced a stroke four months ago. She can walk with a walker and use her strong leg to push herself into a wheelchair. She is very independent and refuses help in washing and dressing herself. Every morning when you go in to see if she needs help, you find her sitting on her weak hand. She says she does not feel it, so it is OK. Explain what you will do to prevent Mrs. Sherman from sitting on her hand, and explain why it is important to protect the weak hand (20 points).

2. Mr. Cash calls for help to the bathroom. You know he has little control of his bladder. If you attend to him immediately, you will help him remain dry and clean. On your way to his room, you see a spilled urinal on the floor. Determine which situation requires attention first. Explain how you would handle both situations and what you expect the results to be (20 points).

3. Mrs. Collins is a resident with rheumatoid arthritis. She tries very hard to care for herself and becomes depressed when she is unable to do the activities of daily living. You deliver her lunch tray. As you are leaving, she says, "I hope I won't have trouble opening these containers." Explain what you think her concern and fear is. Determine how Mrs. Collins can be helped without her feeling helpless. Explain in detail what you will do and why (20 points).

4. Mr. Ramsey doesn't want to get out of bed or dress. He likes to stay in bed. He sometimes asks to have his breakfast tray brought to him. Then he asks to stay in bed and to read. You know that he wants to stay in bed all of the time. Explain how you can convince Mr. Ramsey how important it is to get up and attend activities (20 points).

5. When you are giving Mr. Gammons a back rub, you notice a reddened area on his shoulder and one on his hip. The reddened areas are both on his left side. Explain what steps you can take to be certain that he doesn't get a pressure sore. Write down the reasons why you give back rubs and explain why they are important (20 points).

6. Mr. Stevens is a new resident. When you ask him to get dressed, he refuses. You agree to allow him to rest an additional 20 minutes and ask him to get up again. He still refuses. Explain what you will do to encourage Mr. Stevens to get up and dress. Include in your explanation why it is important that he not be left in bed (20 points).

7. You are helping Ms. Hermans get out of bed. She has been in bed with the flu for three days. While she is sitting on the bedside, you notice that she is very pale and her face has beads of water on it. Her arm feels cool and wet. Explain what you will do for her (20 points).

8. Mr. White is short of breath after bathing and dressing. He still needs to shave and brush his teeth. He uses oxygen continuously and is afraid to have the oxygen turned off. He asks you to position his mirror and plug in his razor while his oxygen is on. Identify the problems in this situation. Explain what you will say to him and how you will assist him with shaving and brushing his teeth (20 points).

9. Mrs. Hughes experienced a stroke many years ago that left her paralyzed on the left side. She is usually out of bed in a wheelchair and in the recreation room. However, the last three days she has been sick to her stomach, so she stayed in bed. When rubbing her back, you notice a red area on her hip from lying on her side. You report it to the charge nurse and ask Mrs. Hughes to stay off her side. Later in the day you see her lying on the side where the red spot was. You also notice the sheets are wrinkled and half off the mattress. Think about the complications of the red hip after just three days in bed. Explain in detail the concerns you have about the red hip. Write the steps you will take to prevent further redness on the skin or other more serious complications (20 points).

10. Mrs. Allen has coarse hairs on her chin. She also has a slight mustache on her upper lip. She becomes irritated when she looks in the mirror. She tells you, "I was always such a pretty girl. Now I look old and ugly. Look at the awful hair on my face. I wish I could just die." Explain the steps you can take to help her. What can you do for her, and what can you say to raise her spirits (20 points)?

There are 200 possible points in this worksheet.

CHECK-OFF SHEET:
18-1 Using an Electronic Thermometer
Name _____   **Date** _____

Directions: Practice this procedure, following each step. When you are ready to have your performance evaluated, give this sheet to your instructor. Review the detailed procedure in your textbook.

Procedure	Pass	Redo	Date Competency Met	Instructor Initials
Student must use Standard Precautions.	☐	☐	_____	_____
Preprocedure				
1. Wash hands	☐	☐	_____	_____
2. Assemble equipment:	☐	☐	_____	_____
a. Plastic thermometer cover/sheath	☐	☐	_____	_____
b. Electronic Thermometer with appropriate probe (blue for oral and axillary; red for rectal)	☐	☐	_____	_____
3. Identify patient. Pull privacy curtain or close the door to provide for the patient' privacy.	☐	☐	_____	_____
4. Explain procedure to patient	☐	☐	_____	_____
5. Need to ask the patient if they have had anything to eat, drink or smoke in the last 15 minutes. If they have, wait 15 minutes to take an oral temperature.	☐	☐	_____	_____
Procedure				
6. Place plastic thermometer cover over probe to prevent contamination.	☐	☐	_____	_____
7. Insert probe in proper position to measure body temperature (blue-tipped probe under tongue or in axilla; red-tipped probe in rectum). If taking axillary temperature, need to hold arm down.	☐	☐	_____	_____
8. Hold probe in place until thermometer indicates reading is complete.	☐	☐	_____	_____
9. Remove plastic sheath and discard it into a biohazardous waste container.	☐	☐	_____	_____
Postprocedure				
10. Record temperature. Health care professionals will record a patient's temperature on their chart. Report elevated temperature to a supervisor.	☐	☐	_____	_____
11. Position patient for comfort. Open curtain or door.	☐	☐	_____	_____
12. Wash hands (follow hand-washing guidelines).	☐	☐	_____	_____
13. Return electronic thermometer to its storage place.				
14. Report any unusual observation immediately.	☐	☐	_____	_____

Check-off Sheet:

18-2 Measuring an Oral Temperature Using a Mercury or Nonmercury Thermometer

Name _____ Date _____

Directions: Practice this procedure, following each step. When you are ready to have your performance evaluated, give this sheet to your instructor. Review the detailed procedure in your textbook.

Procedure	Pass	Redo	Date Competency Met	Instructor Initials
Student must use Standard Precautions.	☐	☐	_____	_____
Preprocedure				
1. Wash hands (follow hand-washing guidelines).	☐	☐	_____	_____
2. Assemble equipment:				
a. Clean oral (reusable or disposable) thermometer	☐	☐	_____	_____
b. Alcohol wipes	☐	☐	_____	_____
c. Watch with second hand	☐	☐	_____	_____
d. Disposable thermometer cover	☐	☐	_____	_____
3. Identify patient and preferred route to be used. Pull privacy curtain or close door.	☐	☐	_____	_____
4. Explain procedure to patient.	☐	☐	_____	_____
Procedure				
5. Apply disposable probe cover.	☐	☐	_____	_____
6. Ask patient whether he or she has been smoking, eating or drinking. If the answer is yes, wait 15 minutes before taking temperature.	☐	☐	_____	_____
7. Place thermometer under tongue and to the side of the mouth.	☐	☐	_____	_____
8. Instruct patient to hold thermometer with closed lips. You might need to help the patient hold the thermometer.	☐	☐	_____	_____
9. Leave in mouth until thermometer indicates reading is complete.	☐	☐	_____	_____
10. Remove from mouth.	☐	☐	_____	_____
11. Remove and discard disposable cover in a biohazardous waste container.	☐	☐	_____	_____
12. Note thermometer reading correctly.	☐	☐	_____	_____
13. Open curtain or door.	☐	☐	_____	_____

Procedure	Pass	Redo	Date Competency Met	Instructor Initials
Postprocedure				
14. Wash thermometer in cool water and dry. Discard thermometer if it is disposable.	☐	☐	_____	_____
15. Wash hands (follow hand-washing guidelines).	☐	☐	_____	_____
16. Record temperature correctly on pad.	☐	☐	_____	_____
17. Report any unusual observation immediately.	☐	☐	_____	_____

Check-off Sheet:

18-3 Measuring a Rectal Temperature

Name _____ **Date** _____

Directions: Practice this procedure, following each step. When you are ready to have your performance evaluated, give this sheet to your instructor. Review the detailed procedure in your textbook.

Procedure	Pass	Redo	Date Competency Met	Instructor Initials
Student must use Standard Precautions.	☐	☐	_____	_____
Preprocedure				
1. Wash hands (follow hand-washing guidelines).	☐	☐	_____	_____
2. Assemble equipment:				
a. Clean rectal (reusable or disposable) thermometer.	☐	☐	_____	_____
b. Alcohol wipes	☐	☐	_____	_____
c. Watch with second hand	☐	☐	_____	_____
d. Lubricant	☐	☐	_____	_____
e. Disposable nonsterile gloves	☐	☐	_____	_____
f. Disposable thermometer cover	☐	☐	_____	_____
3. Identify patient and preferred route to be used.	☐	☐	_____	_____
4. Explain procedure to patient. Pull privacy curtain or close the door.	☐	☐	_____	_____
5. Put on disposable gloves.	☐	☐	_____	_____
Procedure				
6. Remove thermometer from container and apply disposable cover.	☐	☐	_____	_____
7. Lower backrest on bed. Have patient lie on their left side with right leg bent at the knee.	☐	☐	_____	_____
8. Apply lubricant to probe end.	☐	☐	_____	_____
9. Separate buttocks by pulling up on upper buttock.	☐	☐	_____	_____
10. Insert thermometer 1.5 inches into rectum, or 1 to 1.2 inches for an infant. Do not force thermometer.	☐	☐	_____	_____
11. Hold in place until thermometer indicates reading is complete.	☐	☐	_____	_____
12. Remove thermometer. Wipe anal area to remove excess lubricant and any feces. Cover the patient.	☐	☐	_____	_____
13. Remove and discard disposable cover in a biohazardous waste container.	☐	☐	_____	_____
14. Read thermometer correctly. Open curtain or door.	☐	☐	_____	_____

Procedure	Pass	Redo	Date Competency Met	Instructor Initials
Postprocedure				
15. Clean equipment and return to appropriate storage place.	☐	☐	_____	_____
16. Remove and discard disposable gloves.	☐	☐	_____	_____
17. Wash hands.	☐	☐	_____	_____
18. Record temperature correctly. Remember to indicate that it is a rectal temperature with an R.	☐	☐	_____	_____
19. Report any unusual observation immediately.	☐	☐	_____	_____

Check-off Sheet:
18-4 Measuring an Axillary Temperature
Name _____ **Date** _____

Directions: Practice this procedure, following each step. When you are ready to have your performance evaluated, give this sheet to your instructor. Review the detailed procedure in your textbook.

Procedure	Pass	Redo	Date Competency Met	Instructor Initials
Student must use Standard Precautions.	☐	☐	_____	_____
Preprocedure				
1. Wash hands (follow hand-washing procedure).	☐	☐	_____	_____
2. Assemble equipment:				
a. Clean reusable or disposable thermometer	☐	☐	_____	_____
b. Alcohol wipes	☐	☐	_____	_____
c. Watch with second hand	☐	☐	_____	_____
d. Disposable thermometer cover	☐	☐	_____	_____
3. Identify patient and preferred route to be used. Pull privacy curtain or close the door.	☐	☐	_____	_____
4. Explain procedure to patient.	☐	☐	_____	_____
Procedure				
5. Remove thermometer from container and apply disposable cover.	☐	☐	_____	_____
6. Dry the axilla with a towel.	☐	☐	_____	_____
7. Place the thermometer in axilla. Hold the arm close to the body. Leave in place until thermometer indicates reading is complete.	☐	☐	_____	_____
8. Remove the thermometer.	☐	☐	_____	_____
9. Remove and discard disposable cover in biohazardous waste container.	☐	☐	_____	_____
10. Read thermometer correctly. Open curtain or door.	☐	☐	_____	_____
Postprocedure				
11. Clean equipment and return to appropriate storage area.	☐	☐	_____	_____
12. Wash hands (follow hand-washing guidelines).	☐	☐	_____	_____
13. Record temperature correctly. You must indicate it was an axillary temperature.	☐	☐	_____	_____
14. Report any unusual observation immediately.	☐	☐	_____	_____

Check-off Sheet:

18-5 Measuring an Aural (or Tympanic) Temperature

Name _____ Date _____

Directions: Practice this procedure, following each step. When you are ready to have your performance evaluated, give this sheet to your instructor. Review the detailed procedure in your textbook.

Procedure	Pass	Redo	Date Competency Met	Instructor Initials
Student must use Standard Precautions.	☐	☐	_____	_____

Preprocedure

Procedure	Pass	Redo	Date Competency Met	Instructor Initials
1. Determine the device to be used for measuring the patient's temperature. Special devices are available for use in the outer ear canal.	☐	☐	_____	_____
2. Review the patient's graphic record to determine baseline temperature and any recent alterations from baseline.	☐	☐	_____	_____

Procedure

Procedure	Pass	Redo	Date Competency Met	Instructor Initials
3. Wash hands.	☐	☐	_____	_____
4. Explain procedure to patient.	☐	☐	_____	_____
5. Gently pull the ear straight back for children under age 1, or up and back for age 1 or older. Insert the covered probe gently but firmly into the external ear.	☐	☐	_____	_____
6. Activate the device.	☐	☐	_____	_____
7. the temperature reading.	☐	☐	_____	_____
8. Remove the device and discard the probe cover in a biohazardous waste container.	☐	☐	_____	_____

Postprocedure

Procedure	Pass	Redo	Date Competency Met	Instructor Initials
9. Assure that the patient is comfortable and has no further needs before leaving the area.	☐	☐	_____	_____
10. Record the reading on the designated form. Remember to indicate that this was an aural route.	☐	☐	_____	_____
11. Note if the temperature is elevated. Compare the reading with previous temperature readings.	☐	☐	_____	_____
12. If temperature is elevated, communicate that information to the nurse in charge of the patient's care.	☐	☐	_____	_____

Check-off Sheet:

18-6 Counting a Radial Pulse

Name _____ **Date** _____

Directions: Practice this procedure, following each step. When you are ready to have your performance evaluated, give this sheet to your instructor. Review the detailed procedure in your textbook.

Procedure	Pass	Redo	Date Competency Met	Instructor Initials
Student must use Standard Precautions.	☐	☐	_____	_____
Preprocedure				
1. Wash hands (follow hand-washing guidelines).	☐	☐	_____	_____
2. Assemble equipment:				
a. Watch with second hand	☐	☐	_____	_____
b. Pad and pencil	☐	☐	_____	_____
3. Identify patient. Pull privacy curtain or close the door.	☐	☐	_____	_____
4. Explain procedure to patient.	☐	☐	_____	_____
Procedure				
5. Place three fingers on the radial artery—do not use thumb.	☐	☐	_____	_____
6. Count pulse (number of beats or pulsations) for 1 minute.	☐	☐	_____	_____
7. Record pulse rate on pad immediately. Open curtain or door.	☐	☐	_____	_____
Postprocedure				
8. Wash hands (follow hand-washing guidelines).	☐	☐	_____	_____
9. Record pulse rate on chart.	☐	☐	_____	_____
10. Immediately report any unusual observation. Examples include an irregular pulse, a bounding or weak pulse, or a pulse rate less than 60 bpm or more than 100 bpm.	☐	☐	_____	_____

Check-off Sheet:

18-7 Counting an Apical Pulse

Name _____ Date _____

Directions: Practice this procedure, following each step. When you are ready to have your performance evaluated, give this sheet to your instructor. Review the detailed procedure in your textbook.

Procedure	Pass	Redo	Date Competency Met	Instructor Initials
Student must use Standard Precautions.	☐	☐	_____	_____
Preprocedure				
1. Assemble equipment:				
a. Stethoscope	☐	☐	_____	_____
b. Alcohol swabs	☐	☐	_____	_____
2. Wash hands (follow hand-washing guidelines).	☐	☐	_____	_____
3. Identify patient. Pull privacy curtain or close door.	☐	☐	_____	_____
4. Explain procedure to patient.	☐	☐	_____	_____
Procedure				
5. Uncover left side of patient's chest.	☐	☐	_____	_____
6. Locate the apex of the heart between the fifth and sixth rib, about 3 inches to the left of the median line and slightly below the nipple.	☐	☐	_____	_____
7. Place stethoscope over apical region and listen for heart sounds. The apical rate of an infant is easily palpated with the fingertips.	☐	☐	_____	_____
8. Count the beats for 1 minute; note rate, rhythm, and strength of beat.	☐	☐	_____	_____
9. Cover the patient. Open the curtain or door.	☐	☐	_____	_____
10. Record pulse rate on pad.	☐	☐	_____	_____
Postprocedure				
11. Wash hands (follow hand-washing guidelines).	☐	☐	_____	_____
12. Record apical pulse rate on chart. Remember to indicate that it was an apical pulse.	☐	☐	_____	_____
13. Report any unusual observation immediately.	☐	☐	_____	_____

Check-off Sheet:

18-8 Counting Respirations

Name _____ Date _____

Directions: Practice this procedure, following each step. When you are ready to have your performance evaluated, give this sheet to your instructor. Review the detailed procedure in your textbook.

Procedure	Pass	Redo	Date Competency Met	Instructor Initials
Student must use Standard Precautions.	☐	☐	_____	_____
Preprocedure				
1. Wash hands (follow hand-washing guidelines).	☐	☐	_____	_____
2. Assemble equipment:				
a. Watch with second hand	☐	☐	_____	_____
b. Pad and pencil	☐	☐	_____	_____
3. Identify patient. Pull privacy curtain or close door.	☐	☐	_____	_____
4. Explain to the patient that you are going to take their pulse.	☐	☐	_____	_____
Procedure				
5. Relax fingers on pulse point.	☐	☐	_____	_____
6. Observe rise and fall of chest.	☐	☐	_____	_____
7. Count respirations and calculate rate.	☐	☐	_____	_____
8. Note rate, rhythm, and quality of respirations.	☐	☐	_____	_____
Postprocedure				
9. Open curtain or door.	☐	☐	_____	_____
10. Wash hands (follow hand-washing guidelines).	☐	☐	_____	_____
11. Record the respiratory rate accurately. Make sure you take it for 30 seconds and multiply times two. If respirations are irregular, take for one full minute	☐	☐	_____	_____
12. Report any unusual observation immediately. This could include irregular respiration, noisy breathing, and pain with or difficulty breathing.	☐	☐	_____	_____

Check-off Sheet:
18-9 Palpating a Blood Pressure

Name _____ **Date** _____

Directions: Practice this procedure, following each step. When you are ready to have your performance evaluated, give this sheet to your instructor. Review the detailed procedure in your textbook.

Procedure	Pass	Redo	Date Competency Met	Instructor Initials
Student must use Standard Precautions.	☐	☐	_____	_____
Preprocedure				
1. Wash hands (follow hand-washing guidelines).	☐	☐	_____	_____
2. Explain procedure to patient. Pull privacy curtain or close door.	☐	☐	_____	_____
Procedure	☐	☐	_____	_____
3. Select the appropriate cuff for your patient. A cuff that is too small may cause a false-high reading and a cuff that is too large may cause a false-low reading.	☐	☐	_____	_____
4. Support patient's arm, palm side up, on a firm surface.	☐	☐	_____	_____
5. Roll up patient's sleeve above elbow, being careful that it is not too tight.	☐	☐	_____	_____
6. Wrap wide part of cuff around patient's arm directly over brachial artery. Most cuffs have an arrow to position over the brachial artery. The lower edge of cuff should be 1 or 2 inches above bend of elbow.	☐	☐	_____	_____
7. Find radial pulse with your fingertips.	☐	☐	_____	_____
8. Inflate cuff until you can no longer feel radial pulse. Continue to inflate another 30 mm of mercury.	☐	☐	_____	_____
9. Open valve and slowly deflate cuff until you feel the first beat of radial pulse again.	☐	☐	_____	_____
10. Observe mercury or dial reading. This is the placatory systolic pressure. It is recorded, for example, as B/P 130 (P).	☐	☐	_____	_____
11. Deflate cuff rapidly and squeeze out all air.	☐	☐	_____	_____
12. Using your first and second fingers, locate brachial artery. You will feel it pulsating. Place bell or diaphragm of stethoscope directly over artery. You will not hear the pulsation. Do not hold the stethoscope in place with your thumb.	☐	☐	_____	_____
13. Tighten thumbscrew of valve to close it. Turn to the left.	☐	☐	_____	_____

Procedure	Pass	Redo	Date Competency Met	Instructor Initials
14. Hold stethoscope in place and inflate cuff until the dial points to about 30 mm above the palpated B/P.	☐	☐	_____	_____
15. Open valve counterclockwise. Let air out slowly until you hear first beat.	☐	☐	_____	_____
16. At this first sound, note reading on sphygmomanometer. This is the systolic pressure.	☐	☐	_____	_____
17. Continue to release air slowly. Note number on the indicator at which you hear last beat or the sound changes to a dull beat. This is the diastolic pressure.	☐	☐	_____	_____
18. Open valve and release all the air.	☐	☐	_____	_____
19. Remove cuff. Open curtain or door.	☐	☐	_____	_____
Postprocedure				
20. Record time and blood pressure.	☐	☐	_____	_____
21. Clean stethoscope—earpieces and diaphragm.	☐	☐	_____	_____
22. Wash hands.	☐	☐	_____	_____
23. Report any unusual observation immediately.	☐	☐	_____	_____

Check-off Sheet:
18-10 Measuring Blood Pressure

Name _____ **Date** _____

Directions: Practice this procedure, following each step. When you are ready to have your performance evaluated, give this sheet to your instructor. Review the detailed procedure in your textbook.

Procedure	Pass	Redo	Date Competency Met	Instructor Initials
Student must use Standard Precautions.	☐	☐	_____	_____
Preprocedure				
1. Wash hands (follow hand-washing guidelines).	☐	☐	_____	_____
2. Assemble equipment:				
a. Alcohol wipes	☐	☐	_____	_____
b. Sphygmomanometer	☐	☐	_____	_____
c. Stethoscope	☐	☐	_____	_____
d. Pad and pencil	☐	☐	_____	_____
3. Identify patient. Pull privacy curtain or close the door.	☐	☐	_____	_____
4. Explain procedure to patient.	☐	☐	_____	_____
Procedure				
5. Delay obtaining the blood pressure if the patient is in acute pain, has just exercised, or is emotionally upset, unless there is an urgent reason to obtain a blood pressure reading.	☐	☐	_____	_____
6. Select the appropriate arm for application of the cuff. Limbs that have an intravenous infusion, breast or axillary surgery on that side, arteriovenous shunt, or are injured or diseased should not be used.	☐	☐	_____	_____
7. Apply cuff correctly. This should be about one inch above the anticubital space. (Refer to steps 4 and 5 in Procedure 18.9 "Palpating a Blood Pressure".)	☐	☐	_____	_____
8. Clean earpieces on stethoscope.	☐	☐	_____	_____
9. Place earpieces in ears.	☐	☐	_____	_____
10. Locate brachial artery. Place stethoscope over it.	☐	☐	_____	_____
11. Tighten thumbscrew on valve. (Remember the two clues: righty tighty and lefty loosey.)	☐	☐	_____	_____
12. Hold stethoscope in place. Do not use your thumb.	☐	☐	_____	_____
13. Inflate cuff to 170 mm.	☐	☐	_____	_____
14. Open valve. If systolic sound is heard immediately, reinflate cuff to 30 mm mercury above systolic sound.	☐	☐	_____	_____

Procedure	Pass	Redo	Date Competency Met	Instructor Initials
15. Note systolic at first beat.	☐	☐	_____	_____
16. Note diastolic.	☐	☐	_____	_____
17. Open valve and release air.	☐	☐	_____	_____
18. Record time and blood pressure reading on pad. Open curtain or door.	☐	☐	_____	_____
Postprocedure				
19. Wash hands.	☐	☐	_____	_____
20. Wash earpieces on stethoscope.	☐	☐	_____	_____
21. Put away equipment.	☐	☐	_____	_____
22. Record blood pressure in chart.	☐	☐	_____	_____
23. Report any unusual observation immediately.	☐	☐	_____	_____

Check-off Sheet:
18-11 AM Care
Name _____ **Date** _____

Directions: Practice this procedure, following each step. When you are ready to have your performance evaluated, give this sheet to your instructor. Review the detailed procedure in your textbook.

Procedure	Pass	Redo	Date Competency Met	Instructor Initials
Student must use Standard Precautions.	☐	☐	_____	_____
Preprocedure				
1. Wash hands	☐	☐	_____	_____
2. Gently awaken patient.	☐	☐	_____	_____
3. Assemble equipment:				
a. Washcloth and towel	☐	☐	_____	_____
b. Toothbrush and toothpaste	☐	☐	_____	_____
c. Emesis basin	☐	☐	_____	_____
d. Glass of water	☐	☐	_____	_____
e. Denture cup if needed	☐	☐	_____	_____
f. Clean gown if necessary	☐	☐	_____	_____
g. Clean linen if necessary	☐	☐	_____	_____
h. Comb and brush	☐	☐	_____	_____
i. Disposable gloves (two pair)	☐	☐	_____	_____
4. Explain what you plan to do.	☐	☐	_____	_____
5. Provide privacy by pulling privacy curtain.	☐	☐	_____	_____
6. Elevate head of the bed if allowed.	☐	☐	_____	_____
7. Put on disposable gloves.	☐	☐	_____	_____
Procedure				
8. Provide a bedpan or urinal if needed, or escort patient to bathroom.	☐	☐	_____	_____
9. Empty bedpan or urinal, rinse it, and dispose of gloves.	☐	☐	_____	_____
10. Put bedpan or urinal out of sight.	☐	☐	_____	_____
11. Allow patient to wash hands and face.	☐	☐	_____	_____
12. Put on disposable gloves.	☐	☐	_____	_____
13. Assist with oral hygiene.	☐	☐	_____	_____
14. Provide a clean gown if necessary.	☐	☐	_____	_____
15. Smooth sheets if patient remains in bed.	☐	☐	_____	_____

Procedure	Pass	Redo	Date Competency Met	Instructor Initials
16. Transfer to a chair if patient is allowed out of bed.	☐	☐	_____	_____
17. Allow patient to comb hair; assist if necessary.	☐	☐	_____	_____
18. Prepare the overbed table.	☐	☐	_____	_____
a. Clear tabletop.	☐	☐	_____	_____
b. Wipe off.	☐	☐	_____	_____
19. Position overbed table and make sure call bell is within reach if patient is to remain in the room, or transport patient to dining room.	☐	☐	_____	_____

Postprocedure

Procedure	Pass	Redo	Date Competency Met	Instructor Initials
20. Remove and discard gloves.	☐	☐	_____	_____
21. Wash hands.	☐	☐	_____	_____

Check-off Sheet:
18-12 PM Care

Name _____ **Date** _____

Directions: Practice this procedure, following each step. When you are ready to have your performance evaluated, give this sheet to your instructor. Review the detailed procedure in your textbook.

Procedure	Pass	Redo	Date Competency Met	Instructor Initials
Student must use Standard Precautions.	☐	☐	_____	_____
Preprocedure				
1. Wash hands.	☐	☐	_____	_____
2. Tell patient what you are going to do.	☐	☐	_____	_____
3. Provide privacy.	☐	☐	_____	_____
4. Assemble equipment:				
a. Washcloth and towel	☐	☐	_____	_____
b. Toothpaste and toothbrush	☐	☐	_____	_____
c. Glass of water	☐	☐	_____	_____
d. Emesis basin	☐	☐	_____	_____
e. Denture cup, if necessary	☐	☐	_____	_____
f. Night clothes	☐	☐	_____	_____
g. Lotion	☐	☐	_____	_____
h. Linen as needed	☐	☐	_____	_____
i. Disposable gloves	☐	☐	_____	_____
Procedure				
5. Encourage patient to do his or her own care if capable.	☐	☐	_____	_____
6. Assist if unable to do his or her own care.	☐	☐	_____	_____
7. Put on disposable gloves.	☐	☐	_____	_____
8. Provide bedpan or urinal if necessary, or escort to bathroom.	☐	☐	_____	_____
9. Empty bedpan or urinal.	☐	☐	_____	_____
10. Rinse and place in convenient place for night-time use.	☐	☐	_____	_____
11. Remove and dispose of gloves.	☐	☐	_____	_____
12. Wash patient's hands and face.	☐	☐	_____	_____
13. Put on gloves.	☐	☐	_____	_____
14. Provide for oral hygiene.	☐	☐	_____	_____
15. Change gown, if soiled.	☐	☐	_____	_____

Procedure	Pass	Redo	Date Competency Met	Instructor Initials
16. Transfer patient from chair or wheelchair into bed if out of bed.	☐	☐	_____	_____
17. Give back rub with lotion.	☐	☐	_____	_____
18. Observe skin for irritations or breakdown.	☐	☐	_____	_____
19. Smooth the sheets.	☐	☐	_____	_____
20. Change draw sheets if necessary.	☐	☐	_____	_____
21. Provide extra blankets if necessary.	☐	☐	_____	_____
22. Position side rails as ordered after patient is in bed.	☐	☐	_____	_____

Postprocedure

Procedure	Pass	Redo	Date Competency Met	Instructor Initials
23. Remove and discard gloves.	☐	☐	_____	_____
24. Wash hands.	☐	☐	_____	_____
25. Provide fresh drinking water.	☐	☐	_____	_____
26. Place bedside table within patient's reach.	☐	☐	_____	_____
27. Secure call light within patient's reach.	☐	☐	_____	_____

Check-off Sheet:

18-13 Skin Care—Giving a Back Rub

Name _____ Date _____

Directions: Practice this procedure, following each step. When you are ready to have your performance evaluated, give this sheet to your instructor. Review the detailed procedure in your textbook.

Procedure	Pass	Redo	Date Competency Met	Instructor Initials
Student must use Standard Precautions.	☐	☐	_____	_____

CAUTION: Check with team leader for permission to give a back rub.

Preprocedure

1. Wash hands.	☐	☐	_____	_____
2. Assemble equipment				
a. Lotion	☐	☐	_____	_____
b. Powder	☐	☐	_____	_____
c. Towel	☐	☐	_____	_____
d. Washcloth	☐	☐	_____	_____
e. Soap	☐	☐	_____	_____
f. Water (105°F)	☐	☐	_____	_____
g. Disposable gloves	☐	☐	_____	_____
3. Tell patient what you are going to do.	☐	☐	_____	_____
4. Provide privacy by pulling privacy curtains.	☐	☐	_____	_____

Procedure

5. Place lotion container in warm water to help warm it.	☐	☐	_____	_____
6. Raise bed to a comfortable working height.	☐	☐	_____	_____
7. Lower side rail on the side you are working on.	☐	☐	_____	_____
8. Put on disposable gloves.	☐	☐	_____	_____
9. Position patient on side or in prone position.	☐	☐	_____	_____
10. Place a towel along back to protect linen if patient is in a side-lying position.	☐	☐	_____	_____
11. Wash back thoroughly.	☐	☐	_____	_____
12. Rub a small amount of lotion into your hands.	☐	☐	_____	_____
13. Begin at base of spine and apply lotion over entire back.	☐	☐	_____	_____
14. Use firm, long strokes, beginning at buttocks and moving upward to neck and shoulders.	☐	☐	_____	_____

Procedure	Pass	Redo	Date Competency Met	Instructor Initials
15. Use firm pressure as you stroke upward, and light circular strokes returning to buttocks.	☐	☐	_____	_____
16. Use a circular motion over each area (shoulder blades, backbone).	☐	☐	_____	_____
17. Observe skin for irritation or breakdown.	☐	☐	_____	_____
18. Repeat several times (3 to 5 minutes).	☐	☐	_____	_____
19. Dry back.	☐	☐	_____	_____
20. Adjust gown for comfort.	☐	☐	_____	_____
21. Remove towel.	☐	☐	_____	_____
22. Position patient comfortably.	☐	☐	_____	_____
23. Return bed to lowest height.	☐	☐	_____	_____
24. Put up side rail if required.	☐	☐	_____	_____
25. Secure call light in reach of patient.	☐	☐	_____	_____

Postprocedure

Procedure	Pass	Redo	Date Competency Met	Instructor Initials
26. Remove and discard gloves.	☐	☐	_____	_____
27. Wash hands.	☐	☐	_____	_____
28. Record procedure and any observations (e.g., redness, broken areas, dry skin).	☐	☐	_____	_____

Check-off Sheet:

18-14 Giving Special Mouth Care to the Unconscious Patient

Name _____ **Date** _____

Directions: Practice this procedure, following each step. When you are ready to have your performance evaluated, give this sheet to your instructor. Review the detailed procedure in your textbook.

Procedure	Pass	Redo	Date Competency Met	Instructor Initials
Student must use Standard Precautions.	☐	☐	_____	_____
Preprocedure				
1. Wash hands prior to and after administering care.	☐	☐	_____	_____
2. Put on disposable gloves.	☐	☐	_____	_____
Procedure				
3. Assemble equipment within reach—toothbrush, toothpaste, emesis basin, normal saline solution, cup with cool water, towel, mouthwash, sponge toothette, padded tongue blade, irrigating syringe with rubber tip, petroleum jelly, suction catheter with suction apparatus.	☐	☐	_____	_____
4. Provide privacy for the patient. Adjust the height of the bed to a comfortable position for the nurse. Lower the side rail next to the nurse and position the patient on their side with the head of the bed lowered. Place the towel across the patient's chest and emesis basin in position under the chin.	☐	☐	_____	_____
5. Open the patient's mouth and gently insert a padded tongue blade between the back molars if necessary	☐	☐	_____	_____
6. If teeth are present, brush carefully with toothbrush and paste. If dentures are present, remove gently and cleans before replacing. Use a toothette moistened with normal saline to gently cleanse guns, mucous membranes, and tongue.	☐	☐	_____	_____
7. If necessary, use the irrigating syringe with rubber tip and rinse mouth gently with a small amount of water. Position the patient's head to allow for return of water or use suction apparatus to remove the water from the oral cavity.	☐	☐	_____	_____
8. Apply petroleum jelly to the patient's lips.	☐	☐	_____	_____
9 Remove equipment and return the patient to a comfortable position. Raise the siderail and lower the bed.	☐	☐	_____	_____
Postprocedure				
10. Document the nursing assistant's oral assessment and any unusual findings.	☐	☐	_____	_____

Check-off Sheet:
18-15 Oral Hygiene—Self Care
Name _____ **Date** _____

Directions: Practice this procedure, following each step. When you are ready to have your performance evaluated, give this sheet to your instructor. Review the detailed procedure in your textbook.

Procedure	Pass	Redo	Date Competency Met	Instructor Initials
Student must use Standard Precautions.	☐	☐	_____	_____
Preprocedure				
1. Wash hands.	☐	☐	_____	_____
2. Assemble equipment:	☐	☐	_____	_____
a. Toothbrush	☐	☐	_____	_____
b. Toothpaste	☐	☐	_____	_____
c. Mouthwash	☐	☐	_____	_____
d. Cup of water with straw, if needed.	☐	☐	_____	_____
e. Emesis basin	☐	☐	_____	_____
f. Bath towel	☐	☐	_____	_____
h. Tissues	☐	☐	_____	_____
3. Identify patient and explain what you are going to do.	☐	☐	_____	_____
4. Screen patient by pulling privacy curtain around bed.	☐	☐	_____	_____
Procedure				
5. Raise head of bed if patient is allowed to sit up.	☐	☐	_____	_____
6. Place towel over blanket and patient's gown.	☐	☐	_____	_____
7. Place toothbrush, toothpaste, mouthwash, emesis basin, and glass of water on overbed table.	☐	☐	_____	_____
8. Remove overbed table with patient has completed brushing.	☐	☐	_____	_____
9. Put away towel and make patient comfortable.				
10. Put up side rails if required.	☐	☐	_____	_____
11. Secure call bell with patient's reach.	☐	☐	_____	_____
12. Put away all equipment and tidy unit.	☐	☐	_____	_____
Postprocedure				
13. Wash hands.	☐	☐	_____	_____
14. Chart procedure	☐	☐	_____	_____

Check-off Sheet:
18-16 Oral Hygiene—Brushing the Patient's Teeth

Name _____ **Date** _____

Directions: Practice this procedure, following each step. When you are ready to have your performance evaluated, give this sheet to your instructor. Review the detailed procedure in your textbook.

Procedure	Pass	Redo	Date Competency Met	Instructor Initials
Student must use Standard Precautions.	☐	☐	_____	_____
Preprocedure				
1. Wash hands.	☐	☐	_____	_____
2. Assemble equipment:				
a. Toothbrush	☐	☐	_____	_____
b. Toothpaste	☐	☐	_____	_____
c. Mouthwash	☐	☐	_____	_____
d. Cup of water with straw, if needed.	☐	☐	_____	_____
e. Emesis basin	☐	☐	_____	_____
f. Bath towel	☐	☐	_____	_____
g. Tissues	☐	☐	_____	_____
h. Disposable nonsterile gloves	☐	☐	_____	_____
3. Identify patient and explain what you are going to do.	☐	☐	_____	_____
4. Screen patient by pulling privacy curtain around bed.	☐	☐	_____	_____
Procedure				
5. Raise head of bed if patient is allowed to sit up.	☐	☐	_____	_____
6. Place a towel over blanket and patient's gown.	☐	☐	_____	_____
7. Put on gloves	☐	☐	_____	_____
8. Pour water over toothbrush, put toothpaste on brush.				
9. Insert brush into the mouth carefully.	☐	☐	_____	_____
10. Place brush at angle on upper teeth and brush in an up-and-down motion starting at rear of mouth.	☐	☐	_____	_____
11. Repeat on lower teeth.	☐	☐	_____	_____
12. Give patient water to rinse mouth. If necessary, use a straw.	☐	☐	_____	_____
13. Hold emesis basin under chin. Have patient expectorate (spit) water into the basin.	☐	☐	_____	_____
14. Offer tissues to patient to wipe mouth and chin. Discard tissues.	☐	☐	_____	_____

Procedure	Pass	Redo	Date Competency Met	Instructor Initials
15. Provide mouthwash if available. Use emesis basin and tissues as above.	☐	☐	_____	_____
16. Put up side rails before turning away from patient.	☐	☐	_____	_____
17. Return all equipment.	☐	☐	_____	_____
18. Remove gloves and put in hazardous waste.	☐	☐	_____	_____
Postprocedure				
19. Wash hands.	☐	☐	_____	_____
20. Tidy up unit.	☐	☐	_____	_____
21. Secure call bell within patient's reach.	☐	☐	_____	_____
22. Make patient comfortable before leaving the room.	☐	☐	_____	_____
23. Chart procedure and how patient tolerated it.	☐	☐	_____	_____

Check-off Sheet:

18-17 Oral Hygiene—Ambulatory Patient

Name _____ Date _____

Directions: Practice this procedure, following each step. When you are ready to have your performance evaluated, give this sheet to your instructor. Review the detailed procedure in your textbook.

Procedure	Pass	Redo	Date Competency Met	Instructor Initials
Student must use Standard Precautions.	☐	☐	_____	_____
Preprocedure				
1. Wash hands.	☐	☐	_____	_____
2. Tell patient what you are going to do.	☐	☐	_____	_____
Procedure				
3. Set up equipment at sink.	☐	☐	_____	_____
a. Toothbrush	☐	☐	_____	_____
b. Toothpaste	☐	☐	_____	_____
c. Tablets or powder to soak dentures in	☐	☐	_____	_____
d. Towel	☐	☐	_____	_____
e. Glass	☐	☐	_____	_____
Postprocedure				
4. Rinse equipment and put away.	☐	☐	_____	_____
5. Wash hands.	☐	☐	_____	_____

Check-off Sheet:

18-18 Oral Hygiene—Denture Care

Name _____ **Date** _____

Directions: Practice this procedure, following each step. When you are ready to have your performance evaluated, give this sheet to your instructor. Review the detailed procedure in your textbook.

Procedure	Pass	Redo	Date Competency Met	Instructor Initials
Student must use Standard Precautions.	☐	☐	_____	_____
Preprocedure				
1. Wash hands.	☐	☐	_____	_____
2. Assemble equipment:				
a. Tissues	☐	☐	_____	_____
b. Paper towel or gauze squares	☐	☐	_____	_____
c. Mouthwash	☐	☐	_____	_____
d. Disposable denture cup	☐	☐	_____	_____
e. Toothbrush or denture brush	☐	☐	_____	_____
f. Denture paste or toothpowder	☐	☐	_____	_____
g. Towel	☐	☐	_____	_____
h. Disposable nonsterile gloves	☐	☐	_____	_____
i. Emesis basin	☐	☐	_____	_____
3. Identify patient.	☐	☐	_____	_____
4. Explain what you are going to do.	☐	☐	_____	_____
Procedure	☐	☐	_____	_____
5. Pull privacy curtain.	☐	☐	_____	_____
6. Lower side rails.	☐	☐	_____	_____
7. Raise head of bed if allowed.	☐	☐	_____	_____
8. Place towel across patient's chest.	☐	☐	_____	_____
9. Prepare emesis basin by placing tissue, paper towel or washcloth in bottom of basin.	☐	☐	_____	_____
10. Put on gloves.	☐	☐	_____	_____
11. Have patient remove his or her dentures.	☐	☐	_____	_____
12. Remove dentures if patient cannot.	☐	☐	_____	_____
Upper Denture				
a. Explain what you are going to do.	☐	☐	_____	_____
b. Use a gauze square to grip under denture.	☐	☐	_____	_____

Procedure	Pass	Redo	Date Competency Met	Instructor Initials
c. Place your index finger between top ridge of denture and cheek.	☐	☐	_____	_____
d. Gently pull on denture to release suction.	☐	☐	_____	_____
e. Remove upper denture.	☐	☐	_____	_____
Lower Denture				
a. Use a gauze square to grip lower denture.	☐	☐	_____	_____
b. Place your index finger between lower ridge and cheek.	☐	☐	_____	_____
c. Gently pull on denture to release suction.	☐	☐	_____	_____
d. Remove lower denture.	☐	☐	_____	_____
13. Place dentures in lined emesis basin and take to sink or utility room.	☐	☐	_____	_____
14. Remember to pull side rails up if you walk away from the bed.	☐	☐	_____	_____
15. Hold dentures firmly in palm of hand.	☐	☐	_____	_____
16. Put toothpowder or toothpaste on toothbrush.	☐	☐	_____	_____
17. Rinse dentures in cool water.	☐	☐	_____	_____
18. Hold dentures under cold running water and brush dentures on all surfaces until clean.	☐	☐	_____	_____
19. Rinse dentures under cold running water.	☐	☐	_____	_____
20. Remember to rinse denture cup with cold water before placing clean dentures in the cup.	☐	☐	_____	_____
21. Place in denture cup.	☐	☐	_____	_____
22. Place some mouthwash and cool water in cup.	☐	☐	_____	_____
23. Help patient rinse mouth with mouthwash; if food particles are between cheek and gumline, gently swab away with gauze. Clean gums with toothette.	☐	☐	_____	_____
24. Have patient replace dentures.	☐	☐	_____	_____
25. Place dentures in labeled denture cup next to bed, if dentures are to be left out.	☐	☐	_____	_____
26. Rinse equipment and put away.	☐	☐	_____	_____
Postprocedure				
27. Remove gloves; dispose of in hazardous waste.	☐	☐	_____	_____
28. Wash hands.	☐	☐	_____	_____
29. Position patient.	☐	☐	_____	_____
30. Secure call bell within patient's reach.	☐	☐	_____	_____
31. Chart procedure and how it was tolerated.	☐	☐	_____	_____

Check-off Sheet:
18-19 Dental Hygiene—For the Unconscious Patient
Name _____ Date _____

Directions: Practice this procedure, following each step. When you are ready to have your performance evaluated, give this sheet to your instructor. Review the detailed procedure in your textbook.

Procedure	Pass	Redo	Date Competency Met	Instructor Initials
Student must use Standard Precautions.	☐	☐	_____	_____
Preprocedure				
1. Wash hands.	☐	☐	_____	_____
2. Tell patient what you are going to do. When patient is unconscious he or she may hear even if she or she cannot respond.	☐	☐	_____	_____
3. Provide privacy	☐	☐	_____	_____
4. Assemble equipment:				
a. Emesis basin	☐	☐	_____	_____
b. Towel	☐	☐	_____	_____
c. Lemon glycerin swabs	☐	☐	_____	_____
d. Tongue blades	☐	☐	_____	_____
e. 4 x 4 gauze	☐	☐	_____	_____
f. Lip moisturizer	☐	☐	_____	_____
g. Disposable nonsterile gloves	☐	☐	_____	_____
5. Position bed at a comfortable working height.	☐	☐	_____	_____
6. Put on gloves.	☐	☐	_____	_____
Procedure				
7. Position patent's head to side and place towel on bed under patient's cheek and chin.	☐	☐	_____	_____
8. Secure emesis basin under patient's chin.	☐	☐	_____	_____
9. Wrap a tongue blade with a 4 x 4 gauze and slightly moisten. Swab mouth being certain to clean gums, teeth, tongue, and roof of mouth.	☐	☐	_____	_____
10. Apply lip moisturizer to lips and swab mouth with lemon and glycerin if available.	☐	☐	_____	_____
11. Remove towel and reposition patient.	☐	☐	_____	_____
12. Make sure side rails are up and bed is in low position.	☐	☐	_____	_____
13. Discard disposable equipment in hazardous waste.	☐	☐	_____	_____

Procedure	Pass	Redo	Date Competency Met	Instructor Initials
14. Clean basin and put away.	☐	☐	_____	_____
15. Remove gloves and put in hazardous waste.	☐	☐	_____	_____
Postprocedure				
16. Wash hands.	☐	☐	_____	_____
17. Report and document patient's tolerance of procedure.	☐	☐	_____	_____

Check-off Sheet:
18-20 Elimination—Offering the Bedpan

Name _____ Date _____

Directions: Practice this procedure, following each step. When you are ready to have your performance evaluated, give this sheet to your instructor. Review the detailed procedure in your textbook.

Procedure	Pass	Redo	Date Competency Met	Instructor Initials
Student must use Standard Precautions.	☐	☐	_____	_____
Preprocedure				
1. Wash hands.	☐	☐	_____	_____
2. Assemble equipment:				
a. Bedpan with cover	☐	☐	_____	_____
b. Toilet tissue	☐	☐	_____	_____
c. Soap and water	☐	☐	_____	_____
d. Towel and washcloth	☐	☐	_____	_____
e. Disposable nonsterile gloves (two pairs)	☐	☐	_____	_____
3. Ask visitors to wait outside room.	☐	☐	_____	_____
4. Provide privacy for patient with curtain, screen, or door.	☐	☐	_____	_____
5. Put on clean gloves before handling the bedpan.	☐	☐	_____	_____
6. Remove bedpan from storage space.	☐	☐	_____	_____
7. Warm metal bedpans by running water over them and drying.	☐	☐	_____	_____
Procedure				
8. Lower head of bed if it is elevated.	☐	☐	_____	_____
9. Fold top covers back enough to see where to place the pan. Do not expose patient.	☐	☐	_____	_____
10. Ask patient to raise hips off bed. Help support patient by placing your hand at patient's midback.	☐	☐	_____	_____
Roll the patient onto his or her side if the patient is unable to lift the hips.	☐	☐	_____	_____
Place bedpan on buttocks. For a standard bedpan: Position so wider end of pan is aligned with patient's buttocks. For a fracture pan: position bedpan with handle toward the foot of the bed.	☐	☐	_____	_____
Hold in place with one hand and help patient roll back onto bedpan.	☐	☐	_____	_____
11. Slide bedpan into place.	☐	☐	_____	_____

Procedure	Pass	Redo	Date Competency Met	Instructor Initials
12. Cover patient again.	☐	☐	_____	_____
13. Raise head of bed for comfort.	☐	☐	_____	_____
14. Put toilet tissue within patient's reach.	☐	☐	_____	_____
15. Remove gloves.	☐	☐	_____	_____
16. Wash your hands.	☐	☐	_____	_____
17. Leave call light with patient and ask patient to signal when finished.	☐	☐	_____	_____
18. Leave room to provide privacy.	☐	☐	_____	_____
19. Watch for call light to signal patient's readiness to be removed from bedpan.	☐	☐	_____	_____
20. Put on gloves.	☐	☐	_____	_____
21. Assist patient as necessary to ensure cleanliness.	☐	☐	_____	_____
22. Lower head of bed before removing bedpan.	☐	☐	_____	_____
23. Remove bedpan and empty, rinse bedpan and pour rinse into the toilet.	☐	☐	_____	_____
24. Use a paper towel to flush the toilet and the faucet, since still have gloves on.	☐	☐	_____	_____
25. Measure urine if on I & O.	☐	☐	_____	_____
26. Remove gloves and dispose of in biohazardous container.	☐	☐	_____	_____

Postprocedure

Procedure	Pass	Redo	Date Competency Met	Instructor Initials
27. Wash hands.	☐	☐	_____	_____
28. Put on clean gloves	☐	☐	_____	_____
29. Provide washcloth, water, and soap for patient to wash hands.	☐	☐	_____	_____
30. Dispose of soiled washcloth or wipes in proper container.	☐	☐	_____	_____
31. Provide comfort measures for patient.	☐	☐	_____	_____
32. Secure call light in patient's reach, make sure side rails are up and bed is in lowest position.	☐	☐	_____	_____
33. Remove and dispose of gloves in biohazardous container.	☐	☐	_____	_____
34. Wash hands.	☐	☐	_____	_____
35. Open privacy curtain.	☐	☐	_____	_____
36. Chart the following:	☐	☐	_____	_____
a. Bowel movement amount, color, consistency	☐	☐	_____	_____
b. Amount voided if on I & O	☐	☐	_____	_____

Check-off Sheet:

18-21 Elimination—Offering the Urinal

Name _____ Date _____

Directions: Practice this procedure, following each step. When you are ready to have your performance evaluated, give this sheet to your instructor. Review the detailed procedure in your textbook.

Procedure	Pass	Redo	Date Competency Met	Instructor Initials
Student must use Standard Precautions.	☐	☐	_____	_____
Preprocedure				
1. Wash hands.	☐	☐	_____	_____
2. Assemble equipment:	☐	☐	_____	_____
a. Urinal with cover	☐	☐	_____	_____
b. Soap and water	☐	☐	_____	_____
c. Towel and washcloth	☐	☐	_____	_____
d. Disposable nonsterile gloves	☐	☐	_____	_____
3. Ask visitors to wait outside room.	☐	☐	_____	_____
4. Provide privacy for patient.	☐	☐	_____	_____
Procedure				
5. Hand urinal to patient.	☐	☐	_____	_____
6. Place call light at patient's side.	☐	☐	_____	_____
7. Wash your hands.	☐	☐	_____	_____
8. Leave room until patient signals with the call light.	☐	☐	_____	_____
9. Return to room when patient has finished voiding.	☐	☐	_____	_____
10. Put on gloves.	☐	☐	_____	_____
11. Offer washcloth for patient to wash their hands.	☐	☐	_____	_____
12. Place cover over urinal and carry it into the bathroom.	☐	☐	_____	_____
13. Check to see if patient is on I & O or if a urine specimen is needed. (See I & O and specimen collection in this chapter.)	☐	☐	_____	_____
14. Observe urine color, consistency, and odor.	☐	☐	_____	_____
15. Empty into toilet.	☐	☐	_____	_____
16. Use a paper towel to turn on the faucet and flush the toilet, since still have gloves on. Rinse urinal with cold water.	☐	☐	_____	_____

Procedure	Pass	Redo	Date Competency Met	Instructor Initials
Postprocedure				
17. Cover and place in a convenient location for the patient.	☐	☐	_____	_____
18. Remove gloves and place in biohazardous container.	☐	☐	_____	_____
19. Wash hands.	☐	☐	_____	_____
20. Secure call light in reach of patient.	☐	☐	_____	_____
21. Report and document unusual color, odor, or consistency of urine.	☐	☐	_____	_____
22. Record amount if on I & O.	☐	☐	_____	_____

Check-off Sheet:

18-22 Elimination—Bedside Commode

Name _____ **Date** _____

Directions: Practice this procedure, following each step. When you are ready to have your performance evaluated, give this sheet to your instructor. Review the detailed procedure in your textbook.

Procedure	Pass	Redo	Date Competency Met	Instructor Initials
Student must use Standard Precautions.	☐	☐	_____	_____
Preprocedure				
1. Wash hands.	☐	☐	_____	_____
2. Assemble equipment:	☐	☐	_____	_____
a. Bedside commode	☐	☐	_____	_____
b. Toilet tissue	☐	☐	_____	_____
c. Washcloth	☐	☐	_____	_____
d. Warm water	☐	☐	_____	_____
e. Soap	☐	☐	_____	_____
f. Towel	☐	☐	_____	_____
g. Disposable nonsterile gloves	☐	☐	_____	_____
3. Identify patient.	☐	☐	_____	_____
4. Explain what you are going to do.	☐	☐	_____	_____
Procedure				
5. Place commode chair next to bed facing head of bed. Lock wheels!	☐	☐	_____	_____
6. Check to see if receptacle is in place under seat.	☐	☐	_____	_____
7. Provide privacy by pulling privacy curtains.	☐	☐	_____	_____
8. Lower bed to lowest position.	☐	☐	_____	_____
9. Lower side rail				
10. Help patient to sitting position.	☐	☐	_____	_____
11. Help patient swing legs over side of bed.	☐	☐	_____	_____
12. Put on patient's slippers and assist to stand.	☐	☐	_____	_____
13. Have patient place hands on your shoulders.	☐	☐	_____	_____
14. Support under patient's arms, pivot patient to right, and lower to commode. (See the procedure "Transferring—Pivot Transfer from Bed to Wheelchair.")	☐	☐	_____	_____
15. Place call bell within reach.	☐	☐	_____	_____

Procedure	Pass	Redo	Date Competency Met	Instructor Initials
16. Place toilet tissue within reach.	☐	☐	_____	_____
17. Remain nearby if patient seems weak.	☐	☐	_____	_____
18. Return immediately when patient signals.	☐	☐	_____	_____
19. Put on gloves.	☐	☐	_____	_____
20. Assist patient to stand.	☐	☐	_____	_____
21. Clean anus or perineum of patient is unable to help self.	☐	☐	_____	_____
22. Remove gloves and put in hazardous waste.	☐	☐	_____	_____
23. Help patient wash hands. Remember to do this before you stand the patient up.	☐	☐	_____	_____
24. Assist back to bed and position comfortably.	☐	☐	_____	_____
25. Put up side rail if required.	☐	☐	_____	_____
26. Put on gloves.	☐	☐	_____	_____
27. Put down cover on commode chair and remove receptacle.	☐	☐	_____	_____
28. Empty contents, measuring if on I & O.	☐	☐	_____	_____
29. Empty and clean per hospital policy.	☐	☐	_____	_____
30. Remove gloves and put in hazardous waste.	☐	☐	_____	_____

Postprocedure

Procedure	Pass	Redo	Date Competency Met	Instructor Initials
31. Wash hands.	☐	☐	_____	_____
32. Replace equipment and tidy unit.	☐	☐	_____	_____
33. Record the following:	☐	☐	_____	_____
a. Bowel movement:	☐	☐	_____	_____
(1) Amount	☐	☐	_____	_____
(2) Consistency	☐	☐	_____	_____
(3) Color	☐	☐	_____	_____
b. Any unusual observations, such as	☐	☐	_____	_____
(1) Weakness	☐	☐	_____	_____
(2) Discomfort	☐	☐	_____	_____

Check-off Sheet:
18-23 Assisting to Bathroom
Name _____ Date _____

Directions: Practice this procedure, following each step. When you are ready to have your performance evaluated, give this sheet to your instructor. Review the detailed procedure in your textbook.

Procedure	Pass	Redo	Date Competency Met	Instructor Initials
Student must use Standard Precautions.	☐	☐	_____	_____

Preprocedure

1. Establish the baseline function of the patient. Determine the amount of assistance required (one nurse, two nurses).	☐	☐	_____	_____
2. Establish the need for assertive devices such as cane, walker, gait belt.				
3. Assure that the path to be used is clear of obstruction.	☐	☐	_____	_____
4. Explain to the patient what is to be done. Instruct the patient to alert the nurse of any lightheadedness or discomfort.	☐	☐	_____	_____

Procedure

5. Assist the patient to an erect position at the edge of the bed.	☐	☐	_____	_____
6. Pause at the edge of the bed (and again after the patient arises) to ensure that the patient feels steady. You should stand in front of and face the patient. Brace the patient's lower extremities. Place belt around the patient's waist.	☐	☐	_____	_____
7. Elevate the bed to a height that allows the patient's legs to rest firmly on the ground but not to have to lift his body from a low position as the patient rises.	☐	☐	_____	_____
8. With your hands under the gait belt, assist the patient to rise.	☐	☐	_____	_____
9. Patients who are fearful of walking may tend to bend forward and look at their feet. They will need to be reminded to stand erect and hold their head high.	☐	☐	_____	_____

Procedure	Pass	Redo	Date Competency Met	Instructor Initials
10. Guide the patient to the bathroom with one hand under the gait belt at the patient's back and the other hand guiding the patient's free arm. Walk slightly behind and to one side of the patient for the full distance, while holding on to the belt. Assist with lowering the patient onto the toilet seat. For those patients who have functional disabilities, it is advisable to obtain and use an elevated toilet seat. This will enable the patient to sit and rise with the least amount of energy use and the greatest degree of safety.	☐	☐	_____	_____
11. Instruct the patient to on using the nurse call light to call for assistance after toileting is complete.	☐	☐	_____	_____
12. After toileting is complete assist the patient with completing personal hygiene as necessary.	☐	☐	_____	_____
13. Return the patient to the bedside and assist as necessary with positioning the patient back into bed.	☐	☐	_____	_____

Postprocedure

14. Assure that all needs are met and that the patient is comfortable prior to leaving the area.	☐	☐	_____	_____
15. Document in the medical record the patient's level of activity, any problems with independent function, and the level of assistance required.	☐	☐	_____	_____

Check-off Sheet:
18-24 Assist to Dangle, Stand, and Walk

Name _____ **Date** _____

Directions: Practice this procedure, following each step. When you are ready to have your performance evaluated, give this sheet to your instructor. Review the detailed procedure in your textbook.

Procedure	Pass	Redo	Date Competency Met	Instructor Initials
Student must use Standard Precautions.	☐	☐	_____	_____

Preprocedure

Procedure	Pass	Redo	Date Competency Met	Instructor Initials
1. Assess the functional level of the patient. Include the patient when determining the plan of care and goals.	☐	☐	_____	_____
2. Explain the procedure to the patient.	☐	☐	_____	_____
3. Provide privacy for the patient.	☐	☐	_____	_____
4. Ensure a clear path for ambulation.	☐	☐	_____	_____
5. Place a chair midway of the distance to be traveled to facilitate a rest spot if necessary.	☐	☐	_____	_____

Procedure

Procedure	Pass	Redo	Date Competency Met	Instructor Initials
6. Assist the patient to an erect position on the side of the bed. Pause to determine the patient's tolerance of the activity.	☐	☐	_____	_____
7. Place a gait belt around the patient's waist to ensure safety for the patient and the nurse.	☐	☐	_____	_____
8. Stand the patient at the bedside. Pause to determine the patient's tolerance of the activity.	☐	☐	_____	_____
9. With the nurse's nearest hand placed under the gait belt at the patient's back and the other hand grasping the patient's nearest elbow, guide the patient forward. Assess the patient's gait and tolerance of activity as the patient progresses forward.	☐	☐	_____	_____
10. If the patient should faint to begin to fall the nurse can use the gait belt to pull the patient towards the nurse and ease the patient to the ground.	☐	☐	_____	_____
11. Return the patient to the bedside and assist the patient into a chair or back into the bed. Assure that the patient is comfortable and has no further needs.	☐	☐	_____	_____
12. Reassure and encourage the patient to continue the mobility program for increasing functional status.	☐	☐	_____	_____

Postprocedure

Procedure	Pass	Redo	Date Competency Met	Instructor Initials
13. Wash hands.	☐	☐	_____	_____
14. Document in observation note the patient's gait, feet walked and tolerance of activity.	☐	☐	_____	_____

Check-off Sheet:

18-25 Transferring—Pivot Transfer from Bed to Wheelchair

Name _____ Date _____

Directions: Practice this procedure, following each step. When you are ready to have your performance evaluated, give this sheet to your instructor. Review the detailed procedure in your textbook.

Procedure	Pass	Redo	Date Competency Met	Instructor Initials
Student must use Standard Precautions.	☐	☐	_____	_____
Preprocedure				
1. Wash hands.	☐	☐	_____	_____
2. Explain procedure to patient, speaking clearly, slowly and directly, maintaining face-to-face contact whenever possible.	☐	☐	_____	_____
3. Provide for patient's privacy during the procedure, using a curtain screen or door.	☐	☐	_____	_____
4. Make sure that wheels on bed are locked.	☐	☐	_____	_____
5. Lift foot rests or swing leg supports out of way.	☐	☐	_____	_____
6. Position wheelchair alongside bed. (See teacher for directions in working with stroke patients.) Lock wheels.	☐	☐	_____	_____
Procedure				
7. Place bed at safe and appropriate level for the patient. Support patient's back and hips and assist patient to sitting position with feet flat on the floor.	☐	☐	_____	_____
8. Move patient to edge of bed, with legs over side.	☐	☐	_____	_____
9. Before transferring patient, put non-skid footwear on patient and securely fasten.	☐	☐	_____	_____
10. Have patient dangle legs for a few minutes and take slow, deep breaths. Observe for dizziness.	☐	☐	_____	_____
11. Remember to use a gait belt. Stand in front of patient, positioning yourself to ensure your safety and that of your patient during transfer (e.g., knees bent, feet apart, back straight), place belt around patient's waist, and grasp belt.	☐	☐	_____	_____
12. Brace patient's lower extremities to prevent slipping.	☐	☐	_____	_____
13. Count to three (or say other prearranged signal) to alert patient to begin transfer.	☐	☐	_____	_____
14. Support him or her at midriff and ask patient to stand, if patient is not dizzy.	☐	☐	_____	_____

Procedure	Pass	Redo	Date Competency Met	Instructor Initials
15. Once standing, have patient pivot (turn) and hold onto armrest of wheelchair with both arms or one strong arm.	☐	☐	_____	_____
16. Gently ease patient into a sitting position.	☐	☐	_____	_____
17. Position yourself at back of wheelchair. Ask patient to push on the floor with feet as you lift gently under each arm to ease patient into a comfortable position against backrest. Make sure patient's hips are touching the back of the wheelchair and then remove the transfer belt, if used.	☐	☐	_____	_____
18. Return foot rests to normal position and place feet and legs in a comfortable position on rests. Make sure the signaling device is within the patient's reach.	☐	☐	_____	_____
19. Do not leave a patient who requires a postural support until it is in place.	☐	☐	_____	_____
20. Reverse above procedure to return patient to bed.	☐	☐	_____	_____

Postprocedure

21. Wash hands.	☐	☐	_____	_____

Check-off Sheet:

18-26 Transferring—Sliding from Bed to Wheelchair and Back

Name _____ Date _____

Directions: Practice this procedure, following each step. When you are ready to have your performance evaluated, give this sheet to your instructor. Review the detailed procedure in your textbook.

Procedure	Pass	Redo	Date Competency Met	Instructor Initials
Student must use Standard Precautions.	☐	☐	_____	_____
Preprocedure				
1. Wash hands.	☐	☐	_____	_____
2. Assemble equipment: wheelchair with removable arms.	☐	☐	_____	_____
3. Explain the procedure to the patient.	☐	☐	_____	_____
4. Provide privacy for the patient.	☐	☐	_____	_____
Procedure				
5. Position wheelchair at bedside with back parallel to head of bed. Lock wheels. Move foot rests out of the way.	☐	☐	_____	_____
6. Remove wheelchair arm nearest to bedside.	☐	☐	_____	_____
7. Place bed level to chair seat height if possible. Lock bed wheels.	☐	☐	_____	_____
8. Raise head of bed so that patient is in sitting position.	☐	☐	_____	_____
9. Position yourself beside wheelchair and carefully assist patient to slide from bed to wheelchair.	☐	☐	_____	_____
10. Replace wheelchair arm and return foot rests to their normal position.	☐	☐	_____	_____
11. Position patient for comfort and apply postural supports.	☐	☐	_____	_____
Postprocedure				
12. Make sure call bell is within reach.	☐	☐	_____	_____
13. Wash hands.	☐	☐	_____	_____

Check-off Sheet:

18-27 Transferring—Two-Person Lift from Bed to Chair and Back

Name _____ Date _____

Directions: Practice this procedure, following each step. When you are ready to have your performance evaluated, give this sheet to your instructor. Review the detailed procedure in your textbook.

Procedure	Pass	Redo	Date Competency Met	Instructor Initials
Student must use Standard Precautions.	☐	☐	_____	_____
Preprocedure				
1. Wash hands.	☐	☐	_____	_____
2. Assemble equipment: chair.	☐	☐	_____	_____
3. Ask one other person to help.	☐	☐	_____	_____
4. Tell patient what you are going to do.	☐	☐	_____	_____
5. Provide privacy for the patient.	☐	☐	_____	_____
Procedure				
6. Position chair next to bed with back of chair parallel with head of bed. Lock wheels.	☐	☐	_____	_____
7. Position patient near edge of bed. Lock wheels of bed.	☐	☐	_____	_____
8. Position co-worker on side of bed near feet.	☐	☐	_____	_____
9. Position yourself behind chair at head of bed.	☐	☐	_____	_____
10. Place your arms under patient's axillae and clasp your hands together at patient's midchest.	☐	☐	_____	_____
11. Co-worker places hands under patient's upper legs.	☐	☐	_____	_____
12. Count to three. On the count of three, lift patient into chair.	☐	☐	_____	_____
13. Position for comfort and secure postural supports PRN.	☐	☐	_____	_____
Postprocedure				
14. Put call bell within reach of patient.	☐	☐	_____	_____
15. Wash hands.	☐	☐	_____	_____

Check-off Sheet:
18-28 Transferring—Sliding from Bed to Gurney and Back

Name _____ **Date** _____

Directions: Practice this procedure, following each step. When you are ready to have your performance evaluated, give this sheet to your instructor. Review the detailed procedure in your textbook.

Procedure	Pass	Redo	Date Competency Met	Instructor Initials
Student must use Standard Precautions.	☐	☐	_____	_____
Preprocedure				
1. Wash hands.	☐	☐	_____	_____
2. Assemble equipment:	☐	☐	_____	_____
a. Gurney	☐	☐	_____	_____
b. Cover Sheet	☐	☐	_____	_____
3. Ask a co-worker to help.	☐	☐	_____	_____
4. Explain what you are going to do and lock wheels on bed.	☐	☐	_____	_____
5. Provide privacy for the patient.	☐	☐	_____	_____
Procedure				
6. Cover patient with sheet and remove bed covers.	☐	☐	_____	_____
7. Raise bed to gurney height; lower side rail and move patient to side of bed.	☐	☐	_____	_____
8. Loosen draw sheet on both sides so it can be used as a pull sheet.	☐	☐	_____	_____
9. Position gurney next to bed and lock wheels on gurney.	☐	☐	_____	_____
10. Position yourself on outside of gurney—one arm at the head, the other at the hips. Co-worker is on other side of bed.	☐	☐	_____	_____
11. Reach across gurney and securely hold edge of draw sheet. Pull patient onto gurney and cover. (If patient is large, a third person on the opposite side of bed may be necessary.)	☐	☐	_____	_____
12. Position patient for comfort.	☐	☐	_____	_____
13. Secure with safety straps or raise side rails.	☐	☐	_____	_____
Postprocedure				
14. Wash hands.	☐	☐	_____	_____

Check-off Sheet:
18-29 Transferring—Lifting with a Mechanical Lift

Name _____ **Date** _____

Directions: Practice this procedure, following each step. When you are ready to have your performance evaluated, give this sheet to your instructor. Review the detailed procedure in your textbook.

Procedure	Pass	Redo	Date Competency Met	Instructor Initials
Student must use Standard Precautions.	☐	☐	_____	_____
Preprocedure				
1. Wash hands.	☐	☐	_____	_____
2. Gather equipment:	☐	☐	_____	_____
a. Mechanical lift	☐	☐	_____	_____
b. Sheet or blanket for patient comfort.	☐	☐	_____	_____
c. Sling	☐	☐	_____	_____
3. Check all equipment to be sure it is in good working order and that the sling is not damaged or torn.	☐	☐	_____	_____
4. Ask one other person to help.	☐	☐	_____	_____
5. Prepare patient's destination:	☐	☐	_____	_____
a. Chair	☐	☐	_____	_____
b. Gurney	☐	☐	_____	_____
c. Bathtub	☐	☐	_____	_____
d. Shower	☐	☐	_____	_____
6. Lock wheels on bed and explain what you are going to do.	☐	☐	_____	_____
7. Provide privacy for the patient.	☐	☐	_____	_____
Procedure				
8. Roll patient toward you.	☐	☐	_____	_____
9. Place sling on bed behind patient.				
a Position top of sling at shoulders.	☐	☐	_____	_____
b Position bottom of sling under buttocks.	☐	☐	_____	_____
c. Leave enough of sling to support body when the body is rolled back. Fan-fold remaining sling next to body. It will be pulled through when patient is rolled back.	☐	☐	_____	_____
10. Roll patient to other side of bed and pull fan-folded portion of sling flat. Remove all wrinkles and allow patient to lie flat on back.	☐	☐	_____	_____

Procedure	Pass	Redo	Date Competency Met	Instructor Initials
11. Position lift over patient, being sure to broaden base of lift. This stabilizes the lift while raising patient.	☐	☐	_____	_____
12. Raise had of bed to a semi-Flower's position.	☐	☐	_____	_____
13. Attach straps on lift to sling loops. Shorter straps must be attached to shoulder loops. Longer straps are attached to loops at hips. (Important: If you reverse the strap attachment, the patient's head will be lower than his or her hips.)	☐	☐	_____	_____
14. Reassure patient. Let patient know you will keep him or her from falling. Gently raise patient from bed with hand crank or pump handle.	☐	☐	_____	_____
15. Keep patient centered over base of lift as you move lift and patient to his or her destination. (It is helpful to have a helper stand by and steady patient while moving so that patient doesn't swing.)	☐	☐	_____	_____
16. Position patient over chair, commode, bathtub, shower chair, etc. Ask a co-worker to steady chair.	☐	☐	_____	_____
17. Slowly lower patient into chair using foot-pedal positioning.	☐	☐	_____	_____
18. Unhook sling from lift straps and carefully move lift away from patient.	☐	☐	_____	_____
19. Provide all comfort measures for patient.	☐	☐	_____	_____
20. Secure postural supports if necessary.	☐	☐	_____	_____
21. Return lift to storage area.	☐	☐	_____	_____
Postprocedure				
22. Wash hands.	☐	☐	_____	_____
23. Reverse procedure when returning item to bed.	☐	☐	_____	_____

Check-off Sheet:
18-30 Transferring—Moving a Patient on a Gurney or Stretcher
Name _____ Date _____

Directions: Practice this procedure, following each step. When you are ready to have your performance evaluated, give this sheet to your instructor. Review the detailed procedure in your textbook.

Procedure	Pass	Redo	Date Competency Met	Instructor Initials
Student must use Standard Precautions.	☐	☐	_____	_____
Preprocedure				
1. Wash hands.	☐	☐	_____	_____
2. Position bed to gurney height.	☐	☐	_____	_____
3. Lock all the brakes on gurney an bed.	☐	☐	_____	_____
4. Follow the procedure for transferring to and from a gurney.	☐	☐	_____	_____
Procedure				
5. Stand at the patient's head and push the gurney with patient's feet moving first down the hallway.	☐	☐	_____	_____
6. Slow down when turning a corner. Always check the intersection mirrors for traffic.	☐	☐	_____	_____
7. Enter an elevator by standing at patient's head and pulling gurney into elevator. The feet will be the last to enter elevator.	☐	☐	_____	_____
8. Leave elevator by carefully pushing the gurney out of elevator into corridor.	☐	☐	_____	_____
9. Position yourself at patient's feet, and back a patient on a gurney down a hill.	☐	☐	_____	_____
10. Never leave a patient unattended on a gurney.	☐	☐	_____	_____
11. Raise side rails and secure a safety strap.	☐	☐	_____	_____
Postprocedure				
12. Wash hands.	☐	☐	_____	_____

Check-off Sheet:

18-31 Transferring—Moving a Patient in a Wheelchair

Name _____ Date _____

Directions: Practice this procedure, following each step. When you are ready to have your performance evaluated, give this sheet to your instructor. Review the detailed procedure in your textbook.

Procedure	Pass	Redo	Date Competency Met	Instructor Initials
Student must use Standard Precautions.	☐	☐	_____	_____
Preprocedure				
1. Wash hands.	☐	☐	_____	_____
2. Position wheelchair.	☐	☐	_____	_____
3. Lock all brakes on wheelchair and bed.	☐	☐	_____	_____
Procedure				
4. Follow procedure for transferring patient to and from a wheelchair.	☐	☐	_____	_____
5. Push wheelchair carefully into hallway, watching for others who may be near doorway.	☐	☐	_____	_____
6. Move cautiously down hallway, being especially careful at intersections.	☐	☐	_____	_____
7. Always back a patient in a wheelchair over bumps, doorways, and into or out of elevators.	☐	☐	_____	_____
8. Always back a patient in a wheelchair down a hill.	☐	☐	_____	_____
9. Check patient for comfort measure before leaving.	☐	☐	_____	_____
10. Always notify appropriate person that patient has arrived.	☐	☐	_____	_____
Postprocedure				
11. Wash hands.	☐	☐	_____	_____

Check-off Sheet:
18-32 Moving—Helping the Helpless Patient to Move Up in Bed
Name _____ **Date** _____

Directions: Practice this procedure, following each step. When you are ready to have your performance evaluated, give this sheet to your instructor. Review the detailed procedure in your textbook.

Procedure	Pass	Redo	Date Competency Met	Instructor Initials
Student must use Standard Precautions.	☐	☐	_____	_____
Preprocedure				
1. Wash hands.	☐	☐	_____	_____
2. Ask a co-worker to help move patient. (Co-worker will work on opposite side of bed.)	☐	☐	_____	_____
3. Identify patient and explain what you are going to do. (Even if the patient seems unresponsive, he or she may be able to hear.) Provide privacy for the patient.	☐	☐	_____	_____
Procedure				
4. Lock wheels of bed. Raise bed to comfortable working position, and lower side rails.	☐	☐	_____	_____
5. Remove pillow and place it at head of bed or on a chair.	☐	☐	_____	_____
6. Loosen both sides of draw sheet.	☐	☐	_____	_____
7. Roll edges toward side of patient's body.	☐	☐	_____	_____
8. Face head of bed and grasp rolled sheet edge with hand closest to patient.	☐	☐	_____	_____
9. Place your feet 12 inches apart with foot farthest from the edge of bed in a forward position.	☐	☐	_____	_____
10. Place your free hand and arm under patient's neck and shoulders, supporting head.	☐	☐	_____	_____
11. Bend your hips slightly.	☐	☐	_____	_____
12. On the count of three, you and your co-worker will raise patient's hips and back with draw sheet, supporting head and shoulders, and move patient smoothly to head of bed.	☐	☐	_____	_____
13. Replace pillow under patient's head and check for good body alignment.	☐	☐	_____	_____
14. Tighten and tuck in draw sheet and smooth bedding.	☐	☐	_____	_____
15. Raise side rails and lower bed.	☐	☐	_____	_____
Postprocedure				
16. Wash hands.	☐	☐	_____	_____

Check-off Sheet:
18-33 Moving—Assisting Patient to Sit Up in Bed

Name _____ Date _____

Directions: Practice this procedure, following each step. When you are ready to have your performance evaluated, give this sheet to your instructor. Review the detailed procedure in your textbook.

Procedure	Pass	Redo	Date Competency Met	Instructor Initials
Student must use Standard Precautions.	☐	☐	_____	_____
Preprocedure				
1. Wash hands.	☐	☐	_____	_____
2. Identify patient and explain what you are going to do. Provide privacy for patient.	☐	☐	_____	_____
Procedure				
3. Lock bed and lower all the way down.	☐	☐	_____	_____
4. Face head of bed, keeping your outer leg forward.	☐	☐	_____	_____
5. Turn your head away from patient's face.	☐	☐	_____	_____
6. Lock your arm nearest patient with patient's arm. To lock arms, place your arm between patient's arm and body, and hold upper arm near shoulder. Have patient hold back of your upper arm.	☐	☐	_____	_____
7. Support patient's head and shoulder with your other arm.	☐	☐	_____	_____
8. Raise patient to sitting position. Adjust had of bed and pillows.	☐	☐	_____	_____
Postprocedure				
9. Wash hands.	☐	☐	_____	_____

Check-off Sheet:
18-34 Moving—Logrolling
Name _____ **Date** _____

Directions: Practice this procedure, following each step. When you are ready to have your performance evaluated, give this sheet to your instructor. Review the detailed procedure in your textbook.

Procedure	Pass	Redo	Date Competency Met	Instructor Initials
Student must use Standard Precautions.	☐	☐	_____	_____
Preprocedure				
1. Wash hands.	☐	☐	_____	_____
2. Identify patient and explain what you are going to do.	☐	☐	_____	_____
3. Provide privacy by pulling privacy curtain.	☐	☐	_____	_____
Procedure				
4. Lock wheels of bed. Raise bed to a comfortable working position.	☐	☐	_____	_____
5. Lower side rail on side you are working on.	☐	☐	_____	_____
6. Be certain that side rail on opposite side of bed is in up position.	☐	☐	_____	_____
7. Leave pillow under head.	☐	☐	_____	_____
8. Place a pillow lengthwise between patient's legs.	☐	☐	_____	_____
9. Fold patient's arms across chest.	☐	☐	_____	_____
10. Roll patient onto his or her side like a log, turning body as a whole unit, without bending joints.	☐	☐	_____	_____
11. Check for good body alignment.	☐	☐	_____	_____
12. Tighten and tuck in draw sheet and smooth bedding.	☐	☐	_____	_____
13. Tuck pillow behind back for support.	☐	☐	_____	_____
14. Raise side rails and lower bed.	☐	☐	_____	_____
15. Secure call light in patient's reach.	☐	☐	_____	_____
Postprocedure				
16. Wash hands.	☐	☐	_____	_____
17. Chart position of patient and how procedure was tolerated.	☐	☐	_____	_____

Check-off Sheet:

18-35 Moving—Turning Patient Away from You

Name _____ Date _____

Directions: Practice this procedure, following each step. When you are ready to have your performance evaluated, give this sheet to your instructor. Review the detailed procedure in your textbook.

Procedure	Pass	Redo	Date Competency Met	Instructor Initials
Student must use Standard Precautions.	☐	☐	_____	_____
Preprocedure				
1. Wash hands.	☐	☐	_____	_____
2. Identify patient and explain what you are going to do. Provide privacy for the patient.	☐	☐	_____	_____
Procedure				
3. Lock bed and elevate to a comfortable working position.	☐	☐	_____	_____
4. Lower side rail on side you are working from.	☐	☐	_____	_____
5. Have patient bend knees. Cross arms on chest.	☐	☐	_____	_____
6. Place arm nearest head of bed under patient's shoulders and head. Place other hand and forearm under small of the patient's back. Bend your body at hips and knees, keeping your back straight. Pull patient toward you.	☐	☐	_____	_____
7. Place forearms under patient's hips and pull patient toward you.	☐	☐	_____	_____
8. Place one hand under ankles and one hand under knees and move ankles toward you.	☐	☐	_____	_____
9. Cross patient's leg closest to you over other leg at ankles.	☐	☐	_____	_____
a. Bend the patient's farthest arm to his or her head and place the other arm across chest. Cross near leg over the other leg.	☐	☐	_____	_____
b. Place one hand on the patient's shoulder and the other on hip. Turn patient away from you onto her side.	☐	☐	_____	_____
c. Place pillows under her upper arm and leg for support.				
10. Roll patient away from you by placing one hand under hips and one hand under shoulders.	☐	☐	_____	_____
11. Place one hand under patient's shoulders and one hand under patient's head. Draw patient back toward center of bed.	☐	☐	_____	_____

Procedure	Pass	Redo	Date Competency Met	Instructor Initials
12. Place both hands under patient's hips and move hips toward center of bed.	☐	☐	_____	_____
13. Put a pillow behind patient's back to give support and keep patient from falling onto his or her back.	☐	☐	_____	_____
14. Be certain patient is in good alignment.	☐	☐	_____	_____
15. Place upper leg on a pillow for support.	☐	☐	_____	_____
16. Replace side rail on near side of bed and return bed to lowest height.	☐	☐	_____	_____
17. You may place a turning sheet under a helpless or heavy patient to help with turning. Use a folded large sheet or half sheet and place it so that it extends just above shoulders and below hips.	☐	☐	_____	_____

Postprocedure

18. Wash hands.	☐	☐	_____	_____

Check-off Sheet:
18-36 Turning Patient on Side

Name _____ Date _____

Directions: Practice this procedure, following each step. When you are ready to have your performance evaluated, give this sheet to your instructor. Review the detailed procedure in your textbook.

Procedure	Pass	Redo	Date Competency Met	Instructor Initials
Student must use Standard Precautions.	☐	☐	_____	_____
Preprocedure				
1. Wash hands.	☐	☐	_____	_____
2. Explain procedure to patient.	☐	☐	_____	_____
3. Provide privacy for the patient with curtain, screen, or door.	☐	☐	_____	_____
Procedure				
4. Raise the bed to a height that allows the nurse to remain in erect posture while moving patient. Adjust the bed to a flat position or as low as the patient can tolerate. Make sure side rails on side to which patient's body will be turned are raised. Lower the side rail nearest to nurse.	☐	☐	_____	_____
5. Use a pull sheet or pad for moving the patient in order to avoid the effects of friction on the patient's skin integrity.	☐	☐	_____	_____
6. Place the patient's arms across the chest and cross the patient's far leg over the near one. Grasping the pull sheet on the far side of the patient, pull the patient towards the nurse.	☐	☐	_____	_____
7. Slowly roll patient onto side toward raised side rail while supporting patient's body.	☐	☐	_____	_____
8. Place a pillow under the head and the neck to prevent lateral flexion of the neck.	☐	☐	_____	_____
9. Place a pillow behind the patient's back to promote the side lying position. Ensure that the shoulders are aligned with the hips.	☐	☐	_____	_____
10. Place a pillow under the upper arm. The lower arm should be flexed and positioned comfortably. Make sure patient is not lying on their arm.	☐	☐	_____	_____
11. Use one or two pillows as needed to support the leg from the groin to the foot. Avoid having bony prominences resting against hard surfaces.	☐	☐	_____	_____
12. Assure that the two shoulders are aligned with the two hips.	☐	☐	_____	_____

Procedure	Pass	Redo	Date Competency Met	Instructor Initials
13. For the completely immobile patient it is important that passive range of motion exercises be provided during the time used to reposition the patient.	☐	☐	_____	_____
14. Readjust the bed height and position and raise the side rail if appropriate. Put the bed in the lowest position.	☐	☐	_____	_____
15. Assure that the patient is comfortable and has no further needs before leaving the bedside.	☐	☐	_____	_____
16. Put the call signal within the patient's reach.	☐	☐	_____	_____
Postprocedure	☐	☐	_____	_____
17. Wash your hands.	☐	☐	_____	_____

Check-off Sheet:
18-37 Moving—Turning the Patient Toward You

Name _____ **Date** _____

Directions: Practice this procedure, following each step. When you are ready to have your performance evaluated, give this sheet to your instructor. Review the detailed procedure in your textbook.

Procedure	Pass	Redo	Date Competency Met	Instructor Initials
Student must use Standard Precautions.	☐	☐	_____	_____
Preprocedure				
1. Wash hands.	☐	☐	_____	_____
2. Identify patient and explain what you are going to do. Provide privacy for the patient.	☐	☐	_____	_____
Procedure	☐	☐	_____	_____
3. Lock bed and elevate to a comfortable working height.	☐	☐	_____	_____
4. Lower side rail on side you are working from.	☐	☐	_____	_____
5. Cross patient's far leg over leg that is closest to you.	☐	☐	_____	_____
6. Place one hand on patient's far shoulder. Place your other hand on the hip.	☐	☐	_____	_____
7. Brace yourself against side of bed. Roll patient toward you in a slow, gentle, smooth movement.	☐	☐	_____	_____
8. Help patient bring upper leg toward you and bend comfortably (Sims position).	☐	☐	_____	_____
9. Put up side rail. Be certain it is secure.	☐	☐	_____	_____
10. Go to other side of bed and lower side rail.	☐	☐	_____	_____
11. Place hands under patient's shoulders and hips. Pull toward center of bed. This helps maintain side-lying position.	☐	☐	_____	_____
12. Be certain to align patient's body properly.	☐	☐	_____	_____
13. Use pillows to position and support legs if patient is unable to move self.	☐	☐	_____	_____
14. *Check tubing to make certain that it is not caught between legs or pulling in any way if patient has an indwelling catheter.*	☐	☐	_____	_____
15. Tuck a pillow behind patient's back. This forms a roll and prevents patient from rolling backward onto back.	☐	☐	_____	_____
16. Return bed to low position.				
17. Secure call light in patient's reach.	☐	☐	_____	_____
Postprocedure				
18. Wash hands.	☐	☐	_____	_____

Check-off Sheet:
18-38 Applying Restraints
Name _____ **Date** _____

Directions: Practice this procedure, following each step. When you are ready to have your performance evaluated, give this sheet to your instructor. Review the detailed procedure in your textbook.

Procedure	Pass	Redo	Date Competency Met	Instructor Initials
Student must use Standard Precautions.	☐	☐	_____	_____
Preprocedure				
1. Determine the need for restraints and that alternative measures have been attempted.	☐	☐	_____	_____
2. Assess patient's physical condition, behavior and mental status.	☐	☐	_____	_____
Procedure				
3. Determine the agency's policy for application of restraints. Secure a physician's order.	☐	☐	_____	_____
4. Explain the reason for use to patient and family. Clarify how the patient's needs will be met and that the use of restraints is only a temporary measure.	☐	☐	_____	_____
5. Wash your hands.	☐	☐	_____	_____
6. Apply restraints according to manufacturer's directions (each type of restraint may require a different type of application).	☐	☐	_____	_____
a. Choose the least restrictive type of device that allows the greatest degree of mobility.	☐	☐	_____	_____
b. Pad bony prominences. Ensure that two fingers can be inserted between the restraint and the patient's wrist or ankle.	☐	☐	_____	_____
c. Maintain restrained extremity in normal anatomical position.	☐	☐	_____	_____
d. Use a quick release for all restraints.	☐	☐	_____	_____
e. Fasten restraint to bed not side rail.	☐	☐	_____	_____
f. Remove restraint every two hours or according to agency policy and patient need.	☐	☐	_____	_____
g. While removed check for signs of decreased circulation, impaired function of limb, or impaired skin integrity.	☐	☐	_____	_____
h. Perform range-of-motion exercises before reapplying.	☐	☐	_____	_____

Procedure	Pass	Redo	Date Competency Met	Instructor Initials
i. Reevaluate the need for use of physical restraints, alternative measures attempted before reapplying.	☐	☐	_____	_____
j. Document procedure and rationale.	☐	☐	_____	_____
k. Obtain a new physician's order for restraint every 24 hours if continued need.	☐	☐	_____	_____
Postprocedure	☐	☐	_____	_____
7. Assure that patient safely and comfort has been maintained throughout the period that restraints are in place.	☐	☐	_____	_____

Check-off Sheet:
18-39 How to Tie Postural Supports

Name _____ Date _____

Directions: Practice this procedure, following each step. When you are ready to have your performance evaluated, give this sheet to your instructor. Review the detailed procedure in your textbook.

Procedure	Pass	Redo	Date Competency Met	Instructor Initials
Student must use Standard Precautions.	☐	☐	_____	_____
Preprocedure				
1. Wash hands.	☐	☐	_____	_____
Procedure				
2. Assemble equipment: a postural support that has been ordered.	☐	☐	_____	_____
3. Tie a half-bow knot or quick release knot. Tie the same way you tie a bow on a shoe. Once bow is in place, grasp one loop and pull end of tie through knot.	☐	☐	_____	_____
4. Knot can be easily released pulling end of loop.	☐	☐	_____	_____
Postprocedure				
5. Wash hands.	☐	☐	_____	_____

Check-off Sheet:
18-40 Postural Supports: Limb

Name _____ **Date** _____

Directions: Practice this procedure, following each step. When you are ready to have your performance evaluated, give this sheet to your instructor. Review the detailed procedure in your textbook.

Procedure	Pass	Redo	Date Competency Met	Instructor Initials
Student must use Standard Precautions.	☐	☐	_____	_____
Preprocedure				
1. Check for physician's order.	☐	☐	_____	_____
2. Wash hands.	☐	☐	_____	_____
3. Assemble equipment: a limb support.	☐	☐	_____	_____
4. Identify patient. Provide privacy for the patient by curtain, screen, or door.	☐	☐	_____	_____
Procedure				
5. Explain what you are doing to do, even if the patient is confused.	☐	☐	_____	_____
6. Place soft side of limb support against skin. Check to make sure the wrinkles are out.	☐	☐	_____	_____
7. Wrap around limb and put one tie through opening on other end of support (see Figure 18.16a).	☐	☐	_____	_____
8. Gently pull until it fits snugly around limb.	☐	☐	_____	_____
9. Buckle or tie in place so that support stays on limb.	☐	☐	_____	_____
10. Tie out of patient's reach. (See the procedure "How to Tie Postural Supports.")	☐	☐	_____	_____
a. Tie to bed frame (*not side rails*).	☐	☐	_____	_____
b. Tie to wheelchair (*not to stationary chair*).	☐	☐	_____	_____
11. Check for proper alignment and comfort of patient.	☐	☐	_____	_____
12. Check for proper alignment and comfort of patient.	☐	☐	_____	_____
13. Check to be certain that support is snug but does not bind. (*You should be able to put two fingers under edges.*)	☐	☐	_____	_____
14. Place call light where it can be easily reached.	☐	☐	_____	_____
Postprocedure				
15. Wash hands.	☐	☐	_____	_____
16. Circulation under restraint should be checked every 15-30 minutes and documented.	☐	☐	_____	_____

Procedure	Pass	Redo	Date Competency Met	Instructor Initials
17. Check patient frequently and move at least every 2 hours. Restraints should be removed every 2 hours for at least 5-10 minutes.	☐	☐	_____	_____
18. Chart the following:	☐	☐	_____	_____
a. Reason for use of support	☐	☐	_____	_____
b. Type of support used	☐	☐	_____	_____
c. When it was applied	☐	☐	_____	_____
d. When it was released	☐	☐	_____	_____
e. Times of repositioning	☐	☐	_____	_____
f. How patient tolerated it	☐	☐	_____	_____
g. Condition of skin	☐	☐	_____	_____

Check-off Sheet:
18-41 Postural Supports: Mitten

Name _____ Date _____

Directions: Practice this procedure, following each step. When you are ready to have your performance evaluated, give this sheet to your instructor. Review the detailed procedure in your textbook.

Procedure	Pass	Redo	Date Competency Met	Instructor Initials
Student must use Standard Precautions.	☐	☐	_____	_____
Preprocedure				
1. Check for physician's order.	☐	☐	_____	_____
2. Wash hands.	☐	☐	_____	_____
3. Assemble equipment: a soft cloth mitten.	☐	☐	_____	_____
4. Identify patient	☐	☐	_____	_____
5. Explain what you are going to do.	☐	☐	_____	_____
Procedure				
6. Slip mitten on hand with padded side against palm and net on top of hand.	☐	☐	_____	_____
7. Lace mitten.	☐	☐	_____	_____
8. Gently pull until it fits snugly around wrist.	☐	☐	_____	_____
9. Tie with a double knot so that support stays on hand.	☐	☐	_____	_____
10. Check for proper alignment and comfort of patient.	☐	☐	_____	_____
11. Check to be certain knots or wrinkles are not causing pressure.	☐	☐	_____	_____
12. Check to be certain support is snug but does not bind. (*You should be able to put two fingers under edges.*)	☐	☐	_____	_____
13. Place call light where it can be easily reached.	☐	☐	_____	_____
Postprocedure				
14. Wash hands.	☐	☐	_____	_____
15. Check circulation and document every 15-30 minutes.	☐	☐	_____	_____
16. Remove mitten restraint every 2 hours for at least 5-10 minutes.	☐	☐	_____	_____
17. Check patient frequently and move at least every 2 hours.	☐	☐	_____	_____

Procedure	Pass	Redo	Date Competency Met	Instructor Initials
18. Chart the following:	☐	☐	_____	_____
a. Reason for use of support	☐	☐	_____	_____
b. Type of support used	☐	☐	_____	_____
c. When it was applied	☐	☐	_____	_____
d. When it was released	☐	☐	_____	_____
e. Times of repositioning	☐	☐	_____	_____
f. How patient tolerated it	☐	☐	_____	_____
g. Condition of skin	☐	☐	_____	_____

Check-off Sheet:
18-42 Postural Supports: Vest

Name _____ **Date** _____

Directions: Practice this procedure, following each step. When you are ready to have your performance evaluated, give this sheet to your instructor. Review the detailed procedure in your textbook.

Procedure	Pass	Redo	Date Competency Met	Instructor Initials
Student must use Standard Precautions.	☐	☐	_____	_____
Preprocedure				
1. Check for physician's order.	☐	☐	_____	_____
2. Wash hands.	☐	☐	_____	_____
3. Assemble equipment: a vest support.	☐	☐	_____	_____
4. Identify patient	☐	☐	_____	_____
5. Explain what you are going to do.	☐	☐	_____	_____
Procedure				
6. Put arms through armholes of vest with opening to back (see Figure 18.16b)	☐	☐	_____	_____
7. Cross back panels by bringing tie on left side over to right and right tie to left.	☐	☐	_____	_____
8. Carefully smooth material so that there are no wrinkles.	☐	☐	_____	_____
9. Tie where patient cannot reach. (See the procedure "How to Tie Postural Supports.")	☐	☐	_____	_____
a. Tie to bed frame (*not side rails*).	☐	☐	_____	_____
b. Tie to wheelchair (*not stationary chair.*)	☐	☐	_____	_____
10. Check for proper alignment and comfort of patient.	☐	☐	_____	_____
11. Check to be certain that knots or wrinkles are not causing pressure.	☐	☐	_____	_____
12. Check to be certain that support is snug but does not bind. (*You should be able to put two fingers under edges*.)	☐	☐	_____	_____
13. Place call light where it can be easily reached.	☐	☐	_____	_____
Postprocedure				
14. Wash hands.	☐	☐	_____	_____
15. Check skin condition and circulation every 15-30 minutes.	☐	☐	_____	_____

Procedure	Pass	Redo	Date Competency Met	Instructor Initials
16. Remove restraint every 2 hours for at least 5-10 minutes.	☐	☐	_____	_____
17. Check patient frequently and move at least every 2 hours.	☐	☐	_____	_____
18. Chart the following:	☐	☐	_____	_____
a. Reason for use of support	☐	☐	_____	_____
b. Type of support used	☐	☐	_____	_____
c. When it was applied	☐	☐	_____	_____
d. When it was released	☐	☐	_____	_____
e. Times of repositioning	☐	☐	_____	_____
f. How patient tolerated it	☐	☐	_____	_____
g. Condition of skin	☐	☐	_____	_____

Check-off Sheet:
18-43 Giving a Bed Bath
Name _____ **Date** _____

Directions: Practice this procedure, following each step. When you are ready to have your performance evaluated, give this sheet to your instructor. Review the detailed procedure in your textbook.

Procedure	Pass	Redo	Date Competency Met	Instructor Initials
Student must use Standard Precautions.	☐	☐	_____	_____
Preprocedure				
1. Wash hands	☐	☐	_____	_____
2. Assemble equipment				
a. Soap and soap dish	☐	☐	_____	_____
b. Face towel	☐	☐	_____	_____
c. Bath towel. You need at least 2.	☐	☐	_____	_____
d. Washcloth. Will need at least 2.	☐	☐	_____	_____
e. Hospital gown or patient's sleepwear	☐	☐	_____	_____
f. Lotion or powder	☐	☐	_____	_____
g. Nailbrush and emery board	☐	☐	_____	_____
h. Comb and brush	☐	☐	_____	_____
i. Bedpan or urinal and cover	☐	☐	_____	_____
j. Bed linen	☐	☐	_____	_____
k. Bath blanket	☐	☐	_____	_____
l. Bath basin, water at 105° F	☐	☐	_____	_____
m. Disposable nonsterile gloves	☐	☐	_____	_____
3. Place linens on chair in order of use and place towels on overbed table.	☐	☐	_____	_____
4. Identify patient.	☐	☐	_____	_____
5. Explain what you are going to do.	☐	☐	_____	_____
6. Provide for privacy by pulling the privacy screen curtain, or door.	☐	☐	_____	_____
Procedure				
7. Raise bed to a comfortable working height.	☐	☐	_____	_____
8. Offer bedpan or urinal. Empty and rinse before starting bath. Wash your hands. (Remember to wear gloves when handling urine.)	☐	☐	_____	_____
9. Lower headrest and knee gatch (raised knee area/bed) so that bed is flat.	☐	☐	_____	_____

Procedure	Pass	Redo	Date Competency Met	Instructor Initials
10. Lower the side rail only on side where you are working.	☐	☐	_____	_____
11. Put on gloves.	☐	☐	_____	_____
12. Loosen top sheet, blanket, and bedspread. Remove and fold blanket and bedspread, and place over back of chair.	☐	☐	_____	_____
13. Cover patient with a bath blanket.	☐	☐	_____	_____
14. Ask patient to hold bath blanket in place. Remove top sheet by sliding it to foot of bed. *Do not expose patient.* (Place soiled linen in laundry container.)	☐	☐	_____	_____
15. Leave a pillow under patient's head for comfort.	☐	☐	_____	_____
16. Remove patient's gown and place in laundry container. If nightwear belongs to patient, follow hospital policy (i.e., send home with family or to hospital laundry.)	☐	☐	_____	_____
17. To remove gown when the patient has an IV:				
a. Loosen gown from neck.	☐	☐	_____	_____
b. Slip gown from free arm.	☐	☐	_____	_____
c. Be certain that patient is covered with a bath blanket.	☐	☐	_____	_____
d. Slip gown away from body toward arm with IV.	☐	☐	_____	_____
e. Gather gown at arm and slip downward over arm and tubing. *Be careful not to pull on tubing.*	☐	☐	_____	_____
f. Gather material of gown in one hand and slowly draw gown over tip of fingers.	☐	☐	_____	_____
g. Lift IV free of stand with free hand and slip gown over bottle.	☐	☐	_____	_____
h. *Do not lower bottle! Raise gown.*	☐	☐	_____	_____
18. Fill bath basin two-thirds full with warm water. Test water temperature and ensure it is safe and comfortable before bathing patients and adjust if necessary.	☐	☐	_____	_____
19. Help patient move to side of bed nearest you.	☐	☐	_____	_____
20. Fold face towel over upper edge of bath blanket. This will keep it dry.	☐	☐	_____	_____
21. Form a mitten by folding washcloth around your hand.	☐	☐	_____	_____
22. Wash patient's eyes from nose to outside of face. Use different corners of washcloth.	☐	☐	_____	_____

Procedure	Pass	Redo	Date Competency Met	Instructor Initials
23. As patient if he or she wants soap used on the face. Gently wash and rinse face, ears, and neck. Be careful not to get soap in eyes. Dry face with towel, using a blotting motion.	☐	☐	_____	_____
24. To wash patient's arms, shoulders, axilla:				
a. Uncover patient's far arm (one farthest away from you.)	☐	☐	_____	_____
b. Protect bed from becoming wet with a bath towel placed under arm. Wash with long, firm, circular strokes, rinse and dry.	☐	☐	_____	_____
c. Wash and dry armpits (axillae). Apply deodorant and powder.	☐	☐	_____	_____
25. To wash hand:				
a. Place basin of water on towel.	☐	☐	_____	_____
b. Put patient's hand into basin.	☐	☐	_____	_____
c. Wash, rinse, and dry and push back cuticle gently.	☐	☐	_____	_____
26. Repeat on other arm.	☐	☐	_____	_____
27. To wash chest:	☐	☐	_____	_____
a. Place towel lengthwise across patient's chest.	☐	☐	_____	_____
b. Fold bath blanket down to patient's abdomen.	☐	☐	_____	_____
c. Wash chest. Be especially careful to dry skin under female breasts to prevent irritation. Dry area thoroughly.	☐	☐	_____	_____
28. To wash abdomen:				
a. Fold down bath blanket to pubic area.	☐	☐	_____	_____
b. Wash, rinse, and dry abdomen.	☐	☐	_____	_____
c. Pull up bath blanket to keep patient warm.	☐	☐	_____	_____
d. Slide towel out from under bath blanket.	☐	☐	_____	_____
29. To wash thigh, leg, and foot:				
a. Ask patient to flex knee if possible.	☐	☐	_____	_____
b. Fold bath blanket to uncover thigh, leg, and foot of leg farthest from you.	☐	☐	_____	_____
c. Place bath towel under leg to keep bed from getting wet.	☐	☐	_____	_____
d. Place basin on towel and put foot into basin.	☐	☐	_____	_____
e. Wash and rinse thigh, leg, and foot.	☐	☐	_____	_____
f. Dry well between toes. Be careful to support the leg when lifting it.	☐	☐	_____	_____

Procedure	Pass	Redo	Date Competency Met	Instructor Initials
30. Follow same procedure for leg nearest you.	☐	☐	_____	_____
31. Change water. You may need to change water before this time if it is dirty or cold.	☐	☐	_____	_____
32. Raise side rail on opposite side if it is down.	☐	☐	_____	_____
33. To wash back and buttocks:				
a. Help patient turn on side away from you.	☐	☐	_____	_____
b. Have patient move toward center of bed.	☐	☐	_____	_____
c. Place a bath towel lengthwise on bed, under patient's back.	☐	☐	_____	_____
d. Wash, rinse, and dry neck, back, and buttocks.	☐	☐	_____	_____
e. Give patient a back rub. Help patient turn back on their back and make sure they are still covered with a bath blanket. Massage back for at least a minute and a half, giving special attention to shoulder blades, hop bones, and spine. *Observe for reddened areas*. (See the procedure "Skin Care – Giving a Back Rub.")	☐	☐	_____	_____
34. To wash genital area:				
a. Offer patient a clean, soapy washcloth to wash genital area.	☐	☐	_____	_____
b. Give the person a clean, wet washcloth to rinse with and a dry towel to dry with.	☐	☐	_____	_____
35. Clean the genital area thoroughly if patient is unable to help. To clean the genital area:	☐	☐	_____	_____
a. Put a towel or disposable pad under the patient's buttock.	☐	☐	_____	_____
b. When washing a female patient always wipe from front to back.	☐	☐	_____	_____
c. Separate the labia and use a clean area of the wash cloth for each side of the perineal area.	☐	☐	_____	_____
d. When washing a male patient, be sure to wash and dry penis, scrotum, and groin area carefully. Clean the tip of the penis using a circular motion and clean the shaft of the penis from top to bottom. Remember to pull back the foreskin if the patient is not circumcised.	☐	☐	_____	_____
e. Remove towel or disposable pad and discard appropriately.	☐	☐	_____	_____
f. Remove gloves and put in hazardous waste.	☐	☐	_____	_____

Procedure	Pass	Redo	Date Competency Met	Instructor Initials
36. If range of motion is ordered, complete at this time. (See the procedure "Range of Motion.")	☐	☐	_____	_____
37. Put a clean gown on patient.	☐	☐	_____	_____
38. If patient has an IV:				
a. Gather the sleeve on IV side in one hand.	☐	☐	_____	_____
b. Lift bottle free of stand. Do not lower bottle.	☐	☐	_____	_____
c. Slip bottle through sleeve from inside and rehang.	☐	☐	_____	_____
d. Guide gown along the IV tubing to bed.	☐	☐	_____	_____
e. Slip gown over the patient's hand. Be careful not to pull or crimp tubing.	☐	☐	_____	_____
f. Put gown on arm with IV, then on opposite arm.	☐	☐	_____	_____
39. Comb or brush hair.	☐	☐	_____	_____
40. Follow hospital policy for towels and washcloths. Some have you hang them for later use; others have you place them in the laundry containers immediately.	☐	☐	_____	_____
41. Leave patient in a comfortable position and in good body alignment.	☐	☐	_____	_____
42. Place call bell within reach. Replace furniture and tidy unit.	☐	☐	_____	_____
Postprocedure				
43. Wash hands.	☐	☐	_____	_____
44. Chart procedure and how patient tolerated it. Note any unusual skin changes or patient complaints.	☐	☐	_____	_____

Check-off Sheet:
18-44 Giving a Partial Bath (Face, Hands, Axillae, Buttocks, and Genitals)
Name _____ **Date** _____

Directions: Practice this procedure, following each step. When you are ready to have your performance evaluated, give this sheet to your instructor. Review the detailed procedure in your textbook.

Procedure	Pass	Redo	Date Competency Met	Instructor Initials
Student must use Standard Precautions.	☐	☐	_____	_____
Preprocedure				
1. Wash hands	☐	☐	_____	_____
2. Assemble equipment				
a. Soap and soap dish	☐	☐	_____	_____
b. Face towel	☐	☐	_____	_____
c. Bath towel	☐	☐	_____	_____
d. Washcloth	☐	☐	_____	_____
e. Hospital gown or patient's sleepwear	☐	☐	_____	_____
f. Lotion or powder	☐	☐	_____	_____
g. Nailbrush and emery board	☐	☐	_____	_____
h. Comb and brush	☐	☐	_____	_____
i. Bedpan or urinal and cover	☐	☐	_____	_____
j. Bath blanket	☐	☐	_____	_____
k. Bath basin, water at 105° F	☐	☐	_____	_____
l. Clean linen as needed	☐	☐	_____	_____
m. Disposable gloves	☐	☐	_____	_____
3. Identify patient.	☐	☐	_____	_____
4. Explain what you are going to do.	☐	☐	_____	_____
5. Provide for privacy by pulling the privacy screen curtain, or door.	☐	☐	_____	_____
6. Offer bedpan or urinal. Empty and rinse before starting bath. (Wear gloves if handling body fluid.)	☐	☐	_____	_____
7. Raise headrest to a comfortable position, if permitted.	☐	☐	_____	_____
8. Lower side rails if permitted. If they are to remain up, lower only side rail on side where you are working.	☐	☐	_____	_____

Procedure	Pass	Redo	Date Competency Met	Instructor Initials
Procedure				
9. Loosen top sheet, blanket, and bedspread. Remove and fold blanket and bedspread and place over back of chair.	☐	☐	_____	_____
10. Cover patient with a bath blanket	☐	☐	_____	_____
11. Ask patient to hold bath blanket in place. Remove top sheet by sliding it to the foot of bed. *Do not expose patient.* (Place soiled linen in laundry container.)	☐	☐	_____	_____
12. Leave a pillow under the patient's head for comfort.	☐	☐	_____	_____
13. Remove patient's gown and place in laundry container. If nightwear belongs to patient, follow hospital policy (i.e., send home with family or to hospital.)	☐	☐	_____	_____
14. To remove gown when patient has an IV, see the procedure "Giving a Bed Bath."	☐	☐	_____	_____
15. Fill bath basin two-thirds full with warm water and place on overbed table. Test water temperature and ensure it is safe and comfortable before bathing patients; adjust if necessary.	☐	☐	_____	_____
16. Put overbed table where patient can reach it comfortably.	☐	☐	_____	_____
17. Place towel, washcloth, and soap on overbed table.	☐	☐	_____	_____
18. Ask patient to wash as much as he or she is able to and tell the person that you will return to complete bath.	☐	☐	_____	_____
19. Place call bell where patient can reach it easily. Ask patient to signal when ready.	☐	☐	_____	_____
20. Remove glove, wash your hands, and leave unit.	☐	☐	_____	_____
21. When patient signals, return to unit, wash your hands, and put on gloves.	☐	☐	_____	_____
22. Change water. Test water temperature and ensure it is safe and comfortable before bathing patients and adjust if necessary.	☐	☐	_____	_____
23. Complete bathing areas the patient was unable to reach. Make sure that face, hands, axillae, genitals, and buttocks are dry. To wash the genital area:	☐	☐	_____	_____
a. Offer the patient a clean, soapy washcloth to wash genital area. Provide a clean, wet washcloth to rinse with and a dry towel to dry with. If patient is unable to help, you will need to clean the genital area thoroughly.	☐	☐	_____	_____

Procedure	Pass	Redo	Date Competency Met	Instructor Initials
b. When washing a female patient, always wipe from front to back.	☐	☐	_____	_____
c. Separate the labia and use a clean area of the wash cloth for each side of the perineal area..	☐	☐	_____	_____
d. When washing a male patient, be sure to wash and dry penis, scrotum, and groin area carefully. Clean the tip of the penis using a circular motion and clean the shaft of the penis from top to bottom. Remember to pull back the foreskin if the patient is not circumcised.	☐	☐	_____	_____
e. Remove gloves and put in hazardous waste. If range of motion is ordered, complete it at this time. (See the procedure "Range of Motion.".	☐	☐	_____	_____
24. Give a back rub. (See the procedure "Skin Care—Giving a Back Rub.")	☐	☐	_____	_____
25. Put a clean gown on patient.	☐	☐	_____	_____
26. If patient has an IV, see the procedure "Giving a Bed Bath.".	☐	☐	_____	_____
27. Assist patient in applying deodorant and putting on a clean gown.	☐	☐	_____	_____
28. Change bed according to hospital policy. Not all facilities change linen every day.	☐	☐	_____	_____
29. Put up side rails if required.	☐	☐	_____	_____
30. Leave patient in a comfortable position and in good body alignment.	☐	☐	_____	_____

Postprocedure

Procedure	Pass	Redo	Date Competency Met	Instructor Initials
31. Remove and discard gloves.	☐	☐	_____	_____
32. Wash hands.	☐	☐	_____	_____
33. Place call bell within reach. Replace furniture and tidy unit.	☐	☐	_____	_____
34. Chart procedure and how it was tolerated.	☐	☐	_____	_____

Check-off Sheet:
18-45 Tub/Shower Bath

Name _____ **Date** _____

Directions: Practice this procedure, following each step. When you are ready to have your performance evaluated, give this sheet to your instructor. Review the detailed procedure in your textbook.

Procedure	Pass	Redo	Date Competency Met	Instructor Initials
Student must use Standard Precautions.	☐	☐	_____	_____
Preprocedure				
1. Wash hands	☐	☐	_____	_____
2. Assemble equipment on a chair near the tub. Be certain the tub is clean.	☐	☐	_____	_____
a. Bath towels	☐	☐	_____	_____
b. Washcloths	☐	☐	_____	_____
c. Soap	☐	☐	_____	_____
d. Bath thermometer	☐	☐	_____	_____
e. Wash basin	☐	☐	_____	_____
f. Clean gown	☐	☐	_____	_____
g. Bathmat	☐	☐	_____	_____
h. Disinfectant solution	☐	☐	_____	_____
i. Shower chair if necessary	☐	☐	_____	_____
3. Identify patient and explain what you are going to do.	☐	☐	_____	_____
4. Provide privacy by pulling private curtain, screen, or door.	☐	☐	_____	_____
Procedure				
5. Help patient out of bed.	☐	☐	_____	_____
6. Help with robe and slippers.	☐	☐	_____	_____
7. Check with head nurse to see if the patient can ambulate or if a wheelchair or shower chair is needed. If a shower chair is used, always do the following:	☐	☐	_____	_____
a. Cover patient with a bath blanket or sheet so that patient is not exposed in any way.	☐	☐	_____	_____
b. Provide adequate clothing for patient, such as a robe or extra cover.	☐	☐	_____	_____
8. Take patient to shower or tub room.	☐	☐	_____	_____
9. For tub bath, place a towel in bottom of tub to help prevent falling.	☐	☐	_____	_____

Procedure	Pass	Redo	Date Competency Met	Instructor Initials
10. Fill tub with water or adjust shower flow (95-105°F).	☐	☐	_____	_____
11. Help patient undress. Give a male patient a towel to wrap around his midriff.	☐	☐	_____	_____
12. Assist patient into tub or shower. If shower, leave weak patient in shower chair.				
13. Wash patient's back. Observe carefully for reddened areas or breaks in skin.	☐	☐	_____	_____
14. Patient may be left alone to complete genitalia area if feeling strong.	☐	☐	_____	_____
15. Assist patient from tub or shower.	☐	☐	_____	_____
16. Wrap bath towel around patient to prevent chilling.	☐	☐	_____	_____
17. Remove gloves and put in biohazardous container.	☐	☐	_____	_____
18. Assist in drying and dressing.	☐	☐	_____	_____
19. Return to unit and make comfortable. Make sure call button is within patient's reach.	☐	☐	_____	_____
20. Put away equipment.	☐	☐	_____	_____
21. Clean bathtub with disinfectant solution.	☐	☐	_____	_____

Postprocedure

Procedure	Pass	Redo	Date Competency Met	Instructor Initials
22. Wash hands.	☐	☐	_____	_____
23. Chart procedure and how patient tolerated it.	☐	☐	_____	_____

Check-off Sheet:
18-46 Patient Gown Change

Name _____ Date _____

Directions: Practice this procedure, following each step. When you are ready to have your performance evaluated, give this sheet to your instructor. Review the detailed procedure in your textbook.

Procedure	Pass	Redo	Date Competency Met	Instructor Initials
Student must use Standard Precautions.	☐	☐	_____	_____
Preprocedure				
1. Wash hands	☐	☐	_____	_____
2. Assemble equipment: clean patient gown.	☐	☐	_____	_____
3. Tell patient what you are going to do.	☐	☐	_____	_____
4. Provide privacy by pulling private curtain.	☐	☐	_____	_____
5. Put on gloves in case you come in contact with bodily fluids.	☐	☐	_____	_____
Procedure				
6. Untie strings of gown at neck and midback. (It may be necessary to assist patient onto side.)	☐	☐	_____	_____
7. Pull soiled gown out from sides of patient.	☐	☐	_____	_____
8. Unfold clean gown and position over patient.	☐	☐	_____	_____
9. Remove soiled gown one sleeve at a time.	☐	☐	_____	_____
10. Leave soiled gown laying over patient's chest; insert one arm into sleeve of clean gown.	☐	☐	_____	_____
11. Fold soiled gown to one side as clean gown is placed over patient's chest.	☐	☐	_____	_____
12. Insert other arm in empty sleeve of gown.	☐	☐	_____	_____
13. Tie neck string on side of neck.	☐	☐	_____	_____
14. Tie midback tie if patient desires.	☐	☐	_____	_____
15. Remove soiled gown to linen hamper.	☐	☐	_____	_____
16. Slip gown under covers, being careful not to expose patient.	☐	☐	_____	_____
17. Position patient for comfort.	☐	☐	_____	_____
18. Raise side rails when necessary.	☐	☐	_____	_____
19. Place bedside stand and call light in patient's reach.	☐	☐	_____	_____
Postprocedure	☐	☐	_____	_____
20. Remove gloves and put in biohazardous container.	☐	☐	_____	_____
21. Wash hands.	☐	☐	_____	_____

Check-off Sheet:
18-47 Perineal Care

Name _____ Date _____

Directions: Practice this procedure, following each step. When you are ready to have your performance evaluated, give this sheet to your instructor. Review the detailed procedure in your textbook.

Procedure	Pass	Redo	Date Competency Met	Instructor Initials
Student must use Standard Precautions.	☐	☐	_____	_____
Preprocedure				
1. Wash hands	☐	☐	_____	_____
2. Assemble equipment.				
a. Bath blanket	☐	☐	_____	_____
b. Bedpan and cover	☐	☐	_____	_____
c. Basin	☐	☐	_____	_____
d. Solution, water or other if ordered	☐	☐	_____	_____
e. Cotton balls	☐	☐	_____	_____
f. Waterproof protector for bed	☐	☐	_____	_____
g. Disposable gloves	☐	☐	_____	_____
h. Perineal pad and belt if needed	☐	☐	_____	_____
3. Identify patient.	☐	☐	_____	_____
4. Explain what you are going to do.	☐	☐	_____	_____
5. Provide privacy by pulling private curtain.	☐	☐	_____	_____
Procedure				
6. Put warm water in basin.	☐	☐	_____	_____
7. Raise bed to a comfortable working height.	☐	☐	_____	_____
8. Lower side rail.	☐	☐	_____	_____
9. Put on disposable gloves.	☐	☐	_____	_____
10. Remove spread and blanket.	☐	☐	_____	_____
11. Cover patient with bath blanket.	☐	☐	_____	_____
12. Have patient hold top of bath blanket, and fold top sheet to bottom of bed.	☐	☐	_____	_____
13. Place waterproof protector under patient's buttocks.	☐	☐	_____	_____
14. Pull up bath blanket to expose perineal area.	☐	☐	_____	_____

Procedure	Pass	Redo	Date Competency Met	Instructor Initials
15. Provide male and female pericare.	☐	☐	_____	_____
a. Circumcised male: Wipe away from urinary meatus as you wash with soap and water, rinse, and dry in a circular motion. Clean the shaft of the penis from top to bottom.	☐	☐	_____	_____
b. Uncircumcised male: Gently move foreskin back away from tip of penis. Wash as directed in step a. After drying, gently move foreskin back over tip of penis.	☐	☐	_____	_____
c. Female:				
(1) Instruct patient to bend knees with feet flat on bed.	☐	☐	_____	_____
(2) Separate patient's knees.	☐	☐	_____	_____
(3) Separate the labia and wipe from front to back away from the urethra as you wash with soap and water, rinse, and dry. Use a clear part of the washcloth for each stroke.	☐	☐	_____	_____
16. Remove waterproof protector from bed and dispose of gloves.	☐	☐	_____	_____
17. Cover patient with sheet and remove bath blanket.	☐	☐	_____	_____
18. Return top covers.	☐	☐	_____	_____
19. Return bed to lowest position and put up side rails if required.	☐	☐	_____	_____
20. Secure call bell within patient's reach.	☐	☐	_____	_____

Postprocedure

Procedure	Pass	Redo	Date Competency Met	Instructor Initials
21. Clean equipment; dispose of disposable material according to hospital policy.	☐	☐	_____	_____
22. Discard gloves and put in biohazardous container.	☐	☐	_____	_____
23. Wash hands.	☐	☐	_____	_____

Check-off Sheet:

18-48 Shampooing the Hair in Bed

Name _____ **Date** _____

Directions: Practice this procedure, following each step. When you are ready to have your performance evaluated, give this sheet to your instructor. Review the detailed procedure in your textbook.

Procedure	Pass	Redo	Date Competency Met	Instructor Initials
Student must use Standard Precautions.	☐	☐	_____	_____
Preprocedure				
1. Wash hands	☐	☐	_____	_____
2. Assemble equipment.				
a. Chair	☐	☐	_____	_____
b. Basin of water (105°F)	☐	☐	_____	_____
c. Pitcher of water (115°F)	☐	☐	_____	_____
d. Paper or styrofoam cup	☐	☐	_____	_____
e. Large basin	☐	☐	_____	_____
f. Shampoo tray or plastic sheet	☐	☐	_____	_____
g. Waterproof bed protector	☐	☐	_____	_____
h. Pillow with waterproof cover	☐	☐	_____	_____
i. Bath towels	☐	☐	_____	_____
j. Small towel	☐	☐	_____	_____
k. Cotton balls	☐	☐	_____	_____
3. Identify patient.	☐	☐	_____	_____
4. Explain what you are going to do.	☐	☐	_____	_____
5. Provide privacy by pulling private curtain.	☐	☐	_____	_____
Procedure				
6. Raise bed to a comfortable working position.	☐	☐	_____	_____
7. Place a chair at side of bed near patient's head.	☐	☐	_____	_____
8. Place small towel on chair.	☐	☐	_____	_____
9. Place large basin on chair to catch water.	☐	☐	_____	_____
10. Put cotton in patient's ears to keep water out of ears.	☐	☐	_____	_____
11. Have patient move to side of bed with head close to where you are standing.	☐	☐	_____	_____

Procedure	Pass	Redo	Date Competency Met	Instructor Initials
12. Remove pillow from under head. Lower head of bed and remove pillows. Cover pillow with water proof case.	☐	☐	_____	_____
13. Place pillow under patient's back so that when he or she lies down the head will be tilted back.	☐	☐	_____	_____
14. Place bath blanket on bed.	☐	☐	_____	_____
15. Have patient hold top of bath blanket, and pull top covers to foot.	☐	☐	_____	_____
16. Place waterproof protector under head.	☐	☐	_____	_____
17. Put shampoo tray under patient's head (i.e., plastic bag with both ends open).	☐	☐	_____	_____
18. Place end of plastic in large basin.	☐	☐	_____	_____
19. Have patient hold washcloth over eyes.	☐	☐	_____	_____
20. Put basin of water on bedside table with paper cup. Have pitcher of water for extra water. Test water temperature to ensure it is safe and comfortable before wetting patient's hair. Adjust if needed.	☐	☐	_____	_____
21. Brush patient's hair thoroughly.	☐	☐	_____	_____
22. Fill cup with water from basin.	☐	☐	_____	_____
23. Pour water over hair; repeat until completely wet.	☐	☐	_____	_____
24. Apply small amount of shampoo; use both hands to massage the patient's scalp with your fingertips. Be careful not to scratch the scalp with your fingernails.	☐	☐	_____	_____
25. Rinse soap off hair by pouring water from cup over hair. Have patient turn head from side to side. Repeat until completely rinsed.	☐	☐	_____	_____
26. Dry patient's forehead and ears.	☐	☐	_____	_____
27. Remove cotton from ears.	☐	☐	_____	_____
28. Lift patient's head gently and wrap with bath towel.	☐	☐	_____	_____
29. Remove equipment from bed.	☐	☐	_____	_____
30. Change patient's gown and be certain patient is dry.	☐	☐	_____	_____
31. Gently dry patient's hair with towel. (Use a hair dryer if allowed by your facility.)	☐	☐	_____	_____
32. Comb or brush hair and arrange neatly.	☐	☐	_____	_____
33. Remove bath blanket and cover patient with top covers.	☐	☐	_____	_____

Procedure	Pass	Redo	Date Competency Met	Instructor Initials
34. Make patient comfortable.	☐	☐	_____	_____
35. Lower bed to its lowest position.	☐	☐	_____	_____
36. Put up side rail if required.	☐	☐	_____	_____
Postprocedure				
37. Return equipment.	☐	☐	_____	_____
38. Tidy unit.	☐	☐	_____	_____
39. Wash hands.	☐	☐	_____	_____
40. Record procedure.	☐	☐	_____	_____

Check-off Sheet:
18-49 Shampooing in Shower or Tub

Name _____ **Date** _____

Directions: Practice this procedure, following each step. When you are ready to have your performance evaluated, give this sheet to your instructor. Review the detailed procedure in your textbook.

Procedure	Pass	Redo	Date Competency Met	Instructor Initials
Student must use Standard Precautions.	☐	☐	_____	_____
Preprocedure				
1. Wash hands	☐	☐	_____	_____
2. Assemble equipment.				
a. Shampoo	☐	☐	_____	_____
b. Washcloth	☐	☐	_____	_____
c. Towel	☐	☐	_____	_____
d. Cream rinse, if desired	☐	☐	_____	_____
3. Provide privacy by pulling curtain or door.	☐	☐	_____	_____
4. Explain what you are going to do.	☐	☐	_____	_____
Procedure				
5. Instruct patient to tip head back.	☐	☐	_____	_____
6. Wet hair with water, being careful not to get eyes wet.	☐	☐	_____	_____
7. Give patient a washcloth to wipe his or her face as needed.	☐	☐	_____	_____
8. Apply a moderate amount of shampoo to hair.	☐	☐	_____	_____
9. Rinse hair with clean, clear water until shampoo has disappeared.	☐	☐	_____	_____
10. Repeat shampooing procedure a second time. When rinsing, be sure to remove all shampoo.	☐	☐	_____	_____
11. If a cream rinse is used, apply a small amount to hair, paying special attention to ends of hair.	☐	☐	_____	_____
12. Allow rinse to remain on hair for a few seconds before rinsing.	☐	☐	_____	_____
13. Rinse thoroughly with clean, clear water.	☐	☐	_____	_____
14. Towel dry.	☐	☐	_____	_____
15. Gently comb or brush hair to remove tangles.	☐	☐	_____	_____

Procedure	Pass	Redo	Date Competency Met	Instructor Initials
16. Use a hair drying to dry hair.	☐	☐	_____	_____
17. Arrange in an appropriate hairstyle for the patient's age and manner. (Remember that ponytails, pigtails, etc. are not appropriate for a 70-year-old patient.)	☐	☐	_____	_____

Postprocedure

18. Return equipment.	☐	☐	_____	_____
19. Wash hands.	☐	☐	_____	_____
20. Record procedure.	☐	☐	_____	_____

Check-off Sheet:
18-50 Arranging the Hair

Name _____ **Date** _____

Directions: Practice this procedure, following each step. When you are ready to have your performance evaluated, give this sheet to your instructor. Review the detailed procedure in your textbook.

Procedure	Pass	Redo	Date Competency Met	Instructor Initials
Student must use Standard Precautions.	☐	☐	_____	_____
Preprocedure				
1. Wash hands	☐	☐	_____	_____
2. Assemble equipment.				
a. Comb and/or brush	☐	☐	_____	_____
b. Towel	☐	☐	_____	_____
3. Identify patient.	☐	☐	_____	_____
4. Explain what you are going to do.	☐	☐	_____	_____
5. Provide privacy by pulling privacy curtain.	☐	☐	_____	_____
6. Raise bed to a comfortable working height.	☐	☐	_____	_____
Procedure				
7. Assist as needed.	☐	☐	_____	_____
8. If total assistance is needed:				
a. Section the hair, starting at one side, working around to other side.	☐	☐	_____	_____
b. Comb or brush hair thoroughly, being careful not to pull it.	☐	☐	_____	_____
c. Arrange hair neatly.	☐	☐	_____	_____
9. Lower bed to lowest position.	☐	☐	_____	_____
10. Put up side rail if required.	☐	☐	_____	_____
11. Secure call light in patient's reach.	☐	☐	_____	_____
Postprocedure				
12. Clean and replace all equipment.	☐	☐	_____	_____
13. Wash hands.	☐	☐	_____	_____
14. Record procedure and observations (e.g., dry scalp, reddened areas).	☐	☐	_____	_____

Check-off Sheet:

18-51 Nail Care

Name _____ Date _____

Directions: Practice this procedure, following each step. When you are ready to have your performance evaluated, give this sheet to your instructor. Review the detailed procedure in your textbook.

Procedure	Pass	Redo	Date Competency Met	Instructor Initials
Student must use Standard Precautions.	☐	☐	_____	_____
Preprocedure				
1. Wash hands	☐	☐	_____	_____
2. Assemble equipment.				
a. Warm water	☐	☐	_____	_____
b. Orange sticks	☐	☐	_____	_____
c. Emery board	☐	☐	_____	_____
d. Nail clippers				
3. Identify patient and explain the procedure.	☐	☐	_____	_____
4. Provide privacy for the patient by pulling a curtain or closing the door.	☐	☐	_____	_____
5. Test water temperature and ensure it is save and comfortable before immersing patient's fingers in water; adjust if needed.	☐	☐	_____	_____
6. Place basin of water at a comfortable level for patients.	☐	☐	_____	_____
7. Put on gloves.	☐	☐	_____	_____
Procedure				
8. Use slanted edge of orange stick to clean dirt out from under nails. Wipe orangewood stick on towel after each nail and dry patient's hand/fingers, including between fingers.	☐	☐	_____	_____
9. File nails with emery board to shorten. (Clip if permitted by your facility.)	☐	☐	_____	_____
10. Use smooth edge of emery board to smooth.	☐	☐	_____	_____
11. Apply lotion to help condition cuticle.	☐	☐	_____	_____
12. Massage hands and feet with lotion.	☐	☐	_____	_____
13. Make patient comfortable.	☐	☐	_____	_____
14. Raise side rail if required. Make sure call bell is within reach.	☐	☐	_____	_____

Procedure	Pass	Redo	Date Competency Met	Instructor Initials
Postprocedure				
15. Empty, rinse and wipe basin.	☐	☐	_____	_____
16. Return equipment.	☐	☐	_____	_____
17. Remove and dispose of gloves in biohazardous container.	☐	☐	_____	_____
18. Wash hands.	☐	☐	_____	_____
19. Record procedure and any unusual conditions (e.g., hangnails, broken nails).	☐	☐	_____	_____

Check-off Sheet:
18-52 Foot Care

Name _____ **Date** _____

Directions: Practice this procedure, following each step. When you are ready to have your performance evaluated, give this sheet to your instructor. Review the detailed procedure in your textbook.

Procedure	Pass	Redo	Date Competency Met	Instructor Initials
Student must use Standard Precautions.	☐	☐	_____	_____

Preprocedure

Procedure	Pass	Redo	Date Competency Met	Instructor Initials
1. Wash hands	☐	☐	_____	_____
2. Put on disposable gloves.	☐	☐	_____	_____
3. Explain procedure to patient and provide for patient privacy with curtain, screen or door.	☐	☐	_____	_____

Procedure

Procedure	Pass	Redo	Date Competency Met	Instructor Initials
4. Inspect the feet for any problems/change in skin integrity. Check for the presence of pulses and not their strengths. Assess for any patient complaints.	☐	☐	_____	_____
5. Test water temperature and ensure it is safe and comfortable before placing patient's foot in water and adjust if needed.	☐	☐	_____	_____
6. Place basin at a comfortable position on protective barrier.	☐	☐	_____	_____
7. Completely submerge and soak foot in water.	☐	☐	_____	_____
8. Bathe the feet thoroughly in tepid water with a mild soap. Be sure to clean the interdigital areas.	☐	☐	_____	_____
9. Dry the feet thoroughly, paying particular attention to the interdigital areas. Apply lotion to feet but avoid leaving lotion in the interdigital areas as it could provide a moist environment for bacteria and fungal growth. Support foot and ankle throughout the procedure.	☐	☐	_____	_____
10. If nails are overgrown use a file instead of scissors or clippers. If the patient is a diabetic and a file is not sufficient refer the patient to a Podiatrist for further nail care.	☐	☐	_____	_____
11. Empty, rinse and wipe basin and return to proper storage.	☐	☐	_____	_____
12. Dispose of soiled linens in proper container. Remove glove and place in biohazardous container.	☐	☐	_____	_____
13. Make sure the patient is comfortable and the call bell is within reach.	☐	☐	_____	_____

Procedure	Pass	Redo	Date Competency Met	Instructor Initials
14. Discourage the patient from going barefoot. Decreased sensation may allow an injury to occur with the patient noting it.	☐	☐	_____	_____
15. Encourage the patient to use appropriate footwear. Ill fitting shoes may contribute to skin breakdown. All new footwear should be broken in gradually over time. All shoes that are rough or worn or do not provide adequate foot support should be discarded.	☐	☐	_____	_____
16. Clean, dry socks that provide warmth, absorb perspiration and protect the feet should be worn.	☐	☐	_____	_____
Postprocedure	☐	☐	_____	_____
17. Return equipment.	☐	☐	_____	_____
18. Remove and dispose of gloves in biohazardous container.	☐	☐	_____	_____
18. Wash hands.	☐	☐	_____	_____
19. Report any signs of foot problems to the physician. Early interventions will diminish the magnitude of any problems noted.	☐	☐	_____	_____

Check-off Sheet:
18-53 Shaving the Patient

Name _____ Date _____

Directions: Practice this procedure, following each step. When you are ready to have your performance evaluated, give this sheet to your instructor. Review the detailed procedure in your textbook.

Procedure	Pass	Redo	Date Competency Met	Instructor Initials
Student must use Standard Precautions.	☐	☐	_____	_____
Preprocedure				
1. Wash hands	☐	☐	_____	_____
2. Assemble equipment:				
a. Electric shaver or safety razor	☐	☐	_____	_____
b. Shaving lather or an electric preshave lotion	☐	☐	_____	_____
c. Basin of warm water	☐	☐	_____	_____
d. Face towel	☐	☐	_____	_____
e. Mirror	☐	☐	_____	_____
f. Aftershave	☐	☐	_____	_____
g. Disposable gloves	☐	☐	_____	_____
3. Identify patient and explain what you are going to do.	☐	☐	_____	_____
4. Provide privacy by pulling curtains.	☐	☐	_____	_____
Procedure				
5. Raise head of bed if permitted.	☐	☐	_____	_____
6. Place equipment on overbed table.	☐	☐	_____	_____
7. Place a towel over patient's chest.	☐	☐	_____	_____
8. Adjust light so that it shines on patient's face.	☐	☐	_____	_____
9. Shave patient.	☐	☐	_____	_____
a. If you are using a safety razor:				
(1) Put on gloves.	☐	☐	_____	_____
(2) Moisten face and apply lather.	☐	☐	_____	_____
(3) Start in front of ear; hold skin taut and bring razor down over cheek toward chin. Use short firm strokes. Repeat until lather on cheek is removed and skin is smooth.	☐	☐	_____	_____
(4) Repeat on other cheek.	☐	☐	_____	_____
(5) Wash face and neck. Dry thoroughly.	☐	☐	_____	_____
(6) Apply aftershave lotion or powder if desired.	☐	☐	_____	_____
(7) Discard gloves according to facility policy.	☐	☐	_____	_____

Procedure	Pass	Redo	Date Competency Met	Instructor Initials
b. If you are using an electric shaver:				
(1) Put on gloves.	☐	☐	_____	_____
(2) Apply preshave lotion.	☐	☐	_____	_____
(3) Gently shave until beard is removed.	☐	☐	_____	_____
(4) Wash face and neck. Dry thoroughly.	☐	☐	_____	_____
(5) Apply aftershave lotion or powder if desired.	☐	☐	_____	_____
(6) Remove gloves	☐	☐	_____	_____
10. Lower bed if you raised it and make sure side rails are up.	☐	☐	_____	_____
11. Make sure patient is comfortable and call bell is within reach.	☐	☐	_____	_____
Postprocedure	☐	☐	_____	_____
12. Wash hands.	☐	☐	_____	_____
13. Chart procedure and how procedure was tolerated.	☐	☐	_____	_____

Check-off Sheet:
18-54 Postmortem Care

Name _____ Date _____

Directions: Practice this procedure, following each step. When you are ready to have your performance evaluated, give this sheet to your instructor. Review the detailed procedure in your textbook.

Procedure	Pass	Redo	Date Competency Met	Instructor Initials
Student must use Standard Precautions.	☐	☐	_____	_____
Preprocedure				
1. Wash hands	☐	☐	_____	_____
2. Assemble equipment:				
a. Wash basin with warm water	☐	☐	_____	_____
b. Washcloth and towel	☐	☐	_____	_____
c. Shroud/postmortem set:	☐	☐	_____	_____
(1) Sheet or plastic container	☐	☐	_____	_____
(2) Identification tag	☐	☐	_____	_____
(3) Large container for personal belongings	☐	☐	_____	_____
(4) Plastic bag	☐	☐	_____	_____
d. Gurney or morgue cart	☐	☐	_____	_____
e. Nonsterile disposable gloves	☐	☐	_____	_____
3. Close privacy curtains.	☐	☐	_____	_____
4. Put on gloves.	☐	☐	_____	_____
Procedure				
5. Position body in good alignment in supine position.	☐	☐	_____	_____
6. Keep one pillow under head.	☐	☐	_____	_____
7. Straighten arms and legs.	☐	☐	_____	_____
8. Gently close each eye. Do not apply pressure to eyelids.	☐	☐	_____	_____
9. Put dentures in mouth or in a denture cup, put cup inside shroud so that mortician can find.	☐	☐	_____	_____
10. Remove all soiled dressings or clothing.	☐	☐	_____	_____
11. Bathe body thoroughly.	☐	☐	_____	_____
12. Apply clean dressings where needed.	☐	☐	_____	_____

Procedure	Pass	Redo	Date Competency Met	Instructor Initials
13. Attach identification tags to wrists and ankles. Tag is usually placed on the right great toe and also on the outside of shroud. Fill in tags with:	☐	☐	_____	_____
a. Name	☐	☐	_____	_____
b. Sex	☐	☐	_____	_____
c. Hospital ID number	☐	☐	_____	_____
d. Age	☐	☐	_____	_____
14. Place body in a shroud, sheet, or other appropriate container. Do this in the following way:	☐	☐	_____	_____
a. Ask for assistance from a co-worker.	☐	☐	_____	_____
b. Logroll body to one side. Place shroud behind body leaving enough material to support body when rolled back. Fan-fold remaining shroud next to body.	☐	☐	_____	_____
c. Place plastic protection pad under buttocks.	☐	☐	_____	_____
d. Roll body on its back and then to the other side.	☐	☐	_____	_____
e. Pull fan-folded portion of shroud until flat.	☐	☐	_____	_____
f. Roll body on it back.	☐	☐	_____	_____
g. Cover entire body with shroud.	☐	☐	_____	_____
h. Tuck in all loose edges of cover.	☐	☐	_____	_____
i. Position a tie above elbows and below knees and secure around body.	☐	☐	_____	_____
j. Attach ID tag to tie just above elbows.	☐	☐	_____	_____
15. Remove gloves and discard according to facility policy and procedure.	☐	☐	_____	_____
16. Wash hands.	☐	☐	_____	_____
17. Place all personal belongings in a large container. Label container with:	☐	☐	_____	_____
a. Patient's name	☐	☐	_____	_____
b. Age	☐	☐	_____	_____
c. Room number	☐	☐	_____	_____
18. Place list of belongings in container and on patient's chart.	☐	☐	_____	_____

Procedure	Pass	Redo	Date Competency Met	Instructor Initials
19. Follow your facility's procedure for transporting body and belongings through hallways.	☐	☐	_____	_____
20. Remove all linen and other supplies from room.	☐	☐	_____	_____
Postprocedure				
12. Wash hands.	☐	☐	_____	_____
13. Report procedure completed to charge nurse.	☐	☐	_____	_____

Check-off Sheet:

18-55 Making a Closed Bed

Name _____ Date _____

Directions: Practice this procedure, following each step. When you are ready to have your performance evaluated, give this sheet to your instructor. Review the detailed procedure in your textbook.

Procedure	Pass	Redo	Date Competency Met	Instructor Initials
Student must use Standard Precautions.	☐	☐	_____	_____
Preprocedure				
1. Wash hands.	☐	☐	_____	_____
2. Assemble equipment:				
a. Fitted bottom sheet and one large sheet	☐	☐	_____	_____
b. Draw sheet or large pad	☐	☐	_____	_____
c. Blankets as needed	☐	☐	_____	_____
d. Spread	☐	☐	_____	_____
e. Pillow	☐	☐	_____	_____
f. Pillowcase	☐	☐	_____	_____
3. Raise bed to a comfortable working height. Lock wheels on bed.	☐	☐	_____	_____
4. Place a chair at side of bed.	☐	☐	_____	_____
5. Put linen on chair in the order in which you will use it. (First things you will use go on top.)	☐	☐	_____	_____
Procedure				
6. Position mattress at head of bed until it is against head board.	☐	☐	_____	_____
7. Work on one side of bed until that side is completed. Then go to the other side of bed. This saves you time and energy.	☐	☐	_____	_____
8. Tuck edges of fitted bottom sheet under bed.	☐	☐	_____	_____
9. Place pad midway on bed or tuck in draw sheet.	☐	☐	_____	_____
10. Top sheet is folded lengthwise. Place on bed.	☐	☐	_____	_____
a. Place the center fold at center of bed from head to foot.	☐	☐	_____	_____
b. Put large hem at head of bed, even with top of mattress.	☐	☐	_____	_____
c. Open the sheet. Be certain rough edge of hem is facing up.	☐	☐	_____	_____

Procedure	Pass	Redo	Date Competency Met	Instructor Initials
d. Tightly tuck the sheet under at foot of bed.	☐	☐	_____	_____
e. Make a mitered corner at foot of bed.	☐	☐	_____	_____
f. Do not tuck in sheet at side of bed.	☐	☐	_____	_____
11. Blanket is folded lengthwise. Place it on bed.	☐	☐	_____	_____
a. Place center fold of blanket on center of bed from head to foot.	☐	☐	_____	_____
b. Place upper hem 6 inches from top of mattress.	☐	☐	_____	_____
c. Open blanket and tuck it under foot tightly.	☐	☐	_____	_____
d. Make a mitered corner at foot of bed.	☐	☐	_____	_____
e. Do not tuck in at sides of bed.	☐	☐	_____	_____
12. Bedspread is folded lengthwise. Place it on bed.	☐	☐	_____	_____
a. Place center fold in center of bed from head to foot.	☐	☐	_____	_____
b. Place upper hem even with upper edge of mattress.	☐	☐	_____	_____
c. Have rough edge down.	☐	☐	_____	_____
d. Open spread and tuck it under at foot of bed.	☐	☐	_____	_____
e. Make a mitered corner.	☐	☐	_____	_____
f. Do not tuck in at sides.	☐	☐	_____	_____
13. Go to other side of bed. Start with bottom sheet.	☐	☐	_____	_____
a. Pull sheet tight and smooth out all wrinkles.	☐	☐	_____	_____
b. Make a mitered corner at top of bed.	☐	☐	_____	_____
c. Pull draw sheet tight and tuck it in.	☐	☐	_____	_____
d. Straighten out top sheet. Make a mitered corner at foot of bed.	☐	☐	_____	_____
e. Miter foot corners of blanket and bedspread.	☐	☐	_____	_____
14. Fold top hem of spread over top hem of blanket.	☐	☐	_____	_____
15. Fold top hem of sheet back over edge of spread and blanket to form cuff. The hem should be on the underside so that a rough surface does not come in contact with patient's skin and cause irritation.	☐	☐	_____	_____

Procedure	Pass	Redo	Date Competency Met	Instructor Initials
16. Put pillowcase on pillow.	☐	☐	_____	_____
a. Hold pillowcase at center of end seam. Do not tuck pillow under the chin.	☐	☐	_____	_____
b. With your other hand, turn pillowcase back over hand holding end seam.	☐	☐	_____	_____
c. Grasp pillow through case at center of end of pillow.	☐	☐	_____	_____
d. Bring case down over pillow and fit pillow into corners of case.	☐	☐	_____	_____
e. Fold extra material over open end of pillow and place it on bed with open end away from door.	☐	☐	_____	_____
17. Put bed in lowest position.	☐	☐	_____	_____

Postprocedure

Procedure	Pass	Redo	Date Competency Met	Instructor Initials
18. Wash hand.	☐	☐	_____	_____

Check-off Sheet:
18-56 Making an Occupied Bed

Name _____ **Date** _____

Directions: Practice this procedure, following each step. When you are ready to have your performance evaluated, give this sheet to your instructor. Review the detailed procedure in your textbook.

Procedure	Pass	Redo	Date Competency Met	Instructor Initials
Student must use Standard Precautions.	☐	☐	_____	_____
Preprocedure				
1. Wash hands.	☐	☐	_____	_____
2. Assemble equipment:				
a. Draw sheet or large pad	☐	☐	_____	_____
b. Two large sheets or fitted bottom sheet and one large sheet	☐	☐	_____	_____
c. Two pillowcases	☐	☐	_____	_____
d. Blankets as needed	☐	☐	_____	_____
e. Bedspread (if clean one is needed)	☐	☐	_____	_____
f. Pillow	☐	☐	_____	_____
g. Disposable gloves if needed	☐	☐	_____	_____
3. Identify patient and explain what you are going to do.	☐	☐	_____	_____
4. Raise bed to comfortable working height. Lock wheels on bed.	☐	☐	_____	_____
5. Place chair at side of bed.	☐	☐	_____	_____
6. Put linen on chair in order in which you will use it. (First things you will use go on top.)	☐	☐	_____	_____
7. Provide for privacy by pulling privacy curtain.	☐	☐	_____	_____
Procedure				
8. Lower headrest and kneerest until bed is flat, if allowed.	☐	☐	_____	_____
9. Loosen linens on all sides by lifting edge of mattress with one hand and pulling out bedclothes with the other. *Never shake linen: This spreads microorganisms.*	☐	☐	_____	_____
10. Push mattress to top of bed. Ask for assistance if you need it.	☐	☐	_____	_____
11. Remove bedspread and blanket by folding them to the bottom, one at a time. Lift them from center and place over back of chair.	☐	☐	_____	_____

Procedure	Pass	Redo	Date Competency Met	Instructor Initials
12. Place bath blanket or plain sheet over top sheet. Ask patient to hold top edge of clean cover if he or she is able to do so. If patient cannot hold the sheet, tuck it under patient's shoulders.	☐	☐	_____	_____
13. Slide soiled sheet from top to bottom and put in dirty linen container. Be careful not to expose patient.	☐	☐	_____	_____
14. Ask patient to turn toward the opposite side of bed. Have patient hold onto the side rail. Assist patient if he or she needs help. Patient should now be on far side of bed from you.	☐	☐	_____	_____
15. Adjust pillow for patient to make him or her com fortable.	☐	☐	_____	_____
16. Fan-fold soiled draw sheet and bottom sheet close to patient and tuck against patient's back. This leaves the mattress stripped linen.	☐	☐	_____	_____
17. Work on one side of bed until that side is completed. Then go to other side of bed. This saves you time an d energy.	☐	☐	_____	_____
18. Take fitted bottom and fold it lengthwise. Be careful not to let it touch floor.	☐	☐	_____	_____
19. Place sheet on bed, still folded, with fold on middle of mattress.	☐	☐	_____	_____
20. Fold top half of sheet toward patient. Tuck folds again patient's back.	☐	☐	_____	_____
21. Miter corner at head of mattress. Tuck bottom sheet under mattress on your side from head to foot of mattress.	☐	☐	_____	_____
22. Place clean bottom draw sheet or large pad that has been folded in half with fold along middle of mattress. Fold top half of sheet toward patient. Tuck folds against patient's back.	☐	☐	_____	_____
23. Raise side rail and lock in place.	☐	☐	_____	_____
24. Lower side rail on opposite side.	☐	☐	_____	_____
25. Ask patient to roll away from you to other side of bed and onto clean linen. Tell patient that there will be a bump in the middle. (Be careful not to let patient become wrapped up in bath blanket.)	☐	☐	_____	_____
26. Remove old bottom sheet and draw sheet from bed and put into laundry container.	☐	☐	_____	_____

Procedure	Pass	Redo	Date Competency Met	Instructor Initials
27. Pull fresh linen toward edge of mattress. Tuck it under mattress at head of bed.	☐	☐	_____	_____
28. Tuck bottom sheet under mattress from head to foot of mattress. Pull firmly to remove wrinkles.	☐	☐	_____	_____
29. Pull draw sheet very tight and tuck under mattress. If pad used, pull from patient and straighten.	☐	☐	_____	_____
30. Have patient roll on back, or turn patient yourself. Loosen bath blanket as patient turns.	☐	☐	_____	_____
31. Change pillowcase.	☐	☐	_____	_____
a. Hold pillowcase at center of end seam.	☐	☐	_____	_____
b. With your other hand turn pillowcase back over hand, holding end seam.	☐	☐	_____	_____
c. Grasp pillow through case at center of end of pillow.	☐	☐	_____	_____
d. Bring case down over pillow and fit pillow into corners of case.	☐	☐	_____	_____
e. Fold extra material over open end of pillow and place it on bed with open end away from door.	☐	☐	_____	_____
32. Spread clean top sheet over bath blanket with wide hem at the top. Middle of sheet should run along middle of bed with wide hem even with the top of mattress. Ask patient to hold hem of clean sheet. Remove bath blanket by moving it toward foot of bed. Be careful not to expose patient.	☐	☐	_____	_____
33. Tuck clean top sheet under mattress at foot of bed. Make toepleat in top sheet so that patient's feet can move freely. To make a toepleat, make 3-inch fold toward foot of bed in topsheet before tucking in sheet. Tuck in and miter corner.	☐	☐	_____	_____
34. Place blanket over patient, being sure that it covers the shoulders.	☐	☐	_____	_____
35. Place bedspread on bed in same way. Tuck blanket and bedspread under bottom of mattress and miter corners.	☐	☐	_____	_____
36. Make cuff.	☐	☐	_____	_____
a. Fold top hem edge of spread over blanket.	☐	☐	_____	_____
b. Fold top hem of top sheet back over edge of bedspread and blanket, being certain that rough hem is turned down.	☐	☐	_____	_____

388

Procedure	Pass	Redo	Date Competency Met	Instructor Initials
37. Position patient and make comfortable.	☐	☐	_____	_____
38. Put bed in lowest position	☐	☐	_____	_____
39. Open privacy curtains.	☐	☐	_____	_____
40. Raise side rails, if required.	☐	☐	_____	_____
41. Place call light where patient can reach it.	☐	☐	_____	_____
Postprocedure				
42. Tidy unit.	☐	☐	_____	_____
43. Wash hands.	☐	☐	_____	_____
44. Chart linen change and how the patient tolerated procedure.	☐	☐	_____	_____

Check-off Sheet:
18-57 Making an Open Bed

Name _____ Date _____

Directions: Practice this procedure, following each step. When you are ready to have your performance evaluated, give this sheet to your instructor. Review the detailed procedure in your textbook.

Procedure	Pass	Redo	Date Competency Met	Instructor Initials
Student must use Standard Precautions.	☐	☐	_____	_____
Preprocedure				
1. Wash hands.	☐	☐	_____	_____
Procedure				
2. Grasp cuff of bedding in both hands and pull to foot of bed.	☐	☐	_____	_____
3. Fold bedding back on itself toward head of bed. The edge of cuff must meet fold. (This is called fan-folding.)	☐	☐	_____	_____
4. Smooth the hanging sheets on each side into folds.	☐	☐	_____	_____
Postprocedure				
5. Wash hands.	☐	☐	_____	_____

Check-off Sheet:

18-58 Placing a Bed Cradle

Name _____ Date _____

Directions: Practice this procedure, following each step. When you are ready to have your performance evaluated, give this sheet to your instructor. Review the detailed procedure in your textbook.

Procedure	Pass	Redo	Date Competency Met	Instructor Initials
Student must use Standard Precautions.	☐	☐	_____	_____
Preprocedure				
1. Identify the patient requiring a bed cradle. Assess the extremity to be protected. Note any special requirements necessitated by the patient's condition	☐	☐	_____	_____
2. Wash hands.	☐	☐	_____	_____
3. Explain the procedure to the patient.	☐	☐	_____	_____
Procedure				
4. Address any needs for repositioning prior to placing the cradle.	☐	☐	_____	_____
5. Fold down the top covers off of the patient.	☐	☐	_____	_____
6. Place the cradle over the patient's lower extremities	☐	☐	_____	_____
7. Secure the cradle to the bed frame so that it will not collapse on to the patient.	☐	☐	_____	_____
8. Replace the top covers over the top of the cradle	☐	☐	_____	_____
9. Assure that no part of the cradle or the top covers are touching the patient's affected extremity.	☐	☐	_____	_____
Postprocedure				
10. Assure that the patient is comfortable and has no further needs before leaving the area.	☐	☐	_____	_____
11. Wash hands.	☐	☐	_____	_____
12. Document the procedure noting any special findings or needs of the patient.	☐	☐	_____	_____
13. Check the patient frequently to assure the stability of the cradle and the comfort of the patient.	☐	☐	_____	_____

Check-off Sheet:

18-59 Preparing the Patient to Eat

Name _____ **Date** _____

Directions: Practice this procedure, following each step. When you are ready to have your performance evaluated, give this sheet to your instructor. Review the detailed procedure in your textbook.

Procedure	Pass	Redo	Date Competency Met	Instructor Initials
Student must use Standard Precautions.	☐	☐	_____	_____
Preprocedure				
1. Wash hands.	☐	☐	_____	_____
2. Assemble equipment:				
a. Bedpan or urinal	☐	☐	_____	_____
b. Toilet tissue	☐	☐	_____	_____
c. Washcloth	☐	☐	_____	_____
d. Hand towel	☐	☐	_____	_____
3. Assist patient as needed to empty bladder and wash hands and face.	☐	☐	_____	_____
4. Explain that you are getting ready to give patient a meal.	☐	☐	_____	_____
Procedure				
5. Clear bedside table.	☐	☐	_____	_____
6. Position patient for comfort and a convenient eating position.	☐	☐	_____	_____
7. Wash your hands.	☐	☐	_____	_____
8. Identify patient and check name on food tray to ensure that you are delivering the correct diet to patient.	☐	☐	_____	_____
9. Place tray in a convenient position in front of patient.	☐	☐	_____	_____
10. Open containers if patient cannot.	☐	☐	_____	_____
11. If patient is unable to prepare food, do it for patient.	☐	☐	_____	_____
a. Butter the bread	☐	☐	_____	_____
b. Cut meat	☐	☐	_____	_____
c. Season food as necessary	☐	☐	_____	_____
12. Follow the procedure for feeding a patient if patient needs to be fed.	☐	☐	_____	_____
Postprocedure				
13. Wash hands.	☐	☐	_____	_____

Check-off Sheet:

18-60 Preparing the Patient to Eat in the Dining Room

Name _____ Date _____

Directions: Practice this procedure, following each step. When you are ready to have your performance evaluated, give this sheet to your instructor. Review the detailed procedure in your textbook.

Procedure	Pass	Redo	Date Competency Met	Instructor Initials
Student must use Standard Precautions.	☐	☐	_____	_____
Preprocedure				
1. Wash hands.	☐	☐	_____	_____
Procedure				
2. Help patient take care of toileting needs.	☐	☐	_____	_____
3. Assist with handwashing.	☐	☐	_____	_____
4. Take patient to dining room.	☐	☐	_____	_____
5. Position patient in wheelchair at table that is proper height for wheelchair.	☐	☐	_____	_____
6. Be certain patient is sitting in a comfortable position in wheelchair.	☐	☐	_____	_____
7. Provide adaptive feeding equipment if needed.	☐	☐	_____	_____
8. Bring patient tray.	☐	☐	_____	_____
9. Identify patient.	☐	☐	_____	_____
10. Serve tray and remove plate covers.	☐	☐	_____	_____
11. Provide assistance as needed (e.g., cut meat, butter bread, open containers).	☐	☐	_____	_____
12. Remove tray when finished, noting what patient ate.	☐	☐	_____	_____
13. Assist with handwashing and take patient to area of choice.	☐	☐	_____	_____
Postprocedure				
14. Wash hands.	☐	☐	_____	_____
15. Record what patient ate.	☐	☐	_____	_____
16. Record I & O if necessary. (See the section "Measuring Intake and Output" later in the section.	☐	☐	_____	_____

Check-off Sheet:
18-61 Assisting the Patient with Meals
Name _____ **Date** _____

Directions: Practice this procedure, following each step. When you are ready to have your performance evaluated, give this sheet to your instructor. Review the detailed procedure in your textbook.

Procedure	Pass	Redo	Date Competency Met	Instructor Initials
Student must use Standard Precautions.	☐	☐	_____	_____
Preprocedure				
1. Wash hands.	☐	☐	_____	_____
2. Check patient's ID band with name on food tray to ensure that you will be feeding correct diet to patient.	☐	☐	_____	_____
Procedure				
3. Tell patient what food is being served.	☐	☐	_____	_____
4. Ask patient how he or she prefers food to be prepared (e.g., salt, pepper, cream or sugar in coffee).	☐	☐	_____	_____
5. Position patient in a sitting position, as allowed by physician. If ordered to lie flat, turn patient on side.	☐	☐	_____	_____
6. Position yourself in a comfortable manner, facing the patient, so that you won't be rushing patient because you are uncomfortable. (Do not sit on bed.)	☐	☐	_____	_____
7. Cut food into small bite-sized pieces.	☐	☐	_____	_____
8. Place a napkin or small hand towel under patient's chin.	☐	☐	_____	_____
9. Put a flex straw in cold drinks. Hot drinks tend to burn mouth if taken through a straw.	☐	☐	_____	_____
10. Use a spoon to feed patient small to average-sized bites of food. (Encourage patient to help self as much as possible.)	☐	☐	_____	_____
11. Always feed patient at a slow pace. It may take more time for him or her to chew and swallow than you think is necessary.	☐	☐	_____	_____
12. Always be sure that one bite has been swallowed before you give another spoonful to patient.	☐	☐	_____	_____
13. Tell patient what is being served and ask which item he or she prefers first, if patient cannot see food.	☐	☐	_____	_____
14. Offer beverages to patient throughout the meal.	☐	☐	_____	_____
15. Talk with patient during meal.	☐	☐	_____	_____
16. Encourage patient to finish eating, but do not force.	☐	☐	_____	_____

Procedure	Pass	Redo	Date Competency Met	Instructor Initials
17. Assist patient in wiping face as necessary and when patient is finished eating.	☐	☐	_____	_____
18. Observe amount of food eaten.	☐	☐	_____	_____
Postprocedure				
19. Remove tray from room.	☐	☐	_____	_____
20. Position patient for comfort and safety.	☐	☐	_____	_____
21. Place call light in a convenient place.	☐	☐	_____	_____
22. Wash hands.	☐	☐	_____	_____
23. Record amount of food eaten (half, three-fourths, one-fourth, etc.) on chart, and indicate if food was tolerated well or not.	☐	☐	_____	_____

Check-off Sheet:
18-62 Serving Food to the Patient in Bed (Self-Help)

Name _____ Date _____

Directions: Practice this procedure, following each step. When you are ready to have your performance evaluated, give this sheet to your instructor. Review the detailed procedure in your textbook.

Procedure	Pass	Redo	Date Competency Met	Instructor Initials
Student must use Standard Precautions.	☐	☐	_____	_____
Preprocedure				
1. Wash hands.	☐	☐	_____	_____
2. Assemble equipment:				
a. Food tray with diet card	☐	☐	_____	_____
b. Flex straws	☐	☐	_____	_____
c. Towel	☐	☐	_____	_____
Procedure				
3. Assist patient with bedpan or urinal.	☐	☐	_____	_____
4. Place in sitting position if possible.	☐	☐	_____	_____
5. Help patient wash hands and face.	☐	☐	_____	_____
6. Remove unsightly or odor-causing articles.	☐	☐	_____	_____
7. Clean overbed table.	☐	☐	_____	_____
8. Check tray with diet card for:				
a. Patient's name	☐	☐	_____	_____
b. Type of diet	☐	☐	_____	_____
c. Correct foods according to diet (e.g., diabetic, puréed, chopped, regular)	☐	☐	_____	_____
9. Set up tray and help with foods if needed (e.g., cut meat, butter bread, open containers). *Do not add foods to the tray until you check on diet.*	☐	☐	_____	_____
10. Encourage patient to eat all foods on tray.	☐	☐	_____	_____
11. Remove tray when finished and note what patient ate.	☐	☐	_____	_____
12. Help patient wash hands and face.	☐	☐	_____	_____
13. Position patient comfortably and make sure call bell in within reach.	☐	☐	_____	_____

Procedure	Pass	Redo	Date Competency Met	Instructor Initials
Postprocedure				
14. Remove tray.	☐	☐	_____	_____
15. Be certain that water is within reach.	☐	☐	_____	_____
16. Wash hands.	☐	☐	_____	_____
17. Record I & O if required	☐	☐	_____	_____
18. Record amount eaten.	☐	☐	_____	_____

Check-off Sheet:
18-63 Providing Fresh Drinking Water

Name _____ Date _____

Directions: Practice this procedure, following each step. When you are ready to have your performance evaluated, give this sheet to your instructor. Review the detailed procedure in your textbook.

Procedure	Pass	Redo	Date Competency Met	Instructor Initials
Student must use Standard Precautions.	☐	☐	_____	_____
Preprocedure				
1. Identify any patients whose fluids may be restricted as a medical necessity.	☐	☐	_____	_____
2. Wash hands.	☐	☐	_____	_____
3. Assemble equipment: the container to be used for patient's water supply.	☐	☐	_____	_____
Procedure				
4. Collect and discard any of the containers previously used for the patient's water supply.	☐	☐	_____	_____
5. Establish the temperature of water preferred by the patient, i.e., iced, tepid, etc.	☐	☐	_____	_____
6. Provide a clean container and fresh water for the patient.	☐	☐	_____	_____
7. Establish that the patient has no further needs before leaving the bedside.	☐	☐	_____	_____
Postprocedure				
8. Wash hands.	☐	☐	_____	_____

Check-off Sheet:
18-64 Feeding the Helpless Patient

Name _____ **Date** _____

Directions: Practice this procedure, following each step. When you are ready to have your performance evaluated, give this sheet to your instructor. Review the detailed procedure in your textbook.

Procedure	Pass	Redo	Date Competency Met	Instructor Initials
Student must use Standard Precautions.	☐	☐	_____	_____
Preprocedure				
1. Wash hands.	☐	☐	_____	_____
2. Bring patient's tray.	☐	☐	_____	_____
3. Check name on card with patient ID band.	☐	☐	_____	_____
4. Explain to patient what you are gong to do.	☐	☐	_____	_____
Procedure				
5. Sit comfortably, facing patient.	☐	☐	_____	_____
6. Tuck a napkin under patient's chin.	☐	☐	_____	_____
7. Season food the way patient likes it.	☐	☐	_____	_____
8. Use a spoon and fill only half full.	☐	☐	_____	_____
9. Give food from tip, not side of spoon.	☐	☐	_____	_____
10. Name each food as you offer it, if patient cannot see food.	☐	☐	_____	_____
11. Describe position of food on plate (e.g., hot liquids in right corner, peas at the position of 3 o'clock on a clock) if patient cannot see but can feed self.	☐	☐	_____	_____
12. Tell patient if you are offering something that is hot or cold.	☐	☐	_____	_____
13. Use a straw for giving liquid.	☐	☐	_____	_____
14. Feed patient slowly and allow time to chew and swallow. Offer beverages throughout the meal.	☐	☐	_____	_____
15. Note amount eaten and remove tray when finished.	☐	☐	_____	_____
16. Help with washing hands and face.	☐	☐	_____	_____
17. Position patient comfortably and place call bell within reach.	☐	☐	_____	_____
Postprocedure				
18. Wash hands.	☐	☐	_____	_____
19. Record amount eaten and I & O if required. See following pages for directions on recording I & O.	☐	☐	_____	_____

Check-off Sheet:

18-65 Serving Nourishments

Name _____   **Date** _____

Directions: Practice this procedure, following each step. When you are ready to have your performance evaluated, give this sheet to your instructor. Review the detailed procedure in your textbook.

Procedure	Pass	Redo	Date Competency Met	Instructor Initials
Student must use Standard Precautions.	☐	☐	_____	_____
Preprocedure				
1. Wash hands.	☐	☐	_____	_____
2. Assemble equipment:				
a. Nourishment	☐	☐	_____	_____
b. Cup, dish, straw, spoon	☐	☐	_____	_____
c. Napkin	☐	☐	_____	_____
3. Identify patient.	☐	☐	_____	_____
Procedure				
4. Take nourishment to patient.	☐	☐	_____	_____
5. Help if needed.	☐	☐	_____	_____
6. After patient is finished, collect dirty utensils.	☐	☐	_____	_____
Postprocedure				
7. Return utensils to dietary cart or kitchen.	☐	☐	_____	_____
8. Record intake on I & O sheet if required.	☐	☐	_____	_____
9. Wash hands.	☐	☐	_____	_____
10. Record nourishment taken.	☐	☐	_____	_____

Check-off Sheet:
18-66 Measuring Urinary Output

Name _____ Date _____

Directions: Practice this procedure, following each step. When you are ready to have your performance evaluated, give this sheet to your instructor. Review the detailed procedure in your textbook.

Procedure	Pass	Redo	Date Competency Met	Instructor Initials
Student must use Standard Precautions.	☐	☐	_____	_____
Preprocedure				
1. Wash hands.	☐	☐	_____	_____
2. Assemble equipment:				
a. Bedpan, urinal, or special container	☐	☐	_____	_____
b. Graduate or measuring cup	☐	☐	_____	_____
c. Disposable nonsterile gloves	☐	☐	_____	_____
3. Put on gloves.	☐	☐	_____	_____
Procedure				
4. Pour urine into measuring graduate.	☐	☐	_____	_____
5. Place graduate on flat surface and read amount of urine.	☐	☐	_____	_____
6. Observe urine for:				
a. Unusual color	☐	☐	_____	_____
b. Blood	☐	☐	_____	_____
c. Dark color	☐	☐	_____	_____
d. Large amounts of mucus	☐	☐	_____	_____
e. Sediment	☐	☐	_____	_____
7. Save the specimen and report to nurse immediately if you notice any unusual appearance.	☐	☐	_____	_____
8. Discard in toilet if urine is normal. Use a paper towel to flush toilet and turn on faucet.	☐	☐	_____	_____
9. Rinse graduate or pitcher and put away.	☐	☐	_____	_____
Postprocedure				
10. Remove gloves and discard according to facility policy.	☐	☐	_____	_____
11. Wash hands.	☐	☐	_____	_____
12. Record amount of urine in cc's on I & O sheet.	☐	☐	_____	_____

Check-off Sheet:
18-67 Oil Retention Enema

Name _____ Date _____

Directions: Practice this procedure, following each step. When you are ready to have your performance evaluated, give this sheet to your instructor. Review the detailed procedure in your textbook.

Procedure	Pass	Redo	Date Competency Met	Instructor Initials
Student must use Standard Precautions.	☐	☐	_____	_____
Preprocedure				
1. Wash your hands.	☐	☐	_____	_____
2. Assemble equipment:				
a. Prepackaged oil retention enema	☐	☐	_____	_____
b. Bedpan and cover	☐	☐	_____	_____
c. Waterproof bed protector	☐	☐	_____	_____
d. Toilet tissue	☐	☐	_____	_____
e. Towel, basin of water, and soap	☐	☐	_____	_____
f. Disposable gloves	☐	☐	_____	_____
3. Identify patient.	☐	☐	_____	_____
4. Ask visitors to leave the room. Provide privacy with curtain, screen, or door.	☐	☐	_____	_____
5. Explain what you are going to do.	☐	☐	_____	_____
6. Put on gloves.	☐	☐	_____	_____
Procedure				
7. Cover patient with a bath blanket, and fan-fold linen to foot of bed.	☐	☐	_____	_____
8. Put bedpan on foot of bed.	☐	☐	_____	_____
9. Elevate the bed to a comfortable working height and lower the side rail on the side you are working on.	☐	☐	_____	_____
10. Place bed protector under buttocks.	☐	☐	_____	_____
11. Help patient into Sims' position.	☐	☐	_____	_____
12. Tell patient to retain enema as long as possible.	☐	☐	_____	_____
13. Open a prepackaged oil retention enema.	☐	☐	_____	_____
14. Fold the bath blanket back to expose the buttock.	☐	☐	_____	_____
15. Lift patient's upper buttock and expose anus.	☐	☐	_____	_____
16. Tell patient when you are going to insert prelubricated tip into anus. (Instruct patient to take deep breaths and try to relax.) Insert tip 2-4 inches into the rectum.	☐	☐	_____	_____

Procedure	Pass	Redo	Date Competency Met	Instructor Initials
17. Squeeze container slowly and steady until all solution has entered rectum.	☐	☐	_____	_____
18. Remove container; place in original package to be disposed of in contaminated waste according to facility policy and procedure.	☐	☐	_____	_____
19. Instruct patient to remain on side and retain the solution for 30 minutes.	☐	☐	_____	_____
20. Lower the bed and pull the side rail up. Leave the call bell in place.	☐	☐	_____	_____
21. Remove gloves and discard according to facility policy.	☐	☐	_____	_____
22. Check patient every 5 minutes until fluid has been retained for at least 20 minutes. Usually it is at least 30 minutes.	☐	☐	_____	_____
23. Position patient on bedpan or assist to bathroom. Instruct patient not to flush toilet.	☐	☐	_____	_____
24. Raise head of bed, if permitted, if using a bedpan.	☐	☐	_____	_____
25. Place toilet tissue and call bell within easy reach.	☐	☐	_____	_____
26. Stay nearby if patient is in bathroom.	☐	☐	_____	_____
27. Put on gloves.	☐	☐	_____	_____
28. Remove bedpan or assist patient to return to bed. Observe contents of toilet or bedpan for:	☐	☐	_____	_____
a. Color, consistency, unusual materials, odor	☐	☐	_____	_____
b. Amount of return	☐	☐	_____	_____
29. Cover bedpan and dispose of contents. Use paper towel to flush toilet and turn on faucet.	☐	☐	_____	_____
30. Remove gloves and discard in biohazardous container.	☐	☐	_____	_____
31. Replace top sheet and remove bath blanket and plastic bed protector.	☐	☐	_____	_____
32. Give patient soap, water, and towel for hands and face.	☐	☐	_____	_____

Postprocedure

Procedure	Pass	Redo	Date Competency Met	Instructor Initials
33. Wash your hands.	☐	☐	_____	_____
34. Chart the following:	☐	☐	_____	_____
a. Type of enema given	☐	☐	_____	_____
b. Consistency and amount of bowel movement	☐	☐	_____	_____
c. How the procedure was tolerated	☐	☐	_____	_____

Check-off Sheet:
18-68 Prepackaged Enemas
Name _____ **Date** _____

Directions: Practice this procedure, following each step. When you are ready to have your performance evaluated, give this sheet to your instructor. Review the detailed procedure in your textbook.

Procedure	Pass	Redo	Date Competency Met	Instructor Initials
Student must use Standard Precautions.	☐	☐	_____	_____
Preprocedure				
1. Wash your hands.	☐	☐	_____	_____
2. Assemble equipment:				
a. Prepackaged enema	☐	☐	_____	_____
b. Bedpan and cover	☐	☐	_____	_____
c. Waterproof bed protector	☐	☐	_____	_____
d. Toilet tissue	☐	☐	_____	_____
e. Towel, basin of water, and soap	☐	☐	_____	_____
f. Disposable gloves	☐	☐	_____	_____
3. Identify patient.	☐	☐	_____	_____
4. Ask visitors to leave the room.	☐	☐	_____	_____
5. Explain what you are going to do and proved privacy with curtain, screen, or door.	☐	☐	_____	_____
Procedure				
6. Cover patient with a bath blanket, and fan-fold linen to foot of bed.	☐	☐	_____	_____
7. Put on gloves.	☐	☐	_____	_____
8. Raise bed to a comfortable working height and lower side.	☐	☐	_____	_____
9. Place bed protector under buttocks.	☐	☐	_____	_____
10. Put bedpan on foot of bed.	☐	☐	_____	_____
11. Help patient into Sims' position.	☐	☐	_____	_____
12. Fold back blanket and expose buttock.	☐	☐	_____	_____
13. Tell patient to retain enema as long as possible.	☐	☐	_____	_____
14. Open a prepackaged enema.	☐	☐	_____	_____
15. Lift patients upper buttock and expose anus.	☐	☐	_____	_____
16. Tell patient when you are going to insert prelubricated tip into anus. (Have patient take deep breaths and try to relax.)	☐	☐	_____	_____

Procedure	Pass	Redo	Date Competency Met	Instructor Initials
17. Squeeze container until all the solution has entered the rectum.	☐	☐	_____	_____
18. Remove container; place in original package to be disposed of according to facility policy.	☐	☐	_____	_____
19. Remove gloves and dispose of in biohazardous container.	☐	☐	_____	_____
20. Instruct patient to remain on side and retain the solution as long as possible. Have call bell in reach.	☐	☐	_____	_____
21. Put on gloves.				
22. Position patient on bedpan or assist to bathroom. Instruct patient not to flush toilet.	☐	☐	_____	_____
23. Raise head of bed if permitted if using a bedpan.	☐	☐	_____	_____
24. Place toilet tissue and call bell within easy reach.	☐	☐	_____	_____
25. Stay nearby if patient is in bathroom.	☐	☐	_____	_____
26. Remove bedpan or assist patient to return to bed.	☐	☐	_____	_____
27. Observe contents of toilet or bedpan for:				
a. Color, consistency, unusual materials, odor	☐	☐	_____	_____
b. Amount of return	☐	☐	_____	_____
28. Cover bedpan and dispose of contents. Use paper towels to flush toilet and turn on faucet.	☐	☐	_____	_____

Postprocedure

Procedure	Pass	Redo	Date Competency Met	Instructor Initials
29. Remove gloves and dispose of according to facility policy.	☐	☐	_____	_____
30. Replace top sheet and remove bath blanket and plastic bed protector.	☐	☐	_____	_____
31. Give patient soap, water, and towel for hands and face.	☐	☐	_____	_____
32. Wash your hands.	☐	☐	_____	_____
33. Chart the following:				
a. Type of enema given	☐	☐	_____	_____
b. Consistency and amount of bowel movement	☐	☐	_____	_____
c. How the procedure was tolerated	☐	☐	_____	_____

Check-off Sheet:
18-69 Tap Water, Soap Suds, Saline Enemas

Name _____ Date _____

Directions: Practice this procedure, following each step. When you are ready to have your performance evaluated, give this sheet to your instructor. Review the detailed procedure in your textbook.

Procedure	Pass	Redo	Date Competency Met	Instructor Initials
Student must use Standard Precautions.	☐	☐	_____	_____
Preprocedure				
1. Wash your hands.	☐	☐	_____	_____
2. Assemble equipment:	☐	☐	_____	_____
a. Disposable gloves	☐	☐	_____	_____
b. Disposable enema equipment	☐	☐	_____	_____
(1) Plastic container	☐	☐	_____	_____
(2) Tubing	☐	☐	_____	_____
(3) Clamp	☐	☐	_____	_____
(4) Lubricant	☐	☐	_____	_____
c. Enema solution as instructed by the head nurse, e.g.:	☐	☐	_____	_____
(1) Tap water, 700-1000 cc water (105°F)	☐	☐	_____	_____
(2) Soap suds, 700-1000 cc (105°F), one package enema soap	☐	☐	_____	_____
(3) Saline, 700-1000 cc water (105°F), 2 teaspoons salt	☐	☐	_____	_____
d. Bedpan and cover	☐	☐	_____	_____
e. Urinal, if necessary	☐	☐	_____	_____
f. Toilet tissue	☐	☐	_____	_____
g. Waterproof disposable bed protector	☐	☐	_____	_____
h. Paper towel	☐	☐	_____	_____
i. Bath blanket	☐	☐	_____	_____
3. Identify patient	☐	☐	_____	_____
Procedure				
4. Ask visitors to leave room.	☐	☐	_____	_____
5. Tell patient what you are going to do.	☐	☐	_____	_____
6. Attach tubing to irrigation container. Adjust clamp to a position where you can easily open and close it. Close clamp.	☐	☐	_____	_____

Procedure	Pass	Redo	Date Competency Met	Instructor Initials
7. Fill container with warm water (105°F).	☐	☐	_____	_____
a. Add one package enema soap suds enema.	☐	☐	_____	_____
b. Add 2 teaspoons salt for saline enema.	☐	☐	_____	_____
c. For tap water enema, do not add anything.	☐	☐	_____	_____
8. Provide privacy by pulling privacy curtain.				
9. Raise bed to working level and put down side rail on the side you are working on.	☐	☐	_____	_____
10. Cover patient with a bath blanket. Remove upper sheet by fan-folding to foot of bed. *Be careful not to expose patient.*	☐	☐	_____	_____
11. Put on gloves.	☐	☐	_____	_____
12. Put waterproof protector under patient's buttocks.	☐	☐	_____	_____
13. Place bedpan on foot of bed.	☐	☐	_____	_____
14. Place patient in Sims' position.	☐	☐	_____	_____
15. Open clamp on enema tubing and let a small amount of solution run into bedpan. (This eliminates air in tubing and warms tube.) Close clamp.	☐	☐	_____	_____
16. Put a small amount of lubricating jelly on tissue. Lubricate enema tip. Check to be certain that the opening is not plugged.	☐	☐	_____	_____
17. Expose buttocks by folding back bath blanket.	☐	☐	_____	_____
18. Lift the upper buttock to expose anus.				
19. Tell patient when you are going to insert lubricant tip into anus.	☐	☐	_____	_____
20. Hold rectal tube about 5 inches from tip and insert slowly into rectum.	☐	☐	_____	_____
21. Tell patient to breathe deeply through mouth and to try to relax.	☐	☐	_____	_____
22. Raise container 12 to 18 inches above patient's hip.	☐	☐	_____	_____
23. Open clamp and let solution run in slowly. If patient complains of cramps, clamp tubing for a minute and lower bag slightly.	☐	☐	_____	_____
24. When most of solution has flowed into rectum close clamp. Gently withdraw rectal tube. Wrap tubing with paper towel and place into enema can.	☐	☐	_____	_____
25. Ask patient to hold solution as long as possible.	☐	☐	_____	_____
26. Assist patient to bathroom and stay nearby if patient can go to bathroom. Ask patient not to flush toilet.	☐	☐	_____	_____

Procedure	Pass	Redo	Date Competency Met	Instructor Initials
27. Help patient onto bedpan and raise head of bed if permitted.	☐	☐	_____	_____
28. Place call light within reach and check patient every few minutes.	☐	☐	_____	_____
29. Dispose of enema equipment while you are waiting for patient to expel enema. *Follow hospital policy.*	☐	☐	_____	_____
30. Remove bedpan or assist patient back to bed.	☐	☐	_____	_____
31. Observe contents for:				
a. Color, consistency, unusual materials	☐	☐	_____	_____
b. Note amount (i.e., large or small)	☐	☐	_____	_____
32. Cover bedpan and remove bed protector.	☐	☐	_____	_____
33. Remove gloves and dispose of according to facility policy. Wash hands.	☐	☐	_____	_____
34. Replace top sheet and remove bath blanket.	☐	☐	_____	_____
35. Give patient soap, water, and a towel to wash hands.	☐	☐	_____	_____
36. Secure call light in patient's reach.	☐	☐	_____	_____
Postprocedure				
37. Clean and replace all equipment used and wash your hands.	☐	☐	_____	_____
38. Chart the following:	☐	☐	_____	_____
a. Date and time	☐	☐	_____	_____
b. Type of enema given	☐	☐	_____	_____
c. Results (amount, color, consistency) of bowel movement	☐	☐	_____	_____
d. How the procedure was tolerated.	☐	☐	_____	_____

Check-off Sheet:
18-70 Disconnecting an Indwelling Catheter

Name _____ **Date** _____

Directions: Practice this procedure, following each step. When you are ready to have your performance evaluated, give this sheet to your instructor. Review the detailed procedure in your textbook.

Procedure	Pass	Redo	Date Competency Met	Instructor Initials
Student must use Standard Precautions.	☐	☐	_____	_____
Preprocedure				
1. Wash hands.	☐	☐	_____	_____
2. Assemble equipment:				
a. Disinfectant (Can use an alcohol or Betadine swab.)	☐	☐	_____	_____
b. Sterile gauze sponges	☐	☐	_____	_____
c. Sterile cap or plug	☐	☐	_____	_____
d. Disposable gloves	☐	☐	_____	_____
3. Identify patient and provide privacy with curtain, screen, or door.	☐	☐	_____	_____
4. Explain what you are going to do.	☐	☐	_____	_____
5. Put on gloves.	☐	☐	_____	_____
Procedure				
6. Place a towel under the tubing where it connects to the catheter.	☐	☐	_____	_____
7. Disinfect connections between catheter and drainage tubing where it is to be disconnected by applying disinfectant with cotton or gauze.	☐	☐	_____	_____
8. Disconnect catheter and drainage tubing. *Do not allow catheter ends to touch anything!*	☐	☐	_____	_____
9. Insert a sterile plug in end of catheter. Place sterile cap over exposed end of drainage tube.	☐	☐	_____	_____
10. Carefully secure drainage tube to bed.	☐	☐	_____	_____
Postprocedure				
11. Remove gloves and discard according to facility policy.	☐	☐	_____	_____
12. Wash hands.	☐	☐	_____	_____
13. Record procedure. *Reverse procedure to reconnect.*	☐	☐	_____	_____

Check-off Sheet:
18-71 Giving Indwelling Catheter Care

Name _____ Date _____

Directions: Practice this procedure, following each step. When you are ready to have your performance evaluated, give this sheet to your instructor. Review the detailed procedure in your textbook.

Procedure	Pass	Redo	Date Competency Met	Instructor Initials
Student must use Standard Precautions.	☐	☐	_____	_____
Preprocedure				
1. Wash hands.	☐	☐	_____	_____
2. Assemble equipment:				
a. Antiseptic solution or catheter care kits	☐	☐	_____	_____
b. Waterproof bed protector	☐	☐	_____	_____
c. Disposable nonsterile gloves	☐	☐	_____	_____
d. Bath Blanket	☐	☐	_____	_____
3. Identify patient.	☐	☐	_____	_____
4. Explain what you are going to do.	☐	☐	_____	_____
5. Provide privacy by pulling the privacy curtains.	☐	☐	_____	_____
6. Put on gloves. (Some facilities require you use sterile gloves.)				
Procedure				
7. Raise bed to comfortable working level and lower side rail.	☐	☐	_____	_____
8. Put waterproof protector on bed.	☐	☐	_____	_____
9. For female patients, have them bend their knee and drape them with the bath blanket, so that only the perineum is exposed. For males, pull covers back to knee and cover top half of body with bath blanket.	☐	☐	_____	_____
10. Carefully clean perineum.	☐	☐	_____	_____
11. Observe around catheter for sores, leakage, bleeding, or crusting. Report any unusual observation to nurse.	☐	☐	_____	_____
12. For females, separate labia with forefinger and thumb. Apply antiseptic solution around area where catheter enters the urethra. Wipe from front to back and placed used applicator or gauze pad in biohazardous container. Use a clean applicator or gauze solution each time you wipe from back to front.	☐	☐	_____	_____

Procedure	Pass	Redo	Date Competency Met	Instructor Initials
13. For males, pull back foreskin on uncircumcised patient and apply antiseptic to entire area. Wipe from the meatus down the shaft of the penis. Use a clean applicator or gauze with every stroke.	☐	☐	_____	_____
14. Remove gloves and dispose of according to facility policy.	☐	☐	_____	_____
15. Position patient comfortably. Lower bed and raise side rail.	☐	☐	_____	_____
16. Secure call light within patient's reach.	☐	☐	_____	_____
Postprocedure				
17. Wash hands.	☐	☐	_____	_____
18. Record procedure.	☐	☐	_____	_____

Check-off Sheet:
18-72 External Urinary Catheter
Name _____ Date _____

Directions: Practice this procedure, following each step. When you are ready to have your performance evaluated, give this sheet to your instructor. Review the detailed procedure in your textbook.

Procedure	Pass	Redo	Date Competency Met	Instructor Initials
Student must use Standard Precautions.	☐	☐	_____	_____
Preprocedure				
1. Wash hands.	☐	☐	_____	_____
2. Assemble equipment:				
a. Basin warm water	☐	☐	_____	_____
b. Washcloth	☐	☐	_____	_____
c. Towel	☐	☐	_____	_____
d. Waterproof bed protector	☐	☐	_____	_____
e. Gloves	☐	☐	_____	_____
f. Plastic bag	☐	☐	_____	_____
g. Condom with drainage tip	☐	☐	_____	_____
h. Paper towels	☐	☐	_____	_____
3. Identify patient.	☐	☐	_____	_____
4. Explain what you are going to do.	☐	☐	_____	_____
Procedure				
5. Provide privacy by pulling privacy curtain.	☐	☐	_____	_____
6. Raise bed to comfortable working height.	☐	☐	_____	_____
7. Cover patient with bath blanket. Have patient hold top of blanket, and fold cover to bottom of bed.	☐	☐	_____	_____
8. Put on gloves.	☐	☐	_____	_____
9. Place waterproof protector under patient's buttocks.	☐	☐	_____	_____
10. Pull up bath blanket to expose genitals only.	☐	☐	_____	_____
11. Remove condom by rolling gently toward tip of penis.	☐	☐	_____	_____
12. Wash and dry penis.	☐	☐	_____	_____
13. Observe for irritation, open areas, bleeding.	☐	☐	_____	_____
14. Report any unusual observations..	☐	☐	_____	_____

Procedure	Pass	Redo	Date Competency Met	Instructor Initials
15. Check condom for "ready stick" surface. If there is none, apply a thin spray of tincture of benzoin. *Do not spray on head of penis.*	☐	☐	_____	_____
16. Apply new condom and drainage tip to penis by rolling toward base of penis.	☐	☐	_____	_____
17. Reconnect drainage system.	☐	☐	_____	_____
18. Remove and dispose of gloves in biohazardous container.	☐	☐	_____	_____
19. Pull up top bedding and remove bath blanket.	☐	☐	_____	_____
20. Replace equipment.	☐	☐	_____	_____
21. Lower bed to lowest position.	☐	☐	_____	_____
22. Put up side rail if required.	☐	☐	_____	_____
23. Secure call light within patient's reach.	☐	☐	_____	_____

Postprocedure

Procedure	Pass	Redo	Date Competency Met	Instructor Initials
24. Tidy unit.	☐	☐	_____	_____
25. Wash hands.	☐	☐	_____	_____
26. Record procedure.	☐	☐	_____	_____

Check-off Sheet:
18-73 Emptying the Urinary Drainage Bag

Name _____ **Date** _____

Directions: Practice this procedure, following each step. When you are ready to have your performance evaluated, give this sheet to your instructor. Review the detailed procedure in your textbook.

Procedure	Pass	Redo	Date Competency Met	Instructor Initials
Student must use Standard Precautions.	☐	☐	_____	_____
Preprocedure				
1. Wash hands.	☐	☐	_____	_____
2. Identify patient and explain procedure.	☐	☐	_____	_____
3. Provide privacy with curtain, screen, or door.	☐	☐	_____	_____
4. Assemble equipment.				
a. Graduate or measuring cup	☐	☐	_____	_____
b. Disposable gloves	☐	☐	_____	_____
c. Paper towel	☐	☐	_____	_____
d. An alcohol swab	☐	☐	_____	_____
5. Put on disposable gloves.	☐	☐	_____	_____
Procedure				
6. Place towel on floor and set graduate cylinder on top of the towel.	☐	☐	_____	_____
7. Carefully open drain outlet on urinary bag. *Do not allow container outlet to touch floor*! This will introduce microorganisms into bag and can cause infection.	☐	☐	_____	_____
8. Drain bag into graduate and clean drain outlet with alcohol swab. Then reattach drainage outlet securely.	☐	☐	_____	_____
9. Observe urine for:				
a. Dark color	☐	☐	_____	_____
b. Blood	☐	☐	_____	_____
c. Unusual odor	☐	☐	_____	_____
d. Large amount of mucus	☐	☐	_____	_____
e. Sediment	☐	☐	_____	_____

Procedure	Pass	Redo	Date Competency Met	Instructor Initials
10. Report any unusual observations to nurse immediately (do not discard urine).	☐	☐	_____	_____
11. Hold graduate at eye level and read amount of urine on measuring scale.	☐	☐	_____	_____
12. Discard urine if normal. Flush toilet and turn on faucet with paper towel.	☐	☐	_____	_____
13. Rinse graduate and put away.	☐	☐	_____	_____

Postprocedure

14. Remove gloves and discard in hazardous waste.	☐	☐	_____	_____
15. Wash hands.	☐	☐	_____	_____
16. Record amount of urine in cc's on the I & O record.	☐	☐	_____	_____

Check-off Sheet:
18-74 Collect Specimen Under Transmission-Based Precautions

Name _____ Date _____

Directions: Practice this procedure, following each step. When you are ready to have your performance evaluated, give this sheet to your instructor. Review the detailed procedure in your textbook.

Procedure	Pass	Redo	Date Competency Met	Instructor Initials
Student must use Standard Precautions.	☐	☐	_____	_____

Preprocedure

Procedure	Pass	Redo	Date Competency Met	Instructor Initials
1. Collect the equipment necessary for obtaining the specimen (specimen cup, lab tubes, tourniquets, etc.)	☐	☐	_____	_____
2. Wash hands.	☐	☐	_____	_____
3. Put on disposable gloves, gowns, mask, and protective eyewear as may be required depending on the specimen to be collected.	☐	☐	_____	_____

Procedure

Procedure	Pass	Redo	Date Competency Met	Instructor Initials
4. Provide an explanation to the patient regarding the specimen to be collected. Answer any questions the patient may have.	☐	☐	_____	_____
5. Collect the specimen using aseptic or sterile technique as required.	☐	☐	_____	_____
6. Label the specimen with the patient's name, date, and time of collection.	☐	☐	_____	_____
7. Place the specimen in a protective package as prescribed by the institution.	☐	☐	_____	_____
8. Assure that the patient has no further needs.	☐	☐	_____	_____
9. Dispose of any used supplies and any protective items used in the collection of the specimen in the appropriate manner, as determined by your institution.	☐	☐	_____	_____

Postprocedure

Procedure	Pass	Redo	Date Competency Met	Instructor Initials
10. Wash hands.	☐	☐	_____	_____
11. Send the specimen to the laboratory.	☐	☐	_____	_____

Check-off Sheet:

18-75 Routine Urine Specimen

Name _____ Date _____

Directions: Practice this procedure, following each step. When you are ready to have your performance evaluated, give this sheet to your instructor. Review the detailed procedure in your textbook.

Procedure	Pass	Redo	Date Competency Met	Instructor Initials
Student must use Standard Precautions.	☐	☐	_____	_____
Preprocedure				
1. Wash hands.	☐	☐	_____	_____
2. Assemble equipment:				
a. Graduate (pitcher)	☐	☐	_____	_____
b. Bedpan or urinal	☐	☐	_____	_____
c. Urine specimen container	☐	☐	_____	_____
d. Label	☐	☐	_____	_____
e. Paper bag	☐	☐	_____	_____
f. Disposable nonsterile gloves	☐	☐	_____	_____
3. Identify patient.	☐	☐	_____	_____
4. Explain what you are going to do.	☐	☐	_____	_____
5. Label specimen carefully:	☐	☐	_____	_____
a. Patient's name	☐	☐	_____	_____
b. Date	☐	☐	_____	_____
c. Time	☐	☐	_____	_____
d. Room number	☐	☐	_____	_____
6. Provide privacy by pulling privacy curtain.	☐	☐	_____	_____
7. Put on gloves.	☐	☐	_____	_____
8. Have patient void (urinate) into clean bedpan or urinal.	☐	☐	_____	_____
9. Ask patient to put toilet tissue into paper bag.	☐	☐	_____	_____
10. Pour specimen into graduate.	☐	☐	_____	_____
11. Pour from graduate into specimen container until about three-quarters full.	☐	☐	_____	_____
12. Place lid on container.	☐	☐	_____	_____
13. Discard leftover urine.	☐	☐	_____	_____

Procedure	Pass	Redo	Date Competency Met	Instructor Initials
14. Clean and rinse graduate, bedpan, or urinal, and put away.	☐	☐	_____	_____
15. Remove gloves.	☐	☐	_____	_____
16. Position patient comfortably.	☐	☐	_____	_____
17. Assist patient to wash hands.	☐	☐	_____	_____
Postprocedure				
18. Wash hands.	☐	☐	_____	_____
19. Store specimen according to direction for lab pickup.	☐	☐	_____	_____
20. Report and record procedure and observation of specimen.	☐	☐	_____	_____

Check-off Sheet:
18-76 Midstream Clean-Catch Urine, Female

Name _____ Date _____

Directions: Practice this procedure, following each step. When you are ready to have your performance evaluated, give this sheet to your instructor. Review the detailed procedure in your textbook.

Procedure	Pass	Redo	Date Competency Met	Instructor Initials
Student must use Standard Precautions.	☐	☐	_____	_____
Preprocedure				
1. Wash hands.	☐	☐	_____	_____
2. Assemble equipment:				
a. Antiseptic solution or soap and water or towelettes	☐	☐	_____	_____
b. Sterile specimen container	☐	☐	_____	_____
c. Tissues	☐	☐	_____	_____
d. Nonsterile gloves	☐	☐	_____	_____
3. Identify patient.	☐	☐	_____	_____
4. Explain what you are going to do.	☐	☐	_____	_____
Procedure				
5. Label specimen carefully:	☐	☐	_____	_____
a. Patient's name	☐	☐	_____	_____
b. Time obtained	☐	☐	_____	_____
c. Date	☐	☐	_____	_____
6. If patient is on bedrest:				
a. Put on gloves.	☐	☐	_____	_____
b. Lower side rail.	☐	☐	_____	_____
c. Position bedpan under patient.	☐	☐	_____	_____
7. Have patient carefully clean perineal area if able; if not, you will be responsible for cleaning perineum:	☐	☐	_____	_____
a. Wipe with towelette or gauze with antiseptic solution from front to back.	☐	☐	_____	_____
b. Wipe one side and throw away wipe.	☐	☐	_____	_____
c. Use a clean wipe for other side.	☐	☐	_____	_____
d. Use another wipe down center.	☐	☐	_____	_____
e. Then proceed with collecting midstream urine.	☐	☐	_____	_____

Procedure	Pass	Redo	Date Competency Met	Instructor Initials
8. Explain procedure if patient can obtain own specimen.	☐	☐	_____	_____
a. Have patient start to urinate into bedpan/toilet.	☐	☐	_____	_____
b. Allow stream to begin.	☐	☐	_____	_____
c. Stop stream and place specimen container to collect midstream..	☐	☐	_____	_____
d. Remove container before bladder is empty.	☐	☐	_____	_____
9. Wipe perineum, if on bedpan.	☐	☐	_____	_____
10. Remove bedpan.	☐	☐	_____	_____
11. Rinse bedpan and put away.	☐	☐	_____	_____
12. Remove gloves and discard according to facility policy and procedure.	☐	☐	_____	_____
13. Raise side rail.	☐	☐	_____	_____
14. Secure call light in patient's reach.	☐	☐	_____	_____
15. Dispose of equipment. Never handle contaminated equipment without gloves.	☐	☐	_____	_____

Postprocedure

Procedure	Pass	Redo	Date Competency Met	Instructor Initials
16. Wash hands.	☐	☐	_____	_____
17. Record specimen collection.	☐	☐	_____	_____
18. Report any unusual:	☐	☐	_____	_____
a. Color	☐	☐	_____	_____
b. Consistency	☐	☐	_____	_____
c. Odor	☐	☐	_____	_____

Check-off Sheet:
18-77 Midstream Clean-Catch Urine, Male

Name _____ Date _____

Directions: Practice this procedure, following each step. When you are ready to have your performance evaluated, give this sheet to your instructor. Review the detailed procedure in your textbook.

Procedure	Pass	Redo	Date Competency Met	Instructor Initials
Student must use Standard Precautions.	☐	☐	_____	_____
Preprocedure				
1. Wash hands.	☐	☐	_____	_____
2. Assemble equipment:				
a. Antiseptic solution or soap and water or towelettes	☐	☐	_____	_____
b. Sterile specimen container	☐	☐	_____	_____
c. Tissues	☐	☐	_____	_____
d. Disposable gloves				
3. Identify patient.	☐	☐	_____	_____
Procedure				
4. Label specimen:	☐	☐	_____	_____
a. Patient's name	☐	☐	_____	_____
b. Date	☐	☐	_____	_____
c. Time obtained	☐	☐	_____	_____
5. Explain procedure (if possible allow patient to obtain his own specimen).	☐	☐	_____	_____
a. Put on gloves.	☐	☐	_____	_____
b. Cleanse head of penis in a circular motion with towelette or gauze and antiseptic. (If patient is uncircumcised, have him pull back foreskin before cleaning.)	☐	☐	_____	_____
c. Have patient start to urinate into clean bedpan, urinal, or toilet. (If he is uncircumcised have patient pull back foreskin before urinating.)	☐	☐	_____	_____
d. Allow stream to begin.	☐	☐	_____	_____
e. Stop stream and place specimen container to collect midstream.	☐	☐	_____	_____
f. Remove container before bladder is empty.	☐	☐	_____	_____
6. Dispose of equipment according to facility policy.	☐	☐	_____	_____

Procedure	Pass	Redo	Date Competency Met	Instructor Initials
Postprocedure				
7. Remove and discard gloves according to facility policy and procedure.	☐	☐	_____	_____
8. Make patient comfortable and put call bell within reach.	☐	☐	_____	_____
9. Wash hands.	☐	☐	_____	_____
10. Record specimen collection.	☐	☐	_____	_____

Check-off Sheet:
18-78 HemaCombistix

Name _____ **Date** _____

Directions: Practice this procedure, following each step. When you are ready to have your performance evaluated, give this sheet to your instructor. Review the detailed procedure in your textbook.

Procedure	Pass	Redo	Date Competency Met	Instructor Initials
Student must use Standard Precautions.	☐	☐	_____	_____
Preprocedure				
1. Wash hands.	☐	☐	_____	_____
2. Assemble equipment:				
a. Bottle of HemaCombistix	☐	☐	_____	_____
b. Nonsterile gloves	☐	☐	_____	_____
3. Identify patient.	☐	☐	_____	_____
4. Explain what you are going to do.	☐	☐	_____	_____
5. Put on gloves.	☐	☐	_____	_____
Procedure				
6. Secure fresh urine sample form patient.	☐	☐	_____	_____
7. Take urine and reagent to bathroom.	☐	☐	_____	_____
8. Remove cap and place on flat surface. Be sure top side of cap is down.	☐	☐	_____	_____
9. Remove strip from bottle gently. *Do not touch areas of strip with fingers.*	☐	☐	_____	_____
10. Dip reagent stick in urine. Remove immediately.	☐	☐	_____	_____
11. Tap edge of strip on container to remove excess urine.	☐	☐	_____	_____
12. Compare reagent side of test areas with color chart on bottle. Use time intervals that are given on bottle.				
13. Remove gloves and discard both strip and urine specimen according to facility policy and procedure. Need to discard specimen and then take off gloves.	☐	☐	_____	_____
Postprocedure				
14. Replace equipment.	☐	☐	_____	_____
15. Wash hands.	☐	☐	_____	_____
16. Record results.	☐	☐	_____	_____
a. Date and time	☐	☐	_____	_____
b. Name of procedure used	☐	☐	_____	_____
c. Results	☐	☐	_____	_____

Check-off Sheet:
18-79 Straining Urine

Name _____ Date _____

Directions: Practice this procedure, following each step. When you are ready to have your performance evaluated, give this sheet to your instructor. Review the detailed procedure in your textbook.

Procedure	Pass	Redo	Date Competency Met	Instructor Initials
Student must use Standard Precautions.	☐	☐	_____	_____
Preprocedure				
1. Wash hands.	☐	☐	_____	_____
2. Assemble equipment:				
a. Paper strainers or gauze	☐	☐	_____	_____
b. Specimen container and label	☐	☐	_____	_____
c. Bedpan or urinal and cover	☐	☐	_____	_____
d. Laboratory request for analysis of specimen	☐	☐	_____	_____
e. Sign for patient's room or bathroom explaining that all urine must be strained	☐	☐	_____	_____
f. Nonsterile gloves	☐	☐	_____	_____
Procedure				
4. Tell the patient to urinate into a urinal or bedpan and that the nurse assistant must be called to filter each specimen. Tell patient not to put paper in specimen.	☐	☐	_____	_____
5. Put on gloves.	☐	☐	_____	_____
6. Pour voided specimen through a paper strainer or gauze into a measuring container.	☐	☐	_____	_____
7. Place paper or gauze strainer into a dry specimen container if stones or particles are present after pouring urine through.	☐	☐	_____	_____
8. Measure the amount voided and record on intake and output record.	☐	☐	_____	_____
9. Discard urine and container according to facility policy and procedure.	☐	☐	_____	_____
10. Clean urinal or bedpan and put away. Flush toilet and turn faucet on with a paper towel.	☐	☐	_____	_____
11. Remove gloves and discard according to facility policy and procedure.	☐	☐	_____	_____
12. Wash hands.	☐	☐	_____	_____

Procedure	Pass	Redo	Date Competency Met	Instructor Initials
13. Label specimen:	☐	☐	_____	_____
a. Patient's name	☐	☐	_____	_____
b. Date	☐	☐	_____	_____
c. Room number	☐	☐	_____	_____
d. Time	☐	☐	_____	_____
14. Return patient to comfortable position.	☐	☐	_____	_____
15. Place call button within reach of patient.	☐	☐	_____	_____
16. Provide for patient safety by raising side rails when indicated or using postural supports as ordered.	☐	☐	_____	_____

Postprocedure

Procedure	Pass	Redo	Date Competency Met	Instructor Initials
17. Wash hands.	☐	☐	_____	_____
18. Report collection of specimen to supervisor immediately.	☐	☐	_____	_____
19. Record specimen collection.	☐	☐	_____	_____

Check-off Sheet:
18-80 Stool Specimen Collection
Name _____ **Date** _____

Directions: Practice this procedure, following each step. When you are ready to have your performance evaluated, give this sheet to your instructor. Review the detailed procedure in your textbook.

Procedure	Pass	Redo	Date Competency Met	Instructor Initials
Student must use Standard Precautions.	☐	☐	_____	_____
Preprocedure				
1. Wash hands.	☐	☐	_____	_____
2. Assemble equipment:				
a. Stool specimen container with label	☐	☐	_____	_____
b. Wooden tongue depressor	☐	☐	_____	_____
c. Disposable gloves	☐	☐	_____	_____
d. Bedpan and cover	☐	☐	_____	_____
3. Identify patient.	☐	☐	_____	_____
4. Explain what you are going to do.	☐	☐	_____	_____
Procedure				
5. Be certain container is properly labeled with:				
a. Patient's name	☐	☐	_____	_____
b. Time	☐	☐	_____	_____
c. Date	☐	☐	_____	_____
d. Room number	☐	☐	_____	_____
6. Provide privacy by pulling privacy curtains.	☐	☐	_____	_____
7. Put on gloves.	☐	☐	_____	_____
8. Take bedpan into bathroom after patient has had bowel movement.	☐	☐	_____	_____
9. Use tongue depressor to remove about 1 to 2 tablespoons of feces from bedpan.	☐	☐	_____	_____
10. Place in specimen container.	☐	☐	_____	_____
11. Patient's name.	☐	☐	_____	_____
12. Wrap tongue depressor in paper towel and discard as per facility rules.	☐	☐	_____	_____
13. Remove gloves and dispose of according to facility policy.	☐	☐	_____	_____

Procedure	Pass	Redo	Date Competency Met	Instructor Initials
Postprocedure				
14. Wash hands.	☐	☐	_____	_____
15. Follow instruction for storage of specimen for collection by lab.	☐	☐	_____	_____
16. Position patient comfortably with call bell in place.	☐	☐	_____	_____
17. Report and record procedure.	☐	☐	_____	_____

Check-off Sheet:
18-81 Occult Blood Hematest

Name _____ Date _____

Directions: Practice this procedure, following each step. When you are ready to have your performance evaluated, give this sheet to your instructor. Review the detailed procedure in your textbook.

Procedure	Pass	Redo	Date Competency Met	Instructor Initials
Student must use Standard Precautions.	☐	☐	_____	_____
Preprocedure				
1. Wash hands.	☐	☐	_____	_____
2. Assemble equipment:				
a. Hematest Reagent filter paper	☐	☐	_____	_____
b. Hematest Reagent tablet	☐	☐	_____	_____
c. Distilled water	☐	☐	_____	_____
d. Tongue blade	☐	☐	_____	_____
e. Disposable gloves	☐	☐	_____	_____
3. Identify patient.	☐	☐	_____	_____
4. Explain what you are going to do.	☐	☐	_____	_____
5. Put on gloves.	☐	☐	_____	_____
Procedure				
6. Secure stool specimen from patient.	☐	☐	_____	_____
7. Place filter paper on glass or porcelain plate.	☐	☐	_____	_____
8. Use tongue blade to smear a thin streak of fecal material on filter paper.	☐	☐	_____	_____
9. Place Hematest Reagent tablet on smear.	☐	☐	_____	_____
10. Place 1 drop distilled water on tablet.	☐	☐	_____	_____
11. Allow 5 to 10 seconds for water to penetrate tablet.	☐	☐	_____	_____
12. Add second drop, allowing water to run down side of tablet onto filter paper and specimen.	☐	☐	_____	_____
13. Gently tap side of plate to knock water droplets from top of tablet.	☐	☐	_____	_____
14. Observe filter paper for color change (2 minutes). Positive is indicated by blue halo on paper.	☐	☐	_____	_____
15. Dispose of specimen and equipment according to your facility's policy.	☐	☐	_____	_____
16. Remove gloves and dispose of according to your facility's policy.	☐	☐	_____	_____

Procedure	Pass	Redo	Date Competency Met	Instructor Initials
Postprocedure				
17. Wash hands.	☐	☐	_____	_____
18. Report and record results (e.g., date, time, procedure, and results).	☐	☐	_____	_____

Check-off Sheet:

18-82 24-Hour Urine Test

Name _____ Date _____

Directions: Practice this procedure, following each step. When you are ready to have your performance evaluated, give this sheet to your instructor. Review the detailed procedure in your textbook.

Procedure	Pass	Redo	Date Competency Met	Instructor Initials
Student must use Standard Precautions.	☐	☐	_____	_____

Preprocedure

1. Determine the laboratory test and any special requirements associated with the test.

   This could include altering the dietary intake, special collection containers, adding preservatives to the designated container, icing the container, etc. ☐ ☐ _____ _____

2. The nurse should determine if any drugs affect the results of this test. Obtain a history of any drugs that patient is currently taking and advise the laboratory as necessary. ☐ ☐ _____ _____

3. Obtain the appropriate container to be used for urine collection. Label the container with the patient's name, hospital number, date, and time of the urine collection. ☐ ☐ _____ _____

Procedure

4. Explain the procedure to the patient. Provide a means for the patient to collect their urinary output, if the patient is able to participate in the procedure. ☐ ☐ _____ _____

5. Post a sign that all urine is to be collect for a specified time. Assure that all staff providing care for this patient during this period of time are aware of the need to save all urine output. ☐ ☐ _____ _____

6. When initiating the collection the patient will empty his bladder, and this specimen will be discarded. All urine produced after this time will be saved. At the end of the time period, the patient will again empty his bladder and this last specimen will be added to the specimen container. ☐ ☐ _____ _____

7. If any urine is inadvertently discarded during the 24-hour collection, the test must be restarted. ☐ ☐ _____ _____

Postprocedure

8. At the end of the test period, transport the labeled specimen to the laboratory. ☐ ☐ _____ _____

Chapter 19

Therapeutic Techniques and Sports Medicine

Therapeutic Techniques and Sports Medicine

- ● **OBJECTIVES**

  When you have completed this section, you will be able to do the following:

  - ■ Describe the responsibilities of a physical therapy aide.

  - ■ Describe the responsibilities of a sports medicine aide.

  - ■ Define ultraviolet light and name four conditions treated with ultraviolet light.

  - ■ Describe four conditions treated with diathermy.

  - ■ List three conditions commonly treated by ultrasound.

  - ■ Document the most important question to ask a patient when preparing for an ultrasound treatment.

  - ■ Identify two kinds of thermotherapy and the conditions they treat.

  - ■ Identify two ways to give cryotherapy and conditions they treat.

  - ■ Define hydrotherapy and list three reasons hydrotherapy is used.

  - ■ Explain the purpose of range of motion.

- ● **DIRECTIONS**

  1. Complete Worksheet 1.

  2. Complete Worksheets 2 through 4 as assigned.

  3. Demonstrate all procedures.

  4. Prepare responses to each item listed in Chapter Review.

5. When you are confident that you can meet each objective for this section, ask your teacher for the section evaluation.

● EVALUATION METHODS

- Worksheets/Activities
- Class participation
- Written evaluation
- Return demonstrations

● WORKSHEET 1

1. Place an *X* next to the duties of a physical therapy aide (8 points).

_____	Suction the mouth	_____	Prepare equipment
_____	Feed the patient	_____	Prepare hot packs
_____	Clean work area	_____	Give medication
_____	Position patient	_____	Clean equipment
_____	Prepare paraffin baths	_____	Daily census
_____	Fold linen	_____	Assist patient to dress and undress
_____	Take x-rays	_____	Prepare food

2. Describe the responsibilities of a physical therapy aide (5 points).

_____

_____

_____

3. List four conditions for which ultraviolet light treatments are used (4 points).

a. _____

b. _____

c. _____

d. _____

4. List four conditions for which diathermy treatments are often used (4 points).

a. _____

b. _____

c. _____

d. _____

5. Describe in your own words what diathermy treatments do to the treated area (2 points).

   _____

   _____

   _____

6. Explain the physical therapy aide's main responsibility when setting up a patient for a diathermy treatment (5 points).

   _____

   _____

   _____

7. List the three conditions commonly treated by ultrasound (3 points).

   a. _____

   b. _____

   c. _____

8. State the most important question a patient must be asked when being prepared for an ultrasound treatment (1 point).

   _____

   _____

9. Define the following terms (3 points):

   a. hydrotherapy _____

   b. guarding technique_____

   c. guarding belt _____

10. Explain the purpose of range of motion exercises (5 points). _____

   _____

   _____

11. Name two ways range of motion can be done (2 points).

   a. _____

   b. _____

12. Define adaptive devices (2 points). _____

   _____

There are 44 possible points in this worksheet.

● WORKSHEET 2

1. How is a sports medicine aide related to a physical therapy aide (2 points)?

   _____

   _____

   _____

2. List the responsibilities of a sports medicine aide (6 points)?

a. _____

b. _____

c. _____

d. _____

e. _____

f. _____

3. What is the role of massage in sports medicine (2 points)?

_____

_____

_____

There are 10 possible points in this worksheet.

● WORKSHEET 3

1. Define thermotherapy (3 points).

_____

_____

_____

2. Identify two kinds of thermotherapy and how each is given (4 points).

a. _____

b. _____

3. Define cryotherapy (3 points). _____

_____

_____

4. Identify two ways to give cryotherapy and how they are given (4 points).

a. _____

b. _____

There are 14 possible points in this worksheet.

● WORKSHEET 4

1. What is an ambulation device (1 point)? _____

_____

_____

2. List five commonly used ambulation devices (5 points).

a. _____

b. _____

    c. _____

    d. _____

    e. _____

3. What is a transporting device (1 point)? _____

_____

_____

4. List two commonly used transporting devices (2 points).

    a. _____

    b. _____

There are 9 possible points in this worksheet.

CHECK-OFF SHEET:
19-1 Preparing Moist Hot Soaks

Name _____ Date _____

Directions: Practice this procedure, following each step. When you are ready to have your performance evaluated, give this sheet to your instructor. Review the detailed procedure in your textbook.

Procedure	Pass	Redo	Date Competency Met	Instructor Initials
Student must use Standard Precautions.	☐	☐	_____	_____
Preprocedure				
1. Check physician's orders.	☐	☐	_____	_____
2. Wash hands.	☐	☐	_____	_____
3. Assemble equipment:				
a. Hydroculator pad	☐	☐	_____	_____
b. Towel	☐	☐	_____	_____
4. Identify patient.	☐	☐	_____	_____
5. Explain what you will be doing and reassure patient that procedure is painless.	☐	☐	_____	_____
6. Provide privacy.	☐	☐	_____	_____
7. Cover warm hydroculator pad with towel.	☐	☐	_____	_____
8. Expose site to be treated.	☐	☐	_____	_____
9. Position patient for comfort.	☐	☐	_____	_____
Procedure				
10. Apply covered warm hydroculator pad to appropriate site. (Never put warm hydroculator pad directly on the skin, unless it is covered.)	☐	☐	_____	_____
11. Make sure call bell is in reach.	☐	☐	_____	_____
12. Wash hands.	☐	☐	_____	_____
13. Recheck patient frequently—every 5 minutes when heating device is on skin. Look for:	☐	☐	_____	_____
a. Severely reddened areas	☐	☐	_____	_____
b. Irritated areas	☐	☐	_____	_____
c. Painful areas	☐	☐	_____	_____
14. Remove soaks as ordered.	☐	☐	_____	_____
Postprocedure				
15. Position patient for comfort and make sure call bell is in reach.	☐	☐	_____	_____
16. Wash hands.	☐	☐	_____	_____
17. Report and record patient's tolerance of treatment and any changes in condition you observed.	☐	☐	_____	_____

CHECK-OFF SHEET:
19-2 Moist Cryotherapy (Cold) Compress

Name _____ Date _____

Directions: Practice this procedure, following each step. When you are ready to have your performance evaluated, give this sheet to your instructor. Review the detailed procedure in your textbook.

Procedure	Pass	Redo	Date Competency Met	Instructor Initials
Student must use Standard Precautions.	☐	☐	_____	_____
Preprocedure				
1. Check doctor's orders.	☐	☐	_____	_____
2. Wash hands.	☐	☐	_____	_____
3. Assemble equipment:				
a. Cool, wet cloth	☐	☐	_____	_____
b. Plastic cover	☐	☐	_____	_____
c. Dry towel	☐	☐	_____	_____
Procedure	☐	☐	_____	_____
4. Explain procedure to patient.	☐	☐	_____	_____
5. Apply cool, wet cloth to patient as ordered.	☐	☐	_____	_____
6. Cover area with plastic cover.	☐	☐	_____	_____
7. Cover plastic with dry towel.	☐	☐	_____	_____
8. Wash hands.	☐	☐	_____	_____
9. Recheck frequently for:				
a. Coolness of cloth	☐	☐	_____	_____
b. Position	☐	☐	_____	_____
c. Patient's comfort needs (reapply PRN)	☐	☐	_____	_____
10. Remove as ordered.	☐	☐	_____	_____
Postprocedure	☐	☐	_____	_____
11. Dry skin.	☐	☐	_____	_____
12. Dispose of supplies and clean area.	☐	☐	_____	_____
13. Wash hands.	☐	☐	_____	_____
14. Report and document effects of treatment.	☐	☐	_____	_____

CHECK-OFF SHEET:
19-3 Dry Cryotherapy: Ice Bags/Ice Collars

Name _____ Date _____

Directions: Practice this procedure, following each step. When you are ready to have your performance evaluated, give this sheet to your instructor. Review the detailed procedure in your textbook.

Procedure	Pass	Redo	Date Competency Met	Instructor Initials
Student must use Standard Precautions.	☐	☐	_____	_____
Preprocedure				
1. Check physician's orders.	☐	☐	_____	_____
2. Wash hands.	☐	☐	_____	_____
3. Assemble equipment:				
a. Ice bag or commercial cold compress	☐	☐	_____	_____
b. Ice	☐	☐	_____	_____
c. Cover for ice bag	☐	☐	_____	_____
4. Fill bag with ice. (Run water over cubes to soften sharp edges.)	☐	☐	_____	_____
5. Remove air from bag by pressing sides together.	☐	☐	_____	_____
6. Close end and check for leaks.	☐	☐	_____	_____
7. Cover bag with cloth or towel. (Never apply bag directly to skin; it may stick, burn, and tear skin when removed.)	☐	☐	_____	_____
8. Identify patient by checking order and name with patient's armband or patient chart.	☐	☐	_____	_____
Procedure				
9. Explain procedure to patient.	☐	☐	_____	_____
10. Gently position ice bag as ordered. (The metal cap cannot touch the skin.)	☐	☐	_____	_____
11. Secure bag so that it does not move away from affected area.	☐	☐	_____	_____
12. Provide needed comfort measures for patient and make sure call bell is in reach.	☐	☐	_____	_____
13. Wash hands.	☐	☐	_____	_____
14. Return frequently to check for:				
a. Coolness of ice bag	☐	☐	_____	_____
b. Position of ice bag	☐	☐	_____	_____
c. Color of skin (remove ice if skin is white or bluish in color or if patient reports numbness and report)	☐	☐	_____	_____

Procedure	Pass	Redo	Date Competency Met	Instructor Initials
15. Remove ice bag at ordered time.	☐	☐	_____	_____
16. Make sure patient is comfortable and call bell is in reach.	☐	☐	_____	_____
Postprocedure	☐	☐	_____	_____
17. Recheck skin, and report and document effects of treatment.	☐	☐	_____	_____
18. Wash hands.	☐	☐	_____	_____
19. Empty bag, dry, and return to appropriate area for cleaning.	☐	☐	_____	_____

CHECK-OFF SHEET:
19-4 Range of Motion

Name _____ Date _____

Directions: Practice this procedure, following each step. When you are ready to have your performance evaluated, give this sheet to your instructor. Review the detailed procedure in your textbook.

Procedure	Pass	Redo	Date Competency Met	Instructor Initials
Student must use Standard Precautions.	☐	☐	_____	_____
Preprocedure				
1. Wash hands.	☐	☐	_____	_____
2. Assemble equipment:				
a. Sheet or bath blanket	☐	☐	_____	_____
b. Treatment table or bed	☐	☐	_____	_____
c. Good lighting	☐	☐	_____	_____
3. Identify patient.	☐	☐	_____	_____
4. Explain what you are going to do.	☐	☐	_____	_____
5. Ask visitors to wait outside, and provide privacy.	☐	☐	_____	_____
Procedure				
6. Place patient in a supine position on bed or treatment table and cover with sheet or bath blanket. Only expose affected area. Instruct patient to do the following movements at least five times each or to tolerance.	☐	☐	_____	_____
Head Flexion and Extension				
7. Bend head until chin touches chest (flexion), then gently bend backward (extension).	☐	☐	_____	_____
Right/Left Rotation				
8. Turn head to right (right rotation), then turn head to left (left rotation).	☐	☐	_____	_____
Right/Left Lateral Flexion				
9. Move head so that right ear moves toward right shoulder (right lateral flexion), then move head to central position and continue moving head so that left ear moves toward left shoulder (left lateral flexion).	☐	☐	_____	_____
Hyperextension and Extension				
10. Place the pillow under the shoulders and gently support the head in a backward tilt and return to straight position. Readjust pillow under head when finished.	☐	☐	_____	_____

Procedure	Pass	Redo	Date Competency Met	Instructor Initials

Shoulder Flexion and Extension

11. Raise one arm overhead keeping elbow straight. Return to side position. Repeat with other arm. □ □ _____ _____

12. With the shoulder in abduction, flex the elbow and raise the entire arm over the head. □ □ _____ _____

Shoulder Abduction and Adduction

13. Raise arm overhead, then lower, keep arm out to side. Repeat with other arm. □ □ _____ _____

14. With the shoulder in abduction, flex the elbow and raise the arm over the head. □ □ _____ _____

Internal and External Rotation of Shoulder

15. Roll entire arm toward body and away. □ □ _____ _____

Elbow Flexion and Extension

16. Bend one hand and forearm toward shoulder (flexion) and straighten (extension). Repeat with other arm. □ □ _____ _____

Forearm Pronation and Supination

17. Bend arm at elbow and rotate hand toward body (pronation), then rotate away from body (supination). Repeat with other arm. □ □ _____ _____

Wrist Flexion and Extension

18. Bend hand at wrist toward shoulder (flex), then gently force backward past a level position with arm (extension) to below arm level (hyperextension). Repeat with other hand. □ □ _____ _____

Ulnar and Radial Deviation

19. Holding hand straight, move toward thumb (radial deviation), then move hand toward little finger (ulnar deviation). Repeat with other hand. □ □ _____ _____

Finger Flexion and Extension

20. Bend thumb and fingers into hand making a fist (flexion), then open hand by straightening fingers and thumb (extension). Repeat with other hand. □ □ _____ _____

21. Move thumb away from hand (abduct), then toward hand (adduct). Repeat with other hand. □ □ _____ _____

Finger/Thumb Opposition

22. Move thumb toward little finger, touch tips. Touch tip of thumb to each finger. Open hand each time. Repeat with other hand. □ □ _____ _____

Procedure	Pass	Redo	Date Competency Met	Instructor Initials
Finger Adduction and Abduction				
23. Keeping fingers straight, separate them (abduction), then bring them together (adduction).Repeat with other hand.	☐	☐	_____	_____
Hip/Knee Flexion and Extension				
24. Raise leg, bend knee, then return to bed straightening knee. Repeat with other leg.	☐	☐	_____	_____
Straight Leg Raising				
25. Keep knee straight. Slowly raise and lower leg. Repeat with other leg.	☐	☐	_____	_____
Hip Abduction and Adduction				
26. Supporting the knee and ankle, separate legs (abduction), then bring back together (adduction). Then turn both legs so knees face outward. Turn legs so knees face inward.	☐	☐	_____	_____
Lateral and Medial Hip Rotation				
27. Roll leg in a circular fashion away from body and then toward body.	☐	☐	_____	_____
28. Rotate one foot toward other foot (internal rotation), then rotate away from other foot (external rotation). Repeat with other foot.	☐	☐	_____	_____
Ankle Dorsiflexion and Plantar Flexion				
29. Grasp toes while supporting ankle. Move foot so that toes move toward knee (dorsi flexion), then move foot so that toes point away from head(plantar flexion). Repeat with other foot.	☐	☐	_____	_____
Toe Flexion and Extension				
30. Spread toes apart (abduction) on one foot, then bring toes together (adduction). Repeat on other foot.	☐	☐	_____	_____
31. Turn patient in a prone position.	☐	☐	_____	_____
Arm Abduction and Adduction				
32. Move arm toward ceiling; do not bend elbows (hyperextension), then return to bed. Repeat with other arm.	☐	☐	_____	_____
Leg Flexion and Extension				
33. Bend leg so that foot moves toward patient's back (flexion), then straighten leg (extension). Repeat with other leg.	☐	☐	_____	_____
34. Position patient for comfort.	☐	☐	_____	_____

Procedure	Pass	Redo	Date Competency Met	Instructor Initials
Postprocedure				
35. Place bath blanket or sheet in laundry basket.	☐	☐	_____	_____
36. Wash your hands.	☐	☐	_____	_____
37. Report and document patient's tolerance of procedure.	☐	☐	_____	_____

CHECK-OFF SHEET:
19-5 Wrapping/Taping an Ankle
Name _____ **Date** _____

Directions: Practice this procedure, following each step. When you are ready to have your performance evaluated, give this sheet to your instructor. Review the detailed procedure in your textbook.

Procedure	Pass	Redo	Date Competency Met	Instructor Initials
Student must use Standard Precautions.	☐	☐	_____	_____
Preprocedure				
1. Identify the patient and joint which requires the use of a supportive bandage. Check the physician's order for any special instructions. Gather the appropriate bandage.	☐	☐	_____	_____
2. Wash hands. Put on gloves.				
3. Explain the procedure to the patient. Assist the patient to a comfortable position that provides easy access to the affected joint.	☐	☐	_____	_____
Procedure	☐	☐	_____	_____
4. Remove any old bandage and discard. If the bandage is to be reused, it may be unwound by keeping the loose end together and passing it as a ball from one hand to the other while unwinding it. Assess the joint for mobility and pain.	☐	☐	_____	_____
5. Clean the area before reapplying bandage. Make sure skin is dry before re-wrapping.	☐	☐	_____	_____
6. To begin, the free end of the bandage roll is held in place with one hand while the other hand passes the roll around the top middle of the ankle and then around the back of the Achilles tendon. After the bandage is anchored, the roll is passed or tolled around the ankle.	☐	☐	_____	_____
7. After the bandage is anchored, the roll is passed or rolled under the foot and back up the outside of the ankle, taking care to exert equal tension in all turns. There should be even overlapping of one half to two-thirds the width of each bandage, except for the circular turn.	☐	☐	_____	_____
8. The figure-of-eight turn is most effective for use around joints such as the ankle. The figure-of-eight turns consists of making oblique overlapping turns that ascend and descend alternatively.	☐	☐	_____	_____

Procedure	Pass	Redo	Date Competency Met	Instructor Initials
Postprocedure				
9. Assure that the patient is comfortable and has no other needs before leaving the area.	☐	☐	_____	_____
10. Wash hands.	☐	☐	_____	_____
11. Document the appearance of the joint, any discomfort present and the application of the new bandage.	☐	☐	_____	_____

CHECK-OFF SHEET:
19-6 Elastic Hose (Antiembolism Hose)

Name _____ Date _____

Directions: Practice this procedure, following each step. When you are ready to have your performance evaluated, give this sheet to your instructor. Review the detailed procedure in your textbook.

Procedure	Pass	Redo	Date Competency Met	Instructor Initials
Student must use Standard Precautions.	☐	☐	_____	_____
Preprocedure				
1. Wash hands.	☐	☐	_____	_____
2. Select elastic hose. Check to be sure that they are the correct size and length.	☐	☐	_____	_____
3. Identify patient and explain procedure to patient.	☐	☐	_____	_____
4. Provide for patient's privacy.	☐	☐	_____	_____
5. Have patient lie down; expose one leg at a time.	☐	☐	_____	_____
Procedure				
6. Hold the hose with both hand at top and roll toward toe end. Turn stockings inside-out, at least to heel area.	☐	☐	_____	_____
7. Place hose over toes, positioning opening at base of toes unless toes are to be covered. The raised seams should be on outside.	☐	☐	_____	_____
8. Pull top of stocking over foot, heel, and leg. Move patient's foot and leg gently and naturally. Avoid forcing and overextending limbs and joints.	☐	☐	_____	_____
9. Check to be sure that the stocking is applied evenly and smoothly. There must be no wrinkles.	☐	☐	_____	_____
10. Repeat on opposite leg.	☐	☐	_____	_____
Postprocedure				
11. Make patient comfortable, lower bed and raise side rails. Make sure call bell is within reach of patient.	☐	☐	_____	_____
12. Wash hands.	☐	☐	_____	_____
13. Record the following in the medical record:	☐	☐	_____	_____
a. Date and time applied	☐	☐	_____	_____
b. Any skin changes, temperature change, or swelling	☐	☐	_____	_____
14. Remove and reapply at least once every 8 hours, or more often if necessary.	☐	☐	_____	_____

CHECK-OFF SHEET:

19-7 Ambulating with a Gait Belt

Name _____ Date _____

Directions: Practice this procedure, following each step. When you are ready to have your performance evaluated, give this sheet to your instructor. Review the detailed procedure in your textbook.

Procedure	Pass	Redo	Date Competency Met	Instructor Initials
Student must use Standard Precautions.	☐	☐	_____	_____
Preprocedure				
1. Wash hands.	☐	☐	_____	_____
2. Assemble equipment:				
a. Gait belt/walking belt (correct size)	☐	☐	_____	_____
b. Patient's robe	☐	☐	_____	_____
c. Patient's footwear	☐	☐	_____	_____
3. Identify patient.	☐	☐	_____	_____
4. Explain what you are going to do.	☐	☐	_____	_____
5. Provide for privacy and lower side rail.	☐	☐	_____	_____
6. Assist patient to sitting position on side of bed.	☐	☐	_____	_____
7. Encourage patient to take a few deep breaths and ask if he or she feels dizzy. (If dizziness is present, let the patient sit a while before walking.)	☐	☐	_____	_____
8. Assist patient with robe and slippers.	☐	☐	_____	_____
9. Secure gait belt around patient's waist over clothing.	☐	☐	_____	_____
10. Tighten belt and buckle securely. Position buckle/clasp slightly off center. Check to see if patient can breathe easily and that breasts are above the belt.	☐	☐	_____	_____
Procedure				
11. Stand in front of patient with broad base of support.	☐	☐	_____	_____
12. Instruct patient to put hands on your shoulder. Position yourself to ensure the safety of both yourself and the patient during transfer (e.g., knees bent, feet apart, back straight). Place hands under side of belt. Give signal for patient to stand.	☐	☐	_____	_____
13. Ease patient to a standing position and hold handgrip securely at back of belt.	☐	☐	_____	_____
14. Keep your back straight straighten knees as patient stands. Move to position behind patient. Keep one hand on side of belt and other hand should grasp the back of the belt.	☐	☐	_____	_____

Procedure	Pass	Redo	Date Competency Met	Instructor Initials
15. Ambulate patient as ordered.	☐	☐	_____	_____
16. Observe patient for weakness or discomfort.	☐	☐	_____	_____
17. Return patient to room and make comfortable.	☐	☐	_____	_____
18. Remove belt, help take off robe and slippers, position patient in bed, raise side rails, and make sure call bell is in place.	☐	☐	_____	_____
Postprocedure				
19. Document and report patient's tolerance of procedure.	☐	☐	_____	_____
20. Return gait belt to storage area so that it will be available for the next procedure.	☐	☐	_____	_____
21. Wash hands.	☐	☐	_____	_____

CHECK-OFF SHEET:
19-8 Walking with a Cane

Name _____   Date _____

Directions: Practice this procedure, following each step. When you are ready to have your performance evaluated, give this sheet to your instructor. Review the detailed procedure in your textbook.

Procedure	Pass	Redo	Date Competency Met	Instructor Initials
Student must use Standard Precautions.	☐	☐	_____	_____
Preprocedure				
1. Wash hands.	☐	☐	_____	_____
2. Assemble equipment:				
a. Cane in good repair and with rubber tip	☐	☐	_____	_____
b. Patient's footwear	☐	☐	_____	_____
c. Patient's robe	☐	☐	_____	_____
3. Identify patient.	☐	☐	_____	_____
4. Assist patient with shoes and robe.	☐	☐	_____	_____
5. Explain what you are going to do.	☐	☐	_____	_____
6. Provide privacy as appropriate.				
7. Assist to sitting position, feet resting on floor. Secure gait belt snug enough to provide support and loose enough to provide comfort. Place cane in reach.	☐	☐	_____	_____
8. Position patient in a standing position (have a co-worker help you, if necessary).	☐	☐	_____	_____
9. Check height of cane. Top of cane should be at the patient's hip joint.	☐	☐	_____	_____
Procedure				
10. Check arm position at side of body and holding top of cane. Arm should be bent at a 25° to 30°angle.	☐	☐	_____	_____
11. Have patient hold cane in hand on stronger side of body (unaffected side).	☐	☐	_____	_____
12. Assist patient as needed while ambulating:				
a. With cane in hand on stronger side, move cane and weaker foot forward.				
b. Place the body weight forward on cane and move stronger foot forward.	☐	☐	_____	_____
13. When you have completed ordered ambulation, return patient to the starting place.	☐	☐	_____	_____

Procedure	Pass	Redo	Date Competency Met	Instructor Initials
Postprocedure				
14. Provide for patient's comfort.	☐	☐	_____	_____
15. Place cane in proper location. If patient is capable and physician permits ambulation without assistance, leave cane in a convenient place for patient.	☐	☐	_____	_____
16. Wash hands.	☐	☐	_____	_____
17. Report and document patient's tolerance of procedure:				
a. Date	☐	☐	_____	_____
b. Time	☐	☐	_____	_____
c. Ambulated with cane (e.g., 15 minutes in hall)	☐	☐	_____	_____
d. How tolerated	☐	☐	_____	_____
e. Signature and classification	☐	☐	_____	_____

CHECK-OFF SHEET:
19-9 Walking with Crutches

Name _____ Date _____

Directions: Practice this procedure, following each step. When you are ready to have your performance evaluated, give this sheet to your instructor. Review the detailed procedure in your textbook.

Procedure	Pass	Redo	Date Competency Met	Instructor Initials
Student must use Standard Precautions.	☐	☐	_____	_____
Preprocedure				
1. Wash hands.	☐	☐	_____	_____
2. Assemble equipment:				
a. Crutches in good repair with rubber tips	☐	☐	_____	_____
b. Patient's footwear	☐	☐	_____	_____
c. Patient's robe, if necessary	☐	☐	_____	_____
3. Identify patient.	☐	☐	_____	_____
4. Explain what you are going to do.	☐	☐	_____	_____
5. Help patient with shoes and robe. Provide privacy as appropriate.	☐	☐	_____	_____
Procedure				
6. Check fit of crutches to patient.				
a. Have patient stand with crutches in place.	☐	☐	_____	_____
b. Position foot of crutches about 4 inches to side of patient's foot and slightly forward of foot.	☐	☐	_____	_____
c. Check distance between underarm and crutch underarm rest. It should be about 2 inches.	☐	☐	_____	_____
d. Check angle of patient's arm. When hand is on hand rest bar and crutches are in walking position, arms should be at a 30° angle.	☐	☐	_____	_____
7. Remind patient that the hands support most of the body weight.	☐	☐	_____	_____
8. Assist patient to ambulate following gait method ordered. There are a variety of crutch walking gaits:				
a. Three-point gait (beginners)				
(1) One leg is weight-bearing.	☐	☐	_____	_____
(2) Place both crutches forward along with nonweight-bearing foot.	☐	☐	_____	_____
(3) Shift weight to hands on crutches and move weight-bearing foot forward.	☐	☐	_____	_____

Procedure	Pass	Redo	Date Competency Met	Instructor Initials
b. Four-point gait (beginners)				
(1) Both legs are weight-bearing.	☐	☐	_____	_____
(2) Place one crutch forward.	☐	☐	_____	_____
(3) Move foot on opposite side of body forward, parallel with forward crutch.	☐	☐	_____	_____
(4) Place other crutch forward and parallel with first crutch.	☐	☐	_____	_____
(5) Move other foot forward so that it rests next to first foot.	☐	☐	_____	_____
c. Two-point gait (advanced)				
(1) Both legs are weight-bearing.	☐	☐	_____	_____
(2) Place one crutch forward and move opposite foot forward with it.	☐	☐	_____	_____
(3) Place other crutch forward and parallel with first crutch.	☐	☐	_____	_____
(4) Move opposite foot forward so that it is even with other foot.	☐	☐	_____	_____
d. Swing-to gait (arm and shoulder strength are needed)				
(1) One or both legs are weight-bearing.	☐	☐	_____	_____
(2) Balance weight on weight-bearing limb.	☐	☐	_____	_____
(3) Place both crutches forward.	☐	☐	_____	_____
(4) Shift weight to hands on crutches.	☐	☐	_____	_____
(5) Swing both feet forward until parallel with crutches.	☐	☐	_____	_____
e. Swing-through gait (advanced: arm and shoulder strength are needed)				
(1) One or both legs are weight-bearing.				
(2) Balance weight on weight-bearing limb(s).	☐	☐	_____	_____
(3) Place both crutches forward.	☐	☐	_____	_____
(4) Shift weight to hands on crutches.	☐	☐	_____	_____
(5) Swing both feet forward just ahead of crutches.	☐	☐	_____	_____
9. Return to room.	☐	☐	_____	_____
Postprocedure				
10. Ensure that patient is comfortable.	☐	☐	_____	_____
11. Wash hands.	☐	☐	_____	_____

Procedure	Pass	Redo	Date Competency Met	Instructor Initials
12. Record:				
a. Date				
b. Time				
c. Distance ambulated				
d. How tolerated				
e. Signature and classification	☐	☐	_____	_____

CHECK-OFF SHEET:
19-10 Walking with a Walker

Name _____ Date _____

Directions: Practice this procedure, following each step. When you are ready to have your performance evaluated, give this sheet to your instructor. Review the detailed procedure in your textbook.

Procedure	Pass	Redo	Date Competency Met	Instructor Initials
Student must use Standard Precautions.	☐	☐	_____	_____
Preprocedure				
1. Wash hands.	☐	☐	_____	_____
2. Assemble equipment:	☐	☐	_____	_____
a. Walker in good condition	☐	☐	_____	_____
b. Patient's footwear	☐	☐	_____	_____
c. Patient's robe, if necessary	☐	☐	_____	_____
3. Identify patient.	☐	☐	_____	_____
4. Tell patient what you are going to do.	☐	☐	_____	_____
5. Check walker for safety.	☐	☐	_____	_____
6. Help put on proper and safe footwear and robe if necessary.	☐	☐	_____	_____
7. Assist to sitting position with feet resting on the floor.	☐	☐	_____	_____
8. Secure gait belt snug enough to provide support and loose enough to provide comfort. Place walker within reach.	☐	☐	_____	_____
Procedure				
9. Stand patient up with walker. (Ask a co-worker to help if necessary.) Remind patient to stand as straight as possible.	☐	☐	_____	_____
10. Check to see if walker fits patient properly.				
a. Walker's handgrips should be at top of patient's leg or bend of leg at hip joint.	☐	☐	_____	_____
b. Arm should be at a 25 to 30° angle.	☐	☐	_____	_____
11. Gripping gait belt from behind, assist patient to ambulate as ordered. Basic guidelines for walking with a walker are as follows:	☐	☐	_____	_____
a. Patient begins by standing inside walker frame.	☐	☐	_____	_____
b. Patient lifts walker (never slides) and places back legs of walker parallel with toes (never ahead of toes).	☐	☐	_____	_____

Procedure	Pass	Redo	Date Competency Met	Instructor Initials
c. Patient shifts weight onto hands and walker (for balance and support).	☐	☐	_____	_____
d. Patient then walks into walker.	☐	☐	_____	_____
e. Place yourself just to side and slightly behind patient. This position will allow you to observe and be close enough to assist if necessary.	☐	☐	_____	_____
f. Ambulate as ordered, observing for correct use of walker.	☐	☐	_____	_____
12. When you have completed the ordered ambulation, return patient to his or her starting place.	☐	☐	_____	_____
Postprocedure	☐	☐	_____	_____
13. Provide for patient's comfort with call signal in reach.	☐	☐	_____	_____
14. Place walker in proper location. If patient is capable and physician permits ambulation without assistance, leave walker in a convenient place for patient.	☐	☐	_____	_____
15. Wash hands.	☐	☐	_____	_____
16. Report/document patient's tolerance of procedure.	☐	☐	_____	_____
17. Record the following:				
a. Date	☐	☐	_____	_____
b. Time	☐	☐	_____	_____
c. Distance and amount of time ambulated	☐	☐	_____	_____
d. How tolerated	☐	☐	_____	_____
e. Signature and classification	☐	☐	_____	_____

CHECK-OFF SHEET:
19-11 Respiratory Therapy

Name _____ **Date** _____

Directions: Practice this procedure, following each step. When you are ready to have your performance evaluated, give this sheet to your instructor. Review the detailed procedure in your textbook.

Procedure	Pass	Redo	Date Competency Met	Instructor Initials
Student must use Standard Precautions.	☐	☐	_____	_____
Preprocedure				
1. Determine the baseline function of the patient's respiratory system.	☐	☐	_____	_____
2. Consult the physician's orders to determine any specific respiratory treatment prescribed for the patient.	☐	☐	_____	_____
3. Determine the health care professional's responsibility for administering/supporting the treatment.	☐	☐	_____	_____
Procedure				
4. Assess the patient's current respiratory status.	☐	☐	_____	_____
5. Review available documentation to determine when specific respiratory treatments were last delivered, and when they will be due again.	☐	☐	_____	_____
6. Determine what the health care professional's role is to be in assisting/promoting respiratory therapy.	☐	☐	_____	_____
7. Consult with the respiratory therapist for any necessary instructions on the use of equipment or procedures.	☐	☐	_____	_____
8. Encourage the patient to use good pulmonary toileting techniques such as deep breathing, coughing, incentive spirometry.	☐	☐	_____	_____
9. Provide continuous monitoring of the patient's respiratory status so that any decline in function can be addressed early and successfully.	☐	☐	_____	_____
Postprocedure	☐	☐	_____	_____
10. Collaborate with the physician and the respiratory therapist if there is a decline in the patient's respiratory status.	☐	☐	_____	_____
11. Document the respiratory assessment and any ongoing problems and their resolution in the medical chart.	☐	☐	_____	_____

Chapter 20 Medical Assisting and Laboratory Skills

SECTION 20.1 Medical Assisting Skills

- **OBJECTIVES**

    When you have completed this section, you will be able to do the following:

    - Match key terms with their correct meanings.

    - Explain the process of admitting, registering, transferring, and discharging a patient.

    - Measure and record height and weight of an adult, child, and infant.

    - Summarize the importance of measuring the circumference of an infant's head.

    - Explain how to read a visual acuity test and the importance of the results.

    - Compare and identify examination positions by name.

    - List four basic examination techniques and explain their purposes.

- **DIRECTIONS**

    1. Complete Worksheets 1 and 2.

    2. Complete Worksheets 3, 4, and 5 as assigned.

    3. Complete Worksheet/Activity 6 as assigned.

    4. Practice all procedures.

    5. When you are confident that you can meet each objective for this section, ask your teacher for the section evaluation.

- **EVALUATION METHODS**
  - Worksheets/Activities
  - Class participation
  - Written evaluation
  - Practice procedures

- **WORKSHEET 1**

  Write the word that best matches each description on the line provided.

  auscultation

  baseline

  diagnosis

  hydroencephaly

  ophthalmoscope

  otoscope

  _____ 1. Excessive accumulation of cerebrospinal fluid in the brain, often leading to increased brain size and other brain trauma.

  _____ 2. The act of listening, either directly or through a stethoscope or other instrument, to sounds within the body as a method of diagnosis.

  _____ 3. The identification of a disease or condition.

  _____ 4. An instrument used to examine the ears.

  _____ 5. A number, graph, or indication to use as a guideline.

  _____ 6. An instrument used to examine the eyes.

  There are 6 possible points in this worksheet.

- **WORKSHEET 2**

  1. What is the first thing you must assess when admitting a patient (1 point)?

     _____

  2. What should you do if you notice a person is in acute distress while being admitted (2 points)?

     _____

  3. List seven basic procedures that should be followed when a patient is admitted (7 points).

     a. _____

     b. _____

     c. _____

     d. _____

     e. _____

f. _____

g. _____

4. In what color ink should all medical records be written (1 point)? _____

_____

5. What two forms must new patient/patients complete when registering (2 points)?

a. _____

b. _____

6. What should you do when transferring a patient to another area (2 points)?

_____

_____

7. What is required for a patient to be discharged (1 point)?

_____

There are 16 possible points in this worksheet.

● WORKSHEET 3

1. What are two reasons why is it important to measure a patient's weight when admitted (2 points)?

a. _____

b. _____

2. List five types of scales that can be used to weigh a patient (5 points).

a. _____

b. _____

c. _____

d. _____

e. _____

3. What are two ways to measure the height of an adult patient (2 points)?

a. _____

b. _____

4. Why is it important to measure head circumference in infants and toddlers (2 points)?

_____

5. Where do you place the measuring tape when determining head circumference (1 point)?

_____

There are 12 possible points in this worksheet.

● WORKSHEET 4

Match each examination position in Column A to its description in Column B (7 points).

Column A

_____ 1. Dorsal lithotomy position

_____ 2. Fowler's position

_____ 3. Horizontal recumbent (supine) position

_____ 4. Knee-chest position

_____ 5. Left lateral position and left Sims' position

_____ 6. Prone position

_____ 7. Trendelenburg position

Column B

a. This position is used for examination, treatment, and surgical procedures of the ventral (anterior) part of the body (for example, for abdominal pain, removal of stitches in chest).

b. This position is used for minor rectal examinations, enemas, and treatments.

c. This position helps restore blood flow to the brain when the body experiences shock. This position also helps promote drainage of congested lungs.

d. This position relieves patients who are having trouble breathing and allows examination of the anterior and posterior chest.

e. This position is used to examine or perform surgical procedures on the peritoneal and rectal areas.

f. This position is used for rectal examinations and surgical procedures. Some examination tables adjust to support the patient's abdomen and chest.

g. This position is used for examination, treatment, or surgical procedures of the dorsal (back) part of the body.

8. List and describe four basic examination techniques (8 points).

a. Technique: _____

Description: _____

_____

b. Technique: _____

Description: _____

_____

c. Technique: _____

Description: _____

_____

d. Technique: _____

Description: _____

_____

There are 15 possible points in this worksheet.

• WORKSHEET 5

1. Why would a provider perform a vision acuity test (2 points)? _____

_____

2. On what chart is a vision acuity test read (1 point)? _____

_____

3. How is the chart read (2 points)? _____

_____

_____

4. A patient is said to have 20/50 vision. What does each number in the fraction mean (5 points)?

_____

_____

_____

There are 10 possible points in this worksheet.

• WORKSHEET/ACTIVITY 6

Using a doll, demonstrate to classmates how to measure correctly the weight, length, and head circumference of an infant. Give an explanation of what you are doing and why while you take the measurements.

There are 15 possible points in this worksheet/activity.

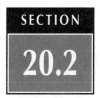

SECTION

20.2 Pharmacology and Medication Administration

• OBJECTIVES

When you have completed this section, you will be able to do the following:

- Match key terms with their correct meanings.
- Match common prescription abbreviations with their meanings.
- Match controlled substances with their assigned schedule level.
- Name four drug reference books.
- Describe methods to ensure safekeeping of medication.
- Write a formula for calculating medication dosage.
- Name six rights of medication administration.
- Recognize the guidelines for preparing and administering medications.
- Demonstrate all procedures in this chapter.

• DIRECTIONS

1. Complete Worksheets 1 and 2.

2. Complete Worksheet 3 as assigned.

3. Complete Worksheet/Activity 4 as assigned.

4. Complete Worksheet 5.

5. Practice all procedures.

6. When you are confident that you can meet each objective for this section, ask your teacher for the section evaluation.

• EVALUATION METHODS

- Worksheets/Activities
- Class participation
- Written evaluation
- Practice procedures

• WORKSHEET 1

Fill in the word from the list that completes each sentence.

antibiotics	formula	PDR
contraceptives	parenteral	topical
diuretics		

1. _____ are substances that slow growth of or destroy microorganisms.

2. Women can use _____ to prevent pregnancy.

3. The use of _____ increases a person's output of urine.

4. Injections that are _____ administered are not in the digestive system.

5. The cream is _____ and should be applied to the surface of the body only.

6. The physician followed the accepted rule, or _____, for determining the dosage.

7. The nurse consulted the _____ to confirm that she was using the correct medication.

There are 7 possible points in this worksheet.

• WORKSHEET 2

Match each prescription abbreviation with its meaning.

_____	**1.** cap	a. international units
_____	**2.** Dil	b. normal saline
_____	**3.** Dr	c. powder
_____	**4.** D/W	d. liter
_____	**5.** fl	e. minim
_____	**6.** Gal	f. right eye
_____	**7.** gt	g. fluid
_____	**8.** IM	h. pint or patient
_____	**9.** IU	i. ointment
_____	**10.** IV	j. milligram
_____	**11.** Kg	k. both eyes
_____	**12.** L	l. ounce
_____	**13.** Liq	m. left eye
_____	**14.** m or min	n. intravenous
_____	**15.** Mcg	o. dilute
_____	**16.** mEq	p. subcutaneous
_____	**17.** Mg	q. capsule
_____	**18.** Ml	r. tincture
_____	**19.** NS	s. dextrose in water
_____	**20.** OD	t. drop
_____	**21.** Oint	u. dram
_____	**22.** OS	v. microgram
_____	**23.** OU	w. liquid
_____	**24.** Oz	x. gallon
_____	**25.** Pt	y. milliliter
_____	**26.** Pulv	z. milliequivalent
_____	**27.** subc	aa. intramuscular
_____	**28.** tinc	bb. kilogram

There are 28 possible points in this worksheet.

• WORKSHEET 3

1. Write each drug in the chart in the column for the appropriate schedule (17 points).

Barbital	Fenethylline	Pentobarbital
Buprenorphine	Heroin	Phendimetrazine
Chlorphentermine	Marijuana	propylhexedrine
Clorazepate	Methadone	Triazolam
Codeine	Midazolam	Tylenol with Codeine
Dihydromorphine	oxycodone	

Schedule I	Schedule II	Schedule III	Schedule IV	Schedule V
The substances in this schedule are those that have no accepted medical use in the United States and have a high abuse potential.	The substances in this schedule have a high abuse potential with severe psychic or physical dependence liability. Schedule II controlled substances consist of certain narcotic, stimulant, and depressant drugs.	The substances in this schedule have an abuse potential less than those in Schedules I and II, and include compounds containing limited quantities of certain narcotic drugs and non-narcotic drugs.	The substances in this schedule have an abuse potential less than those listed in Schedule III.	The substances in this schedule have an abuse potential less than those listed in Schedule IV and consist primarily of preparations containing limited quantities of certain narcotic and stimulant drugs generally for antitussive, anti-diarrheal, and analgesic purposes.

2. List the six parts of a prescription (6 points).

_____

_____

_____

_____

_____

3. Name four drug reference books (4 points).

_____

_____

_____

_____

4. List seven handling procedures to ensure the safekeeping of medications (7 points).

_____

_____

_____

_____

_____

_____

_____

5. Write a formula for calculating medication dosage (5 points).

_____

6. Suppose the physician orders 500 mg of a medication. You have 250-mg tablets of the medication. Use the formula you wrote to figure out how many tablets make up one dose of the medication (5 points).

_____

7. Name six rights of medication administration (6 points).

_____

_____

_____

_____

_____

_____

8. List seven guidelines for preparing and administering medications (7 points).

_____

_____

_____

_____

_____

_____

_____

There are 57 possible points in this worksheet.

● WORKSHEET/ACTIVITY 4

Using the PDR reference book, look up three of the following medications and complete the worksheet (27 points).

Zestril   amitriptyline   ibuprofen

Diflunisal   Veetids   Fiorinal with Codeine 3

Medication #1 _____

  1. Name the resource used _____

  2. Generic name of medication _____

  3. Brand name of medication _____

  4. Color and shape of medication _____

  5. Dosages _____

  6. Frequency of dose _____

  7. Side effects _____

  8. Indications _____

  9. Contraindications _____

Medication #2 _____

  1. Name the resource used _____

  2. Generic name of medication _____

  3. Brand name of medication _____

  4. Color and shape of medication _____

  5. Dosages _____

  6. Frequency of dose _____

  7. Side effects _____

  8. Indications _____

  9. Contraindications _____

Medication #3 _____

1. Name the resource used _____

2. Generic name of medication _____

3. Brand name of medication _____

4. Color and shape of medication _____

5. Dosages _____

6. Frequency of dose _____

7. Side effects _____

8. Indications _____

9. Contraindications _____

● WORKSHEET 5

Match the items in column A with column B. Items in column B may be used more than once (20 points).

Column A

_____ 1. 1,000 ml

_____ 2. 60 mg

_____ 3. 4 mL

_____ 4. 8 pints

_____ 5. 15 mL

_____ 6. 240–250 mL

_____ 7. 0.5 g

_____ 8. 30 g

_____ 9. 250 mL

_____ 10. buccal

_____ 11. inhalation

_____ 12. irrigation

_____ 13. installation

_____ 14. inunction or topical

_____ 15. oral

_____ 16. parenteral

_____ 17. rectal

_____ 18. sublingual

_____ 19. vaginal

_____ 20. 30 mL

Column B

a. 1 fluid ounce.

b. Medication taken by mouth and swallowed.

c. 7 1/2 grains.

d. 8 ounces.

e. Medication applied to skin.

f. 1 grain.

g. Medication applied, inserted, or irrigated into vagina.

h. Medication dropped onto an area.

i. Tablet placed under the tongue to dissolve.

j. 1 L.

k. 8 ounces.

l. 1 gallon.

m. 1/2 ounce.

n. Tablet placed between the gums and cheek.

o. Solution washed through a body cavity or over a membrane.

p. 1 quart.

q. Liquid medications inhaled through respirator, or inhalation device

r. Medicated solution injected into body tissue and absorbed.

s. Medication solutions or suppositories inserted into the rectum.

t. 1 teaspoon, 1 dram, or 60 drops.

u. 1 ounce.

21. How many times must you read a medication label before giving a medication (1 point)? _____

22. When calculating a medication dosage, is it necessary to verify your calculations with a co-worker (1 point)? _____

23. What three things are liquid medications observed for (3 points)?

    a. _____

    b. _____

    c. _____

24. When pouring liquid medication, how is the label protected from drips (1 point)? _____

    _____

25. To achieve an accurate measure of liquid medication, hold the medication cup at _____ level while pouring (1 point).

26. _____ the neck of the bottle before recapping (1 point).

27. Never _____ two or more medications unless ordered (1 point).

28. Never leave medication _____ (1 point).

29. Watch the patient _____ the medication (1 point).

30. Never administer medication prepared by _____ person (1 point).

31. Check with patient for _____ before administering medication (1 point).

32. It is good practice to observe patient for 15 to 20 minutes after administering (4 points):

    a. _____

    b. _____

    c. _____

    d. _____

33. _____ unused or reused medication (1 point).

There are 38 possible points in this worksheet.

Laboratory Skills

- ● OBJECTIVES

    When you have completed this section, you will be able to do the following:

    - ▪ Match key terms with their correct meanings.

    - ▪ Follow 12 general laboratory guidelines.

    - ▪ Practice laboratory safety.

    - ▪ Demonstrate loading and operating an autoclave.

    - ▪ List eight types of specimen studies.

    - ▪ Identify general rules for testing specimen.

    - ▪ Discuss quality control in the laboratory.

    - ▪ Label a diagram of a microscope.

    - ▪ Identify steps to acquire a midstream clean-catch urine specimen for male and female.

    - ▪ Identify seven items learned from a CBC.

    - ▪ Explain why a hematocrit and hemoglobin test are important.

    - ▪ Explain the importance of counting WBCs and RBCs.

- ● DIRECTIONS

    1. Complete Worksheets 1 and 2.

    2. Follow your teacher's directions to complete Worksheet/Activity 3.

    3. Complete Worksheets 4 through 7 as assigned.

    4. Practice all procedures.

    5. Prepare responses to each item listed in Chapter Review.

    6. When you are confident that you can meet each objective for this section, ask your teacher for the section evaluation.

- ● EVALUATION METHODS

    - ▪ Worksheets/Activities

    - ▪ Class participation

    - ▪ Written evaluation

    - ▪ Practice procedures

● WORKSHEET 1

Match each term in Column A with the correct meaning in Column B.

Column A

_____ **1.** reagent

_____ **2.** provider

_____ **3.** binocular

_____ **4.** hazardous

_____ **5.** polycythemia

_____ **6.** acid

_____ **7.** uniformity

_____ **8.** resistant

_____ **9.** agglutination

_____ **10.** monocular

Column B

a. Having one eyepiece.

b. Able to protect itself.

c. Condition of having too much blood.

d. Chemical substance that reacts to the presence of other substances in the blood and urine.

e. Having two eyepieces.

f. Dangerous.

g. Clumping together.

h. Physician, physician assistant, nurse practitioner.

i. A state of being all the same; does not vary.

j. A substance that causes the urine to have a low pH.

There are 10 possible points in this worksheet.

● WORKSHEET 2

1. List twelve general laboratory guidelines (12 points).

_____

_____

_____

_____

_____

_____

_____

_____

_____

_____

_____

_____

2. Fill in the missing words in the list describing protective equipment to be worn (11 points).

a. A _____ lab coat to protect your clothes.

b. Safety _____ to guard your eyes from splashes.

c. Gloves to keep you from being contaminated by _____ material.

d. A rubber apron to protect you from _____ that can spill or splash.

e. Metal tongs when working with _____ objects.

f. Never use your mouth to _____.

g. Do not _____, drink, or apply makeup in the laboratory area.

h. _____ eyes first, then report eye contamination immediately to supervisor for eye treatment.

i. Dispose of all broken glass, _____, or other sharp objects in a sharps container.

j. Do not bend, break, or recap _____.

k. Disinfect counters, surfaces, and equipment _____..

There are 23 possible points in this worksheet.

• WORKSHEET/ACTIVITY 3

Following your teacher's instructions for demonstrating how to load and operate an autoclave.

There are 25 possible points in this worksheet/activity.

• WORKSHEET 4

1. List eight types of specimen studies (8 points).

a. _____

b. _____

c. _____

d. _____

e. _____

f. _____

g. _____

h. _____

2. Identify six basic steps for testing specimen (6 points).

a. _____

b. _____

c. _____

d. _____

e. _____

f. _____

There are 14 possible points in this worksheet.

● **WORKSHEET 5**

1. Label the parts of the microscope below (7 points).

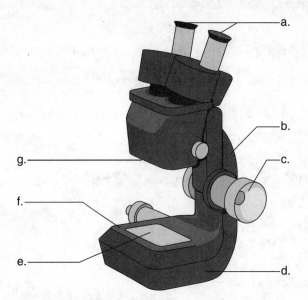

2. The power of the eyepiece is 10X and the power of the objective is 8X. By how many times will the specimen be magnified (2 points)?

_____

There are 9 possible points in this worksheet.

● **WORKSHEET 6**

1. Why might a physician order a clean-catch midstream urine collection? Why (2 points)?

_____

_____

2. Complete the missing steps below to describe the procedure for acquiring a midstream clean-catch urine specimen a female (8 points).

   a. Wash hands.

   b. _____

   c. _____

   d. Take towelette and wipe on side of urinary meatus from front to back.

   e. _____

   f. Repeat with new towelette on other side.

   g. _____

   h. Continue to hold labia open.

   i. _____

   j. Stop stream.

   k. _____

l. Stop stream.

m. _____

n. Empty bladder.

o. Carefully replace lid.

p. _____

q. Transport the specimen to the laboratory within 30 minutes of collection or else refrigerate.

3. Complete the missing steps below to describe the procedure for acquiring a midstream clean-catch urine specimen a male (5 points).

a. _____

b. Remove container lid and place on counter with inside of lid facing up.

c. _____

d. Urinate into toilet. (If uncircumcised, pull back foreskin while urinating.)

e. Allow stream to begin.

f. _____

g. _____

h. Empty bladder into toilet.

i. _____

j. Wipe outside of container with paper towel.

k. Transport the specimen to the laboratory within 30 minutes of collection or else refrigerate.

There are 15 possible points in this worksheet.

• WORKSHEET 7

1. List the four components of blood (4 points).

a. _____

b. _____

c. _____

d. _____

2. Identify seven items learned from a CBC (7 points).

a. _____

b. _____

c. _____

d. _____

e. _____

f. _____

g. _____

3. What is a hematocrit and why is this test important (4 points)?

_____

_____

_____

4. What is a hemoglobin test and why is this test important (4 points)?

_____

_____

_____

5. Why is it important to count WBCs (4 points)?

_____

_____

6. Why is it important to count RBCs (4 points)?

_____

_____

There are 27 possible points in this worksheet.

CHECK-OFF SHEET:
20-1 Admitting a Patient

Name _____ Date _____

Directions: Practice this procedure, following each step. When you are ready to have your performance evaluated, give this sheet to your instructor. Review the detailed procedure in your textbook.

Procedure	Pass	Redo	Date Competency Met	Instructor Initials
Student must use Standard Precautions.	☐	☐	_____	_____
Preprocedure				
1. Wash hands.	☐	☐	_____	_____
2. Assemble equipment:				
a. Admission checklist				
b. Admission pack (may all be disposable depending on facility)				
(1) Bedpan	☐	☐	_____	_____
(2) Urinal	☐	☐	_____	_____
(3) Emesis basin	☐	☐	_____	_____
(4) Wash basin	☐	☐	_____	_____
(5) Tissue	☐	☐	_____	_____
c. Gown or pajamas	☐	☐	_____	_____
d. Portable scale	☐	☐	_____	_____
e. Thermometer	☐	☐	_____	_____
f. Blood pressure cuff	☐	☐	_____	_____
g. Stethoscope	☐	☐	_____	_____
h. Clothing list	☐	☐	_____	_____
i. Envelope for valuables	☐	☐	_____	_____
Procedure				
3. Fan-fold bed covers to foot of bed.	☐	☐	_____	_____
4. Put away patient's equipment.	☐	☐	_____	_____
5. Put gown or pajamas on foot of bed.	☐	☐	_____	_____
6. Greet patient and introduce yourself.	☐	☐	_____	_____
7. Identify patient by looking at arm band and asking name.	☐	☐	_____	_____
8. Introduce patient to roommates.	☐	☐	_____	_____

Procedure	Pass	Redo	Date Competency Met	Instructor Initials
9. Explain	☐	☐	_____	_____
a. How call signal works	☐	☐	_____	_____
b. How bed controls work	☐	☐	_____	_____
c. Hospital regulations	☐	☐	_____	_____
d. What you will be doing to admit him or her	☐	☐	_____	_____
e. How telephone and television work	☐	☐	_____	_____
10. Provide privacy by pulling privacy curtains.	☐	☐	_____	_____
11. Ask patient to put on gown or pajamas.	☐	☐	_____	_____
12. Check weight and height.	☐	☐	_____	_____
13. Help to bed, if ordered. (Check with nurse.)	☐	☐	_____	_____
14. Put side rails up, if required.	☐	☐	_____	_____
15. If patient has valuables:				
a. Make a list of jewelry, money, wallet, and so on	☐	☐	_____	_____
b. Have patient sign in	☐	☐	_____	_____
c. Have relative sign list	☐	☐	_____	_____
d. Either have relative take valuables home or send to cashier's office in valuables envelope	☐	☐	_____	_____
16. Take and record the following:				
a. Temperature, pulse, respiration	☐	☐	_____	_____
b. Blood pressure	☐	☐	_____	_____
c. Urine specimen, if required	☐	☐	_____	_____
17. Complete admission checklist:				
a. Allergies	☐	☐	_____	_____
b. Medications being taken	☐	☐	_____	_____
c. Food preferences and dislikes	☐	☐	_____	_____
d. Any prosthesis	☐	☐	_____	_____
e. Skin condition	☐	☐	_____	_____
f. Handicaps (e.g., deafness, poor sight, lack of movement)	☐	☐	_____	_____
18. Orient patient to meal times, visiting hours, and so on.	☐	☐	_____	_____
19. Ask if patient has any questions regarding the information given.				

Postprocedure

20. Wash hands.	☐	☐	_____	_____
21. Record information according to your facility's policy.	☐	☐	_____	_____

CHECK-OFF SHEET:
20-2 Measuring Weight on Standing Balance Scale
Name _____ Date _____

Directions: Practice this procedure, following each step. When you are ready to have your performance evaluated, give this sheet to your instructor. Review the detailed procedure in your textbook.

Procedure	Pass	Redo	Date Competency Met	Instructor Initials
Student must use Standard Precautions.	☐	☐	_____	_____
Preprocedure				
1. Wash hands.	☐	☐	_____	_____
2. Assemble equipment:	☐	☐	_____	_____
a. Portable balance scale	☐	☐	_____	_____
b. Paper towel	☐	☐	_____	_____
c. Paper and pencil/pen	☐	☐	_____	_____
3. Identify patient.	☐	☐	_____	_____
4. Explain what you are going to do and ask patient if they need to void before you weigh them.	☐	☐	_____	_____
5. Provide privacy with curtain, screen, or door.	☐	☐	_____	_____
Procedure				
6. Take patient to scale or bring scale to patient's room.	☐	☐	_____	_____
7. Place paper towel on platform of scale (with standing scale).	☐	☐	_____	_____
8. Put both weights to the very left on zero.	☐	☐	_____	_____
9. Balance beam pointer must stay steady in middle of balance area.	☐	☐	_____	_____
10. Have patient remove shoes and stand on scale. (Note: the balance bar rises to top of bar guide when pointer is not centered.)	☐	☐	_____	_____
11. While keeping one hand near their back, use the other hand to move large weight to estimated weight of patient.	☐	☐	_____	_____
12. Move small weight to right until balance bar hangs free halfway between upper and lower bar guide.	☐	☐	_____	_____
13. The largest (lower) weight is marked in increments of 50 pounds; the smaller upper weight) is marked in single pounds. The even-numbered pounds are marked with numbers (e.g., 2, 4, 6). The uneven pounds are unmarked long lines and the short line is one-fourth of a pound.	☐	☐	_____	_____

Procedure	Pass	Redo	Date Competency Met	Instructor Initials
14. Write weight down on a notepad.	☐	☐	_____	_____
15. Help patient with shoes and make him or her comfortable.	☐	☐	_____	_____
Postprocedure				
16. Discard towel.	☐	☐	_____	_____
17. Replace scale.	☐	☐	_____	_____
18. Wash your hands.	☐	☐	_____	_____
19. Chart weight. Report any unusual increases or decreases in weight.	☐	☐	_____	_____

CHECK-OFF SHEET:
20-3 Measuring Weight on a Chair Scale
Name _____ **Date** _____

Directions: Practice this procedure, following each step. When you are ready to have your performance evaluated, give this sheet to your instructor. Review the detailed procedure in your textbook.

Procedure	Pass	Redo	Date Competency Met	Instructor Initials
Student must use Standard Precautions.	☐	☐	_____	_____
Preprocedure				
1. Wash hands.	☐	☐	_____	_____
2. Assemble equipment.	☐	☐	_____	_____
a. Balance scale	☐	☐	_____	_____
b. Paper towel	☐	☐	_____	_____
c. Paper and pencil/pen	☐	☐	_____	_____
d. Knock before entering the patient's room	☐	☐	_____	_____
3. Identify patient.	☐	☐	_____	_____
4. Explain what you are going to do and ask patient if they need to void before you weigh them.	☐	☐	_____	_____
5. Provide privacy with curtain, screen, or door.	☐	☐	_____	_____
Procedure				
6. Take patient to scale or bring scale to patient's room.	☐	☐	_____	_____
7. Put both weights to the very left on zero.	☐	☐	_____	_____
8. Balance beam pointer must stay steady in middle of balance area.	☐	☐	_____	_____
9. Have patient remove shoes and move patient to chair at the side of the scale.	☐	☐	_____	_____
10. Place wheelchair on scale and weigh it.	☐	☐	_____	_____
11. Assist patient back into wheelchair. Weigh wheelchair with patient in it.	☐	☐	_____	_____
12. Determine patient weight by subtracting the weight in #10 above with the weigh in #11.	☐	☐	_____	_____
13. Write down weight on a notepad.	☐	☐	_____	_____
14. Help patient with shoes and make him or her comfortable.	☐	☐	_____	_____
Postprocedure				
15. Replace scale.	☐	☐	_____	_____
16. Wash hands.	☐	☐	_____	_____
18. Chart weight. Report any unusual increases or decreases in weight.	☐	☐	_____	_____

CHECK-OFF SHEET:
20-4 Measuring Weight on a Mechanical Lift
Name _____ **Date** _____

Directions: Practice this procedure, following each step. When you are ready to have your performance evaluated, give this sheet to your instructor. Review the detailed pro500cedure in your textbook.

Procedure	Pass	Redo	Date Competency Met	Instructor Initials
Student must use Standard Precautions.	☐	☐	_____	_____
Preprocedure				
1. Wash hands.	☐	☐	_____	_____
2. Assemble equipment:				
a. Mechanical lift	☐	☐	_____	_____
b. Sling	☐	☐	_____	_____
c. Clean sheet	☐	☐	_____	_____
3. Identify patient.	☐	☐	_____	_____
4. Explain what you are going to do.	☐	☐	_____	_____
5. Pull privacy curtain.				
Procedure	☐	☐	_____	_____
6. Lower side rail on side you are working on.	☐	☐	_____	_____
7. Cover sling with clean sheet.	☐	☐	_____	_____
8. Help patient roll on side, and place sling with top at shoulders and bottom at knees.	☐	☐	_____	_____
9. Fan-fold remaining sling.	☐	☐	_____	_____
10. Help patient roll to other side onto half of sling, and pull other half of sling through.	☐	☐	_____	_____
11. Broaden base of lift.	☐	☐	_____	_____
12. Wheel lift to side of bed with base beneath bed.	☐	☐	_____	_____
13. Position lift over patient.	☐	☐	_____	_____
14. Attach sling using chains and hooks provided.	☐	☐	_____	_____
15. Use hand crank or pump handle to raise patient from bed. Make certain that buttocks are not touching bed.	☐	☐	_____	_____
16. Check to be certain that patient is in the center of sling and is safely suspended.	☐	☐	_____	_____

Procedure	Pass	Redo	Date Competency Met	Instructor Initials
17. To weigh patient:				
a. Swing feet and legs over edge of bed; move lift away from bed so that no body part contacts bed.	☐	☐	_____	_____
b. If bed is low enough, raise patient above bed so that no body part contacts bed.	☐	☐	_____	_____
18. Adjust weights until scale is balanced. (See the check-off sheet "Measuring Weight on Standing Balance Scale.")	☐	☐	_____	_____
19. Return patient to bed by reversing steps.	☐	☐	_____	_____
Postprocedure				
20. Replace mechanical lift.	☐	☐	_____	_____
21. Wash hands.	☐	☐	_____	_____
22. Note weight and write on pad.	☐	☐	_____	_____

CHECK-OFF SHEET:
20-5 Measuring Height

Name _____ Date _____

Directions: Practice this procedure, following each step. When you are ready to have your performance evaluated, give this sheet to your instructor. Review the detailed procedure in your textbook.

Procedure	Pass	Redo	Date Competency Met	Instructor Initials
Student must use Standard Precautions.	☐	☐	_____	_____
Preprocedure				
1. Wash hands.	☐	☐	_____	_____
2. Assemble equipment: a. Balance scale with height rod	☐	☐	_____	_____
b. Paper towels	☐	☐	_____	_____
3. Identify patient and explain procedure.	☐	☐	_____	_____
4. Put paper towel on platform of scale.				
5. Explain what you are going to do.				
6. Have patient remove shoes.	☐	☐	_____	_____
Procedure				
7. Raise measuring rod above head.	☐	☐	_____	_____
8. Have patient stand with back against measuring rod.	☐	☐	_____	_____
9. Instruct patient to stand straight, with heels touching measuring rod.	☐	☐	_____	_____
10. Lower measuring rod to rest on patient's head.	☐	☐	_____	_____
11. Check number of inches indicated on rod.	☐	☐	_____	_____
12. Record in inches, centimeters, or feet and inches according to facility policy.	☐	☐	_____	_____
Postprocedure				
13. Help patient with shoes.	☐	☐	_____	_____
14. Chart height.	☐	☐	_____	_____
15. Discard paper towel and wash hands	☐	☐	_____	_____

CHECK-OFF SHEET:
20-6 Measuring Height of Adult/Child (Over 3 Years of Age)

Name _____ **Date** _____

Directions: Practice this procedure, following each step. When you are ready to have your performance evaluated, give this sheet to your instructor. Review the detailed procedure in your textbook.

Procedure	Pass	Redo	Date Competency Met	Instructor Initials
Student must use Standard Precautions.	☐	☐	_____	_____
Preprocedure				
1. Wash hands.	☐	☐	_____	_____
2. Put paper towel on platform of scale.	☐	☐	_____	_____
3. Explain procedure and provide privacy.	☐	☐	_____	_____
Procedure				
4. Raise height-measuring rod on back of scale so that tip of height-measuring rod is above patient's head.	☐	☐	_____	_____
5. Instruct patient to remove shoes.	☐	☐	_____	_____
6. Ask patient to step on to scale so that tip of height-measuring rod is above patient's head.	☐	☐	_____	_____
7. Instruct patient to place heels against back of scale and stand straight.	☐	☐	_____	_____
8. Lift up measuring rod so that it points out above patient's head.	☐	☐	_____	_____
9. Lower rod gently until it rests on patient's head.	☐	☐	_____	_____
10. Assist patient in stepping off scales.	☐	☐	_____	_____
11. Read numbers just above edge of hollow bar of rod at back of scale.	☐	☐	_____	_____
12. Record height on medical record in feet and inches, centimeters, or inches only, according to your provider's policy.	☐	☐	_____	_____
Postprocedure				
13. Discard paper towel.	☐	☐	_____	_____
14. Wash hands.	☐	☐	_____	_____

CHECK-OFF SHEET:

20-7 Measuring the Head Circumference of an Infant/Toddler (Under 3 years of age)

Name _____ Date _____

Directions: Practice this procedure, following each step. When you are ready to have your performance evaluated, give this sheet to your instructor. Review the detailed procedure in your textbook.

Procedure	Pass	Redo	Date Competency Met	Instructor Initials
Student must use Standard Precautions.	☐	☐	_____	_____
Preprocedure				
1. Wash hands.	☐	☐	_____	_____
2. Obtain measuring tape or measuring bar.	☐	☐	_____	_____
3. Identify the patient.	☐	☐	_____	_____
4. Explain the procedure to the patient.	☐	☐	_____	_____
Procedure				
5. Place infant in supine position.	☐	☐	_____	_____
6. Position measuring tape over occipital bone and wrap toward forehead. Bring tape just above ears to the center of the forehead.	☐	☐	_____	_____
7. Record measurement.	☐	☐	_____	_____
Postprocedure	☐	☐	_____	_____
8. Wash hands.	☐	☐	_____	_____

CHECK-OFF SHEET:
20-8 Measuring the Height of an Infant/Toddler

Name _____ Date _____

Directions: Practice this procedure, following each step. When you are ready to have your performance evaluated, give this sheet to your instructor. Review the detailed procedure in your textbook.

Procedure	Pass	Redo	Date Competency Met	Instructor Initials
Student must use Standard Precautions.	☐	☐	_____	_____
Preprocedure				
1. Wash hands.	☐	☐	_____	_____
2. Obtain measuring tape or measuring bar.	☐	☐	_____	_____
Procedure				
3. Place infant in supine position.	☐	☐	_____	_____
4. Place zero mask of tape or measuring bar level with top of infant's head.	☐	☐	_____	_____
5. Ask parent or co-worker to hold top of head gently at zero mask.	☐	☐	_____	_____
6. Gently straighten legs.	☐	☐	_____	_____
7. Read measurement that is level with infant's head.	☐	☐	_____	_____
Postprocedure				
8. Wash hands.	☐	☐	_____	_____

CHECK-OFF SHEET:
20-9 Measuring the Weight of an Infant/Toddler

Name _____ Date _____

Directions: Practice this procedure, following each step. When you are ready to have your performance evaluated, give this sheet to your instructor. Review the detailed procedure in your textbook.

Procedure	Pass	Redo	Date Competency Met	Instructor Initials
Student must use Standard Precautions.	☐	☐	_____	_____
Preprocedure				
1. Wash hands.	☐	☐	_____	_____
2. Assemble equipment.	☐	☐	_____	_____
a. Infant balance scale	☐	☐	_____	_____
b. Towel	☐	☐	_____	_____
c. Growth chart	☐	☐	_____	_____
3. Ask parent to remove infant's clothing.	☐	☐	_____	_____
4. Place clean towel on scale cradle to decrease shock of cold metal against infant.	☐	☐	_____	_____
5. Balance the scale at zero with towel in place.	☐	☐	_____	_____
Procedure				
6. Place infant face up on scale. Keep diaper on towel over infant's genital area in case of elimination.	☐	☐	_____	_____
7. Place one hand over infant (almost touching) to give sense of security.	☐	☐	_____	_____
8. Slide weight easily until scale balances.	☐	☐	_____	_____
9. Read scale in pounds and ounces or in kilograms.	☐	☐	_____	_____
10. Return infant to parent.	☐	☐	_____	_____
Postprocedure				
11. Balance the scale at zero mask.	☐	☐	_____	_____
12. Discard towel.	☐	☐	_____	_____
13. Wash hands.	☐	☐	_____	_____
14. Record weight on growth chart and in patient's chart.	☐	☐	_____	_____

CHECK-OFF SHEET:
20-10 Moving Patient and Belongings to Another Room
Name _____ **Date** _____

Directions: Practice this procedure, following each step. When you are ready to have your performance evaluated, give this sheet to your instructor. Review the detailed procedure in your textbook.

Procedure	Pass	Redo	Date Competency Met	Instructor Initials
Student must use Standard Precautions.	☐	☐	_____	_____
Preprocedure				
1. Wash hands.	☐	☐	_____	_____
2. Assemble equipment:				
a. Patient's chart	☐	☐	_____	_____
b. Nursing care plan	☐	☐	_____	_____
c. Medications	☐	☐	_____	_____
d. Paper bag	☐	☐	_____	_____
3. Identify patient.	☐	☐	_____	_____
4. Explain what you are going to do.	☐	☐	_____	_____
Procedure				
5. Determine location to which patient is being transferred.	☐	☐	_____	_____
6. Gather patient's belongings. (Check admission list.)	☐	☐	_____	_____
7. Determine how patient is to be transported: a. Wheelchair	☐	☐	_____	_____
b. Stretcher	☐	☐	_____	_____
c. Entire bed	☐	☐	_____	_____
d. Ambulate	☐	☐	_____	_____
8. Transport patient to new unit.	☐	☐	_____	_____
9. Introduce to staff on new unit.	☐	☐	_____	_____
10. Introduce to new roommate.	☐	☐	_____	_____
11. Make patient comfortable.	☐	☐	_____	_____
12. Put away belongings.	☐	☐	_____	_____
13. Put away belongings.	☐	☐	_____	_____
Postprocedure				
14. Wash hands.	☐	☐	_____	_____
15. Give transferred medications, care plan, and chart to nurse.	☐	☐	_____	_____

Procedure	Pass	Redo	Date Competency Met	Instructor Initials
16. Before leaving unit, record the following: a. Date and time of transfer	☐	☐	_____	_____
b. How transported (e.g., wheelchair)	☐	☐	_____	_____
c. How transfer was tolerated by patient	☐	☐	_____	_____
17. Return to original unit and report completion of transfer.	☐	☐	_____	_____

CHECK-OFF SHEET:
20-11 Discharging a Patient

Name _____ Date _____

Directions: Practice this procedure, following each step. When you are ready to have your performance evaluated, give this sheet to your instructor. Review the detailed procedure in your textbook.

Procedure	Pass	Redo	Date Competency Met	Instructor Initials
Student must use Standard Precautions.	☐	☐	_____	_____
Preprocedure				
1. Check chart for discharge order.	☐	☐	_____	_____
2. Wash hands.	☐	☐	_____	_____
3. Identify patient.	☐	☐	_____	_____
4. Explain what you are going to do.	☐	☐	_____	_____
5. Provide privacy by pulling the privacy curtain.	☐	☐	_____	_____
Procedure				
6. Check with the patient's nurse regarding discharge status prior to continuing process. The nurse will need to:	☐	☐	_____	_____
a. Remove any tethers such as IV lines or indwelling catheters.	☐	☐	_____	_____
b. Review the patient's medication list, especially new medications and their use.	☐	☐	_____	_____
c. Notify the patient of any follow up appointments to be scheduled or already scheduled with the physician, or for follow up lab or diagnostics.	☐	☐	_____	_____
d. Inform the patient of any restriction of activity or diet.	☐	☐	_____	_____
7. Help patient dress.	☐	☐	_____	_____
8. Collect patient's belongings.	☐	☐	_____	_____
9. Check belongings against admission list.	☐	☐	_____	_____
10. Secure and return valuables:				
a. Verify with patient that all valuables are present.	☐	☐	_____	_____
b. Have patient sign for them.	☐	☐	_____	_____
11. Check to see if patient has medications to take home.	☐	☐	_____	_____
12. Check to see if any equipment is to be taken home.	☐	☐	_____	_____
13. Help patient into wheelchair.	☐	☐	_____	_____
14. Help patient into car.	☐	☐	_____	_____

Procedure	Pass	Redo	Date Competency Met	Instructor Initials
Postprocedure				
15. Return to unit:				
a. Remove all items left in unit.	☐	☐	_____	_____
b. Clean unit according to your facility's policy.	☐	☐	_____	_____
16. Wash hands.	☐	☐	_____	_____
17. Record discharge:				
a. Date and time	☐	☐	_____	_____
b. Method of transport	☐	☐	_____	_____
c. Whom patient left with	☐	☐	_____	_____

CHECK-OFF SHEET:
20-12 Horizontal Recumbent (Supine) Position
Name _____ **Date** _____

Directions: Practice this procedure, following each step. When you are ready to have your performance evaluated, give this sheet to your instructor. Review the detailed procedure in your textbook.

Procedure	Pass	Redo	Date Competency Met	Instructor Initials
Student must use Standard Precautions.	☐	☐	_____	_____
Preprocedure				
1. Wash hands.	☐	☐	_____	_____
2. Explain to patient what you are going to do.	☐	☐	_____	_____
Procedure				
3. Assist patient with gown.	☐	☐	_____	_____
4. Determine any problems associated with placing the patient in this position, such as increased respiratory distress, etc.	☐	☐	_____	_____
5. Assist patient to a position of lying flat on his or her back with arms at side in good alignment, with a small pillow under the head.	☐	☐	_____	_____
6. Drape cover so that he or she is not exposed, leaving all edges of a drape loose.	☐	☐	_____	_____
Postprocedure				
7. After exam, assist patient off the table and with dressing if needed.	☐	☐	_____	_____
8. Wash hands.	☐	☐	_____	_____

CHECK-OFF SHEET:
20-13 Fowler's Position

Name _____ **Date** _____

Directions: Practice this procedure, following each step. When you are ready to have your performance evaluated, give this sheet to your instructor. Review the detailed procedure in your textbook.

Procedure	Pass	Redo	Date Competency Met	Instructor Initials
Student must use Standard Precautions.	☐	☐	_____	_____
Preprocedure				
1. Wash hands.	☐	☐	_____	_____
2. Explain to patient what you are going to do.	☐	☐	_____	_____
3. Assist patient with gown.	☐	☐	_____	_____
Procedure				
4. Determine any problems associated with placing the patient in this position, such as increase in back pain, etc.	☐	☐	_____	_____
5. Assist patient to a position lying flat on his or her back in good alignment with a small pillow under their head.	☐	☐	_____	_____
6. Keep patient covered so that he or she is not exposed.	☐	☐	_____	_____
7. Knees may bend slightly.	☐	☐	_____	_____
8. Adjust backrest to the correct position according to patient's or physician's needs.	☐	☐	_____	_____
9. Drape cover so that patient is not exposed, leaving all edges of drape free.	☐	☐	_____	_____
Postprocedure				
10. After exam, assist patient off table and with dressing.	☐	☐	_____	_____
11. Wash hands.	☐	☐	_____	_____

CHECK-OFF SHEET:
20-14 Trendelenburg Position

Name _____ Date _____

Directions: Practice this procedure, following each step. When you are ready to have your performance evaluated, give this sheet to your instructor. Review the detailed procedure in your textbook.

Procedure	Pass	Redo	Date Competency Met	Instructor Initials
Student must use Standard Precautions.	☐	☐	_____	_____
Preprocedure				
1. Wash hands.	☐	☐	_____	_____
2. Explain to patient what you are going to do.	☐	☐	_____	_____
3. Assist patient with gown.	☐	☐	_____	_____
4. Determine any problems associated with placing the patient in this position, such as increase in back pain, etc.	☐	☐	_____	_____
5. Assist patient to a position lying flat on his or her back in good alignment.	☐	☐	_____	_____
Procedure				
6. Drape cover so that he or she is not exposed, leaving all edges of drape loose.	☐	☐	_____	_____
7. Lower the head of the table until the body is at a 45 degree angle. Legs may be bent or extended.	☐	☐	_____	_____
8. Reassure patient that he or she will not slide off table. Remain with patient at all times.	☐	☐	_____	_____
Postprocedure				
9. After exam, assist patient off table and with dressing.	☐	☐	_____	_____
10. Wash hands.	☐	☐	_____	_____

CHECK-OFF SHEET:
20-15 Dorsal Lithotomy Position
Name _____ **Date** _____

Directions: Practice this procedure, following each step. When you are ready to have your performance evaluated, give this sheet to your instructor. Review the detailed procedure in your textbook.

Procedure	Pass	Redo	Date Competency Met	Instructor Initials
Student must use Standard Precautions.	☐	☐	_____	_____
Preprocedure				
1. Wash hands.	☐	☐	_____	_____
2. Explain to patient what you are going to do.	☐	☐	_____	_____
3. Assist patient with gown.	☐	☐	_____	_____
Procedure				
4. Determine any problems associated with placing the patient in this position, such as increase in back pain, etc.	☐	☐	_____	_____
5. Assist patient to a position lying flat on his or her back with arms at side.	☐	☐	_____	_____
6. Place pillow under head.	☐	☐	_____	_____
7. Cover patient so he or she is not exposed.	☐	☐	_____	_____
8. Gently assist patient to bend knees	☐	☐	_____	_____
9. Separate legs by placing each foot flat on bed about 2 feet apart or in stirrups attached to examination table.	☐	☐	_____	_____
10. Move patient's hips to edge of end of table when stirrups are available.	☐	☐	_____	_____
11. Drape with half-size sheet positioned with one corner toward head and opposite corners between legs. Secure side corner around legs.	☐	☐	_____	_____
12. Remain with patient.	☐	☐	_____	_____
Postprocedure				
13. After exam, assist patient off table and with dressing.	☐	☐	_____	_____
14. Wash hands.	☐	☐	_____	_____

CHECK-OFF SHEET:
20-16 Prone Position

Name _____ Date _____

Directions: Practice this procedure, following each step. When you are ready to have your performance evaluated, give this sheet to your instructor. Review the detailed procedure in your textbook.

Procedure	Pass	Redo	Date Competency Met	Instructor Initials
Student must use Standard Precautions.	☐	☐	_____	_____
Preprocedure				
1. Wash hands.	☐	☐	_____	_____
2. Explain to patient what you are going to do.	☐	☐	_____	_____
3. Assist patient to a position lying flat on his or her back.	☐	☐	_____	_____
Procedure				
4. Determine any problems associated with placing patient in this position, such as increased pain or respiratory distress.	☐	☐	_____	_____
5. Turn patient toward self.	☐	☐	_____	_____
6. Position patient on the abdomen with arms flexed by head.	☐	☐	_____	_____
7. Position head to side on small pillow.	☐	☐	_____	_____
8. Cover patient so that he or she is not exposed and let drape hang loosely.	☐	☐	_____	_____
Postprocedure				
9. After exam, assist patient off the table and with dressing.	☐	☐	_____	_____
10. Wash hands.	☐	☐	_____	_____

CHECK-OFF SHEET:
20-17 Left Lateral Position and Left Sims Position

Name _____ Date _____

Directions: Practice this procedure, following each step. When you are ready to have your
performance evaluated, give this sheet to your instructor. Review the detailed procedure in your
textbook.

Procedure	Pass	Redo	Date Competency Met	Instructor Initials
Student must use Standard Precautions.	☐	☐	_____	_____
Preprocedure				
1. Wash hands.	☐	☐	_____	_____
2. Explain to patient what you are going to do.	☐	☐	_____	_____
3. Assist patient to a position lying flat on his or her back.	☐	☐	_____	_____
Procedure				
4. Determine any problems associated with placing patient in this position, such as increased pain or respiratory distress.	☐	☐	_____	_____
5. Assist patient to a position lying flat on his or her back.	☐	☐	_____	_____
6. Cover patient so that he or she is not exposed.	☐	☐	_____	_____
7. Assist patient to turn onto left side.	☐	☐	_____	_____
8. Position patient's left arm slightly behind him or her on bed and bend right arm in front of the body.	☐	☐	_____	_____
9. Turn head to side on small pillow.	☐	☐	_____	_____
10. Gently bend both knees.	☐	☐	_____	_____
11. Place right leg slightly forward of left leg for lateral position.	☐	☐	_____	_____
12. Bend right knee toward chest for Sim's position.	☐	☐	_____	_____
13. Drape with one sheet; make sure drape is hung loosely.	☐	☐	_____	_____
Postprocedure				
14. After exam, assist patient off table and with dressing.	☐	☐	_____	_____
15. Wash hands.	☐	☐	_____	_____

CHECK-OFF SHEET:
20-18 Knee Chest Position

Name _____ Date _____

Directions: Practice this procedure, following each step. When you are ready to have your performance evaluated, give this sheet to your instructor. Review the detailed procedure in your textbook.

Procedure	Pass	Redo	Date Competency Met	Instructor Initials
Student must use Standard Precautions.	☐	☐	_____	_____
Preprocedure				
1. Wash hands.	☐	☐	_____	_____
2. Explain to patient what you are going to do.	☐	☐	_____	_____
3. Assist patient to a position lying flat on his or her back.	☐	☐	_____	_____
Procedure				
4. Determine any problems associated with placing patient in this position, such as increased pain or respiratory distress.	☐	☐	_____	_____
5. Assist patient to a position lying flat on his or her back.	☐	☐	_____	_____
6. Instruct patient to raise hips upward by kneeling on both knees.	☐	☐	_____	_____
7. Rest patient's head and shoulders on a pillow.	☐	☐	_____	_____
9. Flex arms slightly and have them at the side of their head.	☐	☐	_____	_____
10. Drape with one sheet; make sure drape is hung loosely.	☐	☐	_____	_____
Postprocedure				
11. After exam, assist patient off table and with dressing.	☐	☐	_____	_____
12. Wash hands.	☐	☐	_____	_____

CHECK-OFF SHEET:
20-19 Testing Visual Acuity: Snellen Chart

Name _____ Date _____

Directions: Practice this procedure, following each step. When you are ready to have your performance evaluated, give this sheet to your instructor. Review the detailed procedure in your textbook.

Procedure	Pass	Redo	Date Competency Met	Instructor Initials
Student must use Standard Precautions.	☐	☐	_____	_____
Preprocedure				
1. Wash hands.	☐	☐	_____	_____
2. Assure that the Snellen Chart is at patient's eye level and that the tape for them to stand on is 20 feet from the chart.	☐	☐	_____	_____
3. Identify patient.	☐	☐	_____	_____
4. Explain procedure to patient.	☐	☐	_____	_____
Procedure				
5. Position patient 20 feet (6 meters) from Snellen chart. Have patient stand with heel on 20 foot mark.	☐	☐	_____	_____
6. Instruct patient to keep both eyes open during testing. Ask them to remove corrective lenses.	☐	☐	_____	_____
7. Ask patient to cover left eye with an occlude and read smallest line of letters that he or she can see.	☐	☐	_____	_____
8. Use a pointer and point to letters in the row in random order. Do not cover the letter or symbol with the pointer.	☐	☐	_____	_____
9. Record the distance patient is from the chart compared to the size of letters patient can see clearly (e.g., 20/20, 20/30, 20/40).	☐	☐	_____	_____
10. Repeat test with right eye covered.	☐	☐	_____	_____
11. Repeat test, allowing patient to use both eyes.	☐	☐	_____	_____
12. Repeat each test with patient wearing glasses (if he or she has prescription lenses).	☐	☐	_____	_____
Postprocedure				
13. Wash hands	☐	☐	_____	_____

CHECK-OFF SHEET:
20-20 Using the *Physician's Desk Reference (PDR)*

Name _____ **Date** _____

Directions: Practice this procedure, following each step. When you are ready to have your performance evaluated, give this sheet to your instructor. Review the detailed procedure in your textbook.

Procedure	Pass	Redo	Date Competency Met	Instructor Initials
Student must use Standard Precautions.	☐	☐	_____	_____
Preprocedure				
1. Identify the name of the manufacturer by going to Section 5; compare the tablet with pictures to identify the medication.	☐	☐	_____	_____
a. Wallace is the manufacturer.	☐	☐	_____	_____
b. Turn to the page where Wallace pills are displayed.	☐	☐	_____	_____
c. Match the pill with pictures of pills displayed.	☐	☐	_____	_____
d. A yellow oval pill marked "Wallace 200" matches "Soma Compound with Codeine 200 mg" in the display.	☐	☐	_____	_____
2. Turn to Section 2, the pink pages, Find "Soma Compound with Codeine 200 mg." Two page numbers are listed.	☐	☐	_____	_____
a. The first page number refers to Section 5, the picture of the medication.	☐	☐	_____	_____
b. The second page number refers to Section 6 and provides product information.	☐	☐	_____	_____
3. Turn to the page number indicated in Section 6 to find specific drug information.	☐	☐	_____	_____
a. Description of drug	☐	☐	_____	_____
b. Clinical pharmacology				
c. Indications and usage (describes the reasons for using the drug)	☐	☐	_____	_____
d. Contraindications (reasons not to give this drug)	☐	☐	_____	_____
e. Warnings	☐	☐	_____	_____
f. Precautions	☐	☐	_____	_____
g. Dosage and administration	☐	☐	_____	_____
h. How supplied	☐	☐	_____	_____
i. Storage recommendations	☐	☐	_____	_____

Procedure	Pass	Redo	Date Competency Met	Instructor Initials
4. Go to Section 1 for more information about a drug. Find the manufacturer:	☐	☐	_____	_____
a. Wallace Laboratories is listed with the W's in the alphabetical list.	☐	☐	_____	_____
b. Write requests for information using the address supplied.	☐	☐	_____	_____
c. Call for assistant using the professional services telephone number or night and weekend emergency number if available.	☐	☐	_____	_____

CHECK-OFF SHEET:
20-21 Using a Microscope

Name _____ Date _____

Directions: Practice this procedure, following each step. When you are ready to have your performance evaluated, give this sheet to your instructor. Review the detailed procedure in your textbook.

Procedure	Pass	Redo	Date Competency Met	Instructor Initials
Student must use Standard Precautions.	☐	☐	_____	_____
Preprocedure				
1. Assemble equipment.	☐	☐	_____	_____
a. Microscope	☐	☐	_____	_____
b. Lens paper	☐	☐	_____	_____
c. Slides and slide cover	☐	☐	_____	_____
d. Specimen	☐	☐	_____	_____
e. Oil if using oil immersion	☐	☐	_____	_____
f. Gloves if specimens have been contaminated by blood or body fluids	☐	☐	_____	_____
2. Wash hands.	☐	☐	_____	_____
3. Place specimen on clean slide.	☐	☐	_____	_____
4. Add required solution.	☐	☐	_____	_____
5. Drop clean slide cover over specimen. Hold cover at an angle and let it drop. Make sure there are no air bubbles between the slide and cover slip. If there are bubbles, must do again.	☐	☐	_____	_____
6. Clean eyepiece with lens paper.	☐	☐	_____	_____
7. Clean objectives with lens paper.	☐	☐	_____	_____
8. Turn on illuminating light.	☐	☐	_____	_____
9. Open iris diaphragm.	☐	☐	_____	_____
10. Turn revolving nosepiece to low-power objective.	☐	☐	_____	_____
Procedure				
11. Place slide on stage under slide clips. Avoid getting finger prints on the slide.	☐	☐	_____	_____
12. Turn coarse adjustment knob to move objective close to slide. Do not look into eyepieces while doing this, as you could crack the slide.	☐	☐	_____	_____
13. Look into eyepiece and slowly turn coarse adjustment to move tube upward until you focus specimen.	☐	☐	_____	_____

Procedure	Pass	Redo	Date Competency Met	Instructor Initials
14. Turn fine-adjustment knob until specimen is clear and focused.	☐	☐	_____	_____
15. Continue steps 12 through 14 using higher objectives until you have best possible focus for specimen.	☐	☐	_____	_____
16. Observe specimen. If setup is for technician or physician, tell that person that slide is ready.	☐	☐	_____	_____
Postprocedure				
17. Remove slide after it is read.	☐	☐	_____	_____
18. Discard slide according to procedure in your facility.	☐	☐	_____	_____
19. Clean lens and objective with lens paper.	☐	☐	_____	_____
20. Turn off illuminating light.	☐	☐	_____	_____
21. Put cover back on microscope.	☐	☐	_____	_____
22. Wash hands.	☐	☐	_____	_____
23. Fill out lab slips according to your facility's policies.	☐	☐	_____	_____

CHECK-OFF SHEET:
20-22 Using Reagent Strips to Test Urine
Name _____ Date _____

Directions: Practice this procedure, following each step. When you are ready to have your performance evaluated, give this sheet to your instructor. Review the detailed procedure in your textbook.

Procedure	Pass	Redo	Date Competency Met	Instructor Initials
Student must use Standard Precautions.	☐	☐	_____	_____
Preprocedure				
1. Wash hands.	☐	☐	_____	_____
2. Assemble equipment.	☐	☐	_____	_____
a. Reagent strips and bottle	☐	☐	_____	_____
b. Laboratory report slip	☐	☐	_____	_____
c. Watch	☐	☐	_____	_____
d. Urine specimen	☐	☐	_____	_____
e. Disposable nonsterile gloves	☐	☐	_____	_____
3. Complete laboratory slip.	☐	☐	_____	_____
a. Name	☐	☐	_____	_____
b. Sex	☐	☐	_____	_____
c. Age	☐	☐	_____	_____
d. Physician	☐	☐	_____	_____
e. Date	☐	☐	_____	_____
f. Type of test	☐	☐	_____	_____
4. Put on gloves.	☐	☐	_____	_____
Procedure				
5. Hold specimen to light and observe:	☐	☐	_____	_____
a. Color	☐	☐	_____	_____
b. Clarity	☐	☐	_____	_____
6. Write color and clarity on lab slip.	☐	☐	_____	_____
7. Open reagent jar and remove one strip.	☐	☐	_____	_____
a. Note expiration date. Do not use if expired.				
b. Replace jar cover immediately.	☐	☐	_____	_____
8. Hold strip by clear end and immerse in urine.	☐	☐	_____	_____
9. Remove strip immediately by pulling gently over lip of tube to remove excess urine.	☐	☐	_____	_____

Procedure	Pass	Redo	Date Competency Met	Instructor Initials
10. Hold strip in horizontal position to prevent mixing of chemicals.	☐	☐	_____	_____
11. Hold strip close to color blocks on bottle label and match carefully. Note time.	☐	☐	_____	_____
12. Read strip at time indicated and record results.	☐	☐	_____	_____
13. Discard reagent strip in biohazard waste.	☐	☐	_____	_____
Postprocedure				
14. Clean and replace equipment.	☐	☐	_____	_____
15. Remove gloves.	☐	☐	_____	_____
16. Wash hands.	☐	☐	_____	_____
17. Record required information.	☐	☐	_____	_____
18. Report any abnormal results to supervisor immediately.	☐	☐	_____	_____

CHECK-OFF SHEET:
20-23 Measuring Specific Gravity with Urinometer

Name _____ **Date** _____

Directions: Practice this procedure, following each step. When you are ready to have your performance evaluated, give this sheet to your instructor. Review the detailed procedure in your textbook.

Procedure	Pass	Redo	Date Competency Met	Instructor Initials
Student must use Standard Precautions.	☐	☐	_____	_____
Preprocedure				
1. Wash hands.	☐	☐	_____	_____
2. Assemble equipment.	☐	☐	_____	_____
a. Disposable gloves	☐	☐	_____	_____
b. Glass cylinder (5 inches high)	☐	☐	_____	_____
c. Urinometer (This is a float with a stem that is calibrated in thousands: 1.000, 1.001, 1.002, etc.)	☐	☐	_____	_____
d. Fresh urine specimen. Do not refrigerate	☐	☐	_____	_____
3. Put on gloves.	☐	☐	_____	_____
Procedure				
4. Pour urine into cylinder to about one inch from the top.	☐	☐	_____	_____
5. Place urinometer in urine.	☐	☐	_____	_____
6. Spin urinometer gently. You must not touch side or bottom.	☐	☐	_____	_____
7. Place cylinder with lower line of meniscus at eye level.	☐	☐	_____	_____
8. Read specific gravity:				
a. Look at point where lowest part of meniscus crosses urinometer scale.	☐	☐	_____	_____
b. Read gauge on nearest line.	☐	☐	_____	_____
9. Record reading to enter in computer or on lab slip.	☐	☐	_____	_____
10. Discard urine according to facility's contaminated waste policy.	☐	☐	_____	_____
11. Rinse urinometer with water and dry.	☐	☐	_____	_____
12. Rinse cylinder with water and dry.	☐	☐	_____	_____
13. Remove gloves and discard in contaminated waste.	☐	☐	_____	_____
Postprocedure				
14. Wash hands.	☐	☐	_____	_____
15. Record specific gravity in computer or on lab list.	☐	☐	_____	_____
16. Document according to facility procedure.	☐	☐	_____	_____

CHECK-OFF SHEET:
20-24 Measuring Specific Gravity with Refractometer
Name _____ **Date** _____

Directions: Practice this procedure, following each step. When you are ready to have your performance evaluated, give this sheet to your instructor. Review the detailed procedure in your textbook.

Procedure	Pass	Redo	Date Competency Met	Instructor Initials
Student must use Standard Precautions.	☐	☐	_____	_____
Preprocedure				
1. Wash hands.	☐	☐	_____	_____
2. Assemble equipment:	☐	☐	_____	_____
a. Disposable gloves	☐	☐	_____	_____
b. Refractometer	☐	☐	_____	_____
c. Distilled water	☐	☐	_____	_____
d. Fresh urine sample Do not refrigerate.	☐	☐	_____	_____
e. Will need eye dropper or pipette to get drop of water and/or urine	☐	☐	_____	_____
3. Put on gloves.	☐	☐	_____	_____
Procedure				
4. Place one drop of distilled water on the glass plate.	☐	☐	_____	_____
5. Close lid.	☐	☐	_____	_____
6. Look through eyepiece to read specific gravity.	☐	☐	_____	_____
7. Transfer one drop of well-mixed urine onto glass plate of refractometer.	☐	☐	_____	_____
8. Close lid.	☐	☐	_____	_____
9. Look through eyepiece to read specific gravity.	☐	☐	_____	_____
10. Record reading to enter in computer or on lab slip.				
11. Discard urine according to facility's contaminated waste policy.	☐	☐	_____	_____
Postprocedure				
12. Clean refractometer according to manufacturer's directions.	☐	☐	_____	_____
13. Remove gloves and discard in contaminated waste.	☐	☐	_____	_____
14. Wash hands.	☐	☐	_____	_____
15. Record specific gravity in computer or on lab list.	☐	☐	_____	_____

CHECK-OFF SHEET:
20-25 Centrifuging a Urine Sample

Name _____ **Date** _____

Directions: Practice this procedure, following each step. When you are ready to have your performance evaluated, give this sheet to your instructor. Review the detailed procedure in your textbook.

Procedure	Pass	Redo	Date Competency Met	Instructor Initials
Student must use Standard Precautions.	☐	☐	_____	_____
Preprocedure				
1. Wash hands.	☐	☐	_____	_____
2. Assemble equipment.	☐	☐	_____	_____
a. Centrifuge	☐	☐	_____	_____
b. Two centrifuge tubes	☐	☐	_____	_____
c. Microscope slide (number slide)	☐	☐	_____	_____
d. Coverslip	☐	☐	_____	_____
e. Pipette	☐	☐	_____	_____
f. Disposable nonsterile gloves	☐	☐	_____	_____
g. Urine specimen. It's best to use the first voiding in AM , as it is more concentrate	☐	☐	_____	_____
3. Fill in lab slip:	☐	☐	_____	_____
a. Name	☐	☐	_____	_____
b. Date	☐	☐	_____	_____
c. Time	☐	☐	_____	_____
4. Put on gloves.	☐	☐	_____	_____
Procedure				
5. Mix urine to suspend sediment by rolling specimen container gently between your hands.	☐	☐	_____	_____
6. Pour 10 mL of urine into centrifuge tube.	☐	☐	_____	_____
7. Put tube with urine into centrifuge.	☐	☐	_____	_____
8. Pour 10 mL of water into second centrifuge tube.	☐	☐	_____	_____
9. Place in centrifuge opposite the tube with urine. This is very important for balance.	☐	☐	_____	_____
10. Secure centrifuge lid.	☐	☐	_____	_____
11. Set centrifuge timer for 4 to 5 minutes. (Allow it to stop on its own.)	☐	☐	_____	_____
12. Remove tube with urine.	☐	☐	_____	_____

Procedure	Pass	Redo	Date Competency Met	Instructor Initials
13. Carefully invert urine centrifuge tube quickly over sink to pour 9 mL of urine into sink.	☐	☐	_____	_____
14. Turn tube right side up immediately. (About 1.0 cc will remain in tube.)	☐	☐	_____	_____
15. Mix sediment by snapping end of centrifuge tube with finger or gently shaking.	☐	☐	_____	_____
16. Pipette 1 drop of urine on numbered slide. A pipette works by creating a vacuum above the liquid-holding chamber and then selectively releasing this vacuum to draw up and dispense liquid.	☐	☐	_____	_____
17. Put on coverslip. (Redo if air bubbles appear under coverslip.)	☐	☐	_____	_____
18. Put slide on microscope stage.				
19. Use 10_ objective with coarse adjustment to focus on slide. Watch while moving course adjustment, so that slide does not break.	☐	☐	_____	_____
20. Adjust light source.	☐	☐	_____	_____
21. Follow your facility's policy for reading slide. (If setup is for technician, tell him or her that slide is ready.)	☐	☐	_____	_____
22. Remove slide after it is read.	☐	☐	_____	_____
23. Discard slide according to facility procedure.	☐	☐	_____	_____
24. Clean lens and objective with lens paper.	☐	☐	_____	_____
25. Cover microscope.	☐	☐	_____	_____

Postprocedure

26. Clean equipment and replace equipment.	☐	☐	_____	_____
27. Remove gloves, and dispose of according to facility policy.	☐	☐	_____	_____
28. Wash hands.	☐	☐	_____	_____
29. Record results if you read the specimen.	☐	☐	_____	_____
30. Document according to facility procedure.	☐	☐	_____	_____

CHECK-OFF SHEET:
20-26 Midstream Clean-Catch Urine-Female
Name _____ Date _____

Directions: Practice this procedure, following each step. When you are ready to have your performance evaluated, give this sheet to your instructor. Review the detailed procedure in your textbook.

Procedure	Pass	Redo	Date Competency Met	Instructor Initials
Student must use Standard Precautions.	☐	☐	_____	_____
Preprocedure				
1. Wash hands.	☐	☐	_____	_____
2. Assemble equipment.	☐	☐	_____	_____
a. Sterile urine container for clean catch	☐	☐	_____	_____
b. Label	☐	☐	_____	_____
c. Disposable antiseptic towelettes	☐	☐	_____	_____
d. Disposable nonsterile gloves: wear if you handle cup with specimen	☐	☐	_____	_____
Procedure				
3. Label container.	☐	☐	_____	_____
4. Instruct patient to:	☐	☐	_____	_____
a. Wash hands.	☐	☐	_____	_____
b. Remove container lid and place on counter with inside of lid facing up.	☐	☐	_____	_____
c. Separate labia to expose meatus.	☐	☐	_____	_____
d. Take towelette and wipe on side of urinary meatus from front to back.	☐	☐	_____	_____
e. Dispose of towelette.				
f. Repeat with new towelette on other side.	☐	☐	_____	_____
g. Wipe directly over meatus with new towelette.	☐	☐	_____	_____
h. Continue to hold labia open.	☐	☐	_____	_____
i. Urinate small amount into toilet.	☐	☐	_____	_____
j. Stop stream.	☐	☐	_____	_____
k. Place sterile container under meatus and void into container (60 cc).	☐	☐	_____	_____
l. Stop stream.	☐	☐	_____	_____
m. Remove container carefully.	☐	☐	_____	_____
n. Empty bladder.	☐	☐	_____	_____

Procedure	Pass	Redo	Date Competency Met	Instructor Initials
o. Carefully replace lid.	☐	☐	_____	_____
p. Wipe outside of container with paper towel.	☐	☐	_____	_____
q. Transport the specimen to the laboratory within 30 minutes of collection or else refrigerate.	☐	☐	_____	_____
5. Put on gloves.	☐	☐	_____	_____
6. Finish testing as ordered (e.g., dipstick, set up microscopic exam, drug test).	☐	☐	_____	_____

Postprocedure

7. Document procedure according to facility procedure.	☐	☐	_____	_____
8. Wash hands.	☐	☐	_____	_____

CHECK-OFF SHEET:
20-27 Midstream Clean-Catch Urine, Male

Name _____   **Date** _____

Directions: Practice this procedure, following each step. When you are ready to have your performance evaluated, give this sheet to your instructor. Review the detailed procedure in your textbook.

Procedure	Pass	Redo	Date Competency Met	Instructor Initials
Student must use Standard Precautions.	☐	☐	_____	_____
Preprocedure				
1. Wash hands.	☐	☐	_____	_____
2. Assemble equipment.	☐	☐	_____	_____
a. Sterile urine container for clean catch	☐	☐	_____	_____
b. Label	☐	☐	_____	_____
c. Disposable antiseptic towelettes	☐	☐	_____	_____
d. Disposable nonsterile gloves: wear if you handle cup with specimen	☐	☐	_____	_____
Procedure				
3. Label container.	☐	☐	_____	_____
4. Instruct patient to:	☐	☐	_____	_____
a. Wash hands.	☐	☐	_____	_____
b. Remove container lid and place on counter with inside of lid facing up.	☐	☐	_____	_____
c. Cleanse head of penis in a circular motion with towelett				
e. (If uncircumcised, pull back foreskin before cleaning.)	☐	☐	_____	_____
d. Urinate into toilet. (If uncircumcised, pull back foreskin while urinating.)	☐	☐	_____	_____
e. Allow stream to being.				
f. Stop stream and place specimen container to collect midstream. (Fill about half way full or 60 mL.)	☐	☐	_____	_____
g. Remove container before bladder is empty.	☐	☐	_____	_____
h. Empty bladder into toilet.				
i. Carefully replace lid.	☐	☐	_____	_____
j. Wipe outside of container with paper towel.	☐	☐	_____	_____
k. Transport the specimen to the laboratory within 30 minutes of collection or else refrigerate.	☐	☐	_____	_____

Procedure	Pass	Redo	Date Competency Met	Instructor Initials
5. Put on gloves.	☐	☐	_____	_____
6. Finish testing as ordered (e.g., dip stick, set up microscopic exam, drug test).	☐	☐	_____	_____
Postprocedure				
7. Document procedure according to facility procedure.	☐	☐	_____	_____
8. Wash hands.	☐	☐	_____	_____

CHECK-OFF SHEET:
20-28 Collecting Urine from an Infant

Name _____ Date _____

Directions: Practice this procedure, following each step. When you are ready to have your performance evaluated, give this sheet to your instructor. Review the detailed procedure in your textbook.

Procedure	Pass	Redo	Date Competency Met	Instructor Initials
Student must use Standard Precautions.	☐	☐	_____	_____
Preprocedure				
1. Wash hands.	☐	☐	_____	_____
2. Assemble equipment.	☐	☐	_____	_____
a. Specimen container	☐	☐	_____	_____
b. Disposable urine collector (small plastic bag with opening and sticky area)	☐	☐	_____	_____
c. Disposable nonsterile gloves	☐	☐	_____	_____
3. Identify patient.	☐	☐	_____	_____
4. Explain to parents what you are going to do.	☐	☐	_____	_____
5. Tell child what you are going to do even if you think that he or she is too young to understand. Children often understand.	☐	☐	_____	_____
Preprocedure				
6. Put on gloves.	☐	☐	_____	_____
7. Remove diaper.	☐	☐	_____	_____
8. Make certain that skin is clean and dry in genital area.	☐	☐	_____	_____
9. Remove outside cover that is around opening of bag. This has a sticky area that is applied to vulva or around penis. Place over vulva or penis (at top right).	☐	☐	_____	_____
10. Replace diaper.	☐	☐	_____	_____
11. Remove gloves and dispose of according to facility procedure.	☐	☐	_____	_____
12. Check every half hour to see if bag has urine in it.	☐	☐	_____	_____
13. Remove bag when specimen is collected.	☐	☐	_____	_____
14. Rinse, clean, and dry genital area.	☐	☐	_____	_____
15. Replace diaper.	☐	☐	_____	_____
16. Put specimen in specimen container for lab.	☐	☐	_____	_____

Procedure	Pass	Redo	Date Competency Met	Instructor Initials
17. Label with:				
a. Patient's name	☐	☐	_____	_____
b. Time of collection	☐	☐	_____	_____
c. Date	☐	☐	_____	_____
d. Room number	☐	☐	_____	_____
18. Record collection of specimen.	☐	☐	_____	_____
19. Wash hands.	☐	☐	_____	_____

Chapter 21 Patient and Employee Safety

SECTION

21.1 **General Safety and Injury and Illness Prevention**

- **OBJECTIVES**

    When you have completed this section, you will be able to do the following:

    - Match key terms to their correct meanings.

    - Define *OSHA* and explain the agency's role in safety.

    - Differentiate between IIPP, hazard communication, and exposure control.

    - Name places to find information about hazards in a facility.

    - Explain the health care worker's role in maintaining a safe workplace.

    - Discuss the employer's role in maintaining a safe workplace.

    - Identify 14 general safety rules.

    - Summarize the importance of safety in a health care environment.

- **DIRECTIONS**

    1. Complete Worksheet 1.

    2. Complete Worksheets 2 and 3 as assigned.

    3. Complete Worksheets/Activities 4 through 6 as assigned.

    4. Complete Worksheets 7 and 8 as assigned.

    5. When you are confident that you can meet each objective for this section, ask your teacher for the section evaluation.

- ## EVALUATION METHODS
  - Worksheets/Activities
  - Class participation
  - Written evaluation

- ## WORKSHEET 1

  Define each of the following vocabulary words.

  1. Abreast _____
  2. Biohazard _____
  3. Comply _____
  4. Environment _____
  5. Frayed _____
  6. Implement _____
  7. Horseplay _____
  8. Malfunctioning _____
  9. Mandates _____
  10. Shock _____

  There are 10 possible points in this worksheet.

- ## WORKSHEET 2

  1. What is OSHA (1 point)? _____
  _____

  2. Explain the agency's role in safety (3 points).
     a. _____
     b. _____
     c. _____

  3. What does IIPP stand for (1 point)? _____
  _____

  4. Every employer must establish an injury and illness prevention program. As an employee, you are responsible for understanding the injury and illness prevention program in your facility. What are your specific responsibilities (6 points)?
     a. _____
     b. _____
     c. _____
     d. _____
     e. _____
     f. _____

5. Explain the ergonomic program (1 point). _____

_____

_____

There are 12 possible points in this worksheet.

• WORKSHEET 3

1. Every employer must have a hazard communication program. Put an *X* next to the information that is mandated (6 points).

_____ a. Chemicals or hazards in the environment

_____ b. How to use the telephone in an emergency

_____ c. Where chemicals or hazards are stored and used

_____ d. How to interpret chemical labels and hazard signs

_____ e. The names of the dangerous chemicals in the environment

_____ f. Methods and equipment for cleaning chemical spills

_____ g. Where important medications are stored

_____ h. Personal protective equipment and its storage location

_____ i. The hazard communication system

_____ j. How to write an incident report

2. Define *biohazard* (1 point). _____

_____

3. What must the employee know about the hazard communication system (6 points)?

a. _____

b. _____

c. _____

d. _____

e. _____

f. _____

4. Explain the hazard communication program (1 point). _____

_____

_____

5. What is a material safety data sheet, or MSDS (1 point)? _____

_____

_____

6. Put an *X* next to the information that must be on a material safety data sheet (10 points). Refer to the MSDS in your textbook.

_____ a. Spill or leak procedures

_____ b. Special precautions

_____ c. Table of contents

_____ d. Product identification

_____ e. How to use the product

_____ f. Cost of product

_____ g. Hazardous ingredients of mixtures

_____ h. Physical data

_____ i. Telephone number of the nearest fire department

_____ j. Health hazard data

_____ k. Protection information and control measures

_____ l. Fire and explosion

_____ m. How to perform CPR

_____ n. Emergency and first aid procedures

_____ o. Name and address of your facility's director

_____ p. Reactivity data

7. Write the name of the section on an MSDS where you will find the following information (3 points).

a. How to clean up a spill _____

b. How and where to store the product _____

c. What protective wear to use when working with the product _____

_____

8. List the two hazard categories, and explain each one (4 points).

a. _____

b. _____

There are 32 possible points in this worksheet.

• WORKSHEET/ACTIVITY 4

Get together with three or four classmates and select a safety procedure or issue to demonstrate and explain to the class. For example, you might choose body mechanics and good posture for lifting, patient restraints, or ambulation devices. Have some demonstrate as others describe and explain the procedure and the issues involved.

There are 65 possible points in this worksheet/activity.

• WORKSHEET/ACTIVITY 5

1. Where should you look for hazard communications (5 points)?

a. _____

b. _____

c. _____

d. _____

e. _____

2. Find all the places in your facility where safety information is available. List these places below (50 points).

_____

_____

3. When you find the material safety data sheets, choose two products and read the MSDSs for these products. Fill in the information below for each product (20 points).

	Product 1	**Product 2**
Product identification		
Health hazard data		
Protection information and control measures		
Spill or leak procedures		
Fire and explosion		
Hazardous ingredients of mixtures		
Emergency and first aid procedures		
Special precautions		
Reactivity data		
Physical data		

There are 75 possible points in this worksheet/activity.

• WORKSHEET/ACTIVITY 6

Read the labels on two products that are used in your facility. Use the information on the labels to answer the following questions.

1. What is the name of the product (2 points)?

a. Product 1: _____

b. Product 2: _____

2. Does the label tell you what precautions to take when using the product (2 points)?

a. Product 1: _____

b. Product 2: _____

3. What chemicals are listed on the label (2 points)?

   a. Product 1: _____

   b. Product 2: _____

4. What should you do if the product gets on your skin or in your eyes (2 points)?

   a. Product 1: _____

   b. Product 2: _____

5. How should you clean up a spill (2 points)?

   a. Product 1: _____

   b. Product 2: _____

6. What do you do if you breathe the fumes (2 points)?

   a. Product 1: _____

   b. Product 2: _____

7. What personal protective equipment do you need when using this product (2 points)?

   a. Product 1: _____

   b. Product 2: _____

8. Explain why the labeling of products is important (1 point). _____

_____

_____

There are 15 possible points in this worksheet/activity.

● WORKSHEET 7

1. Explain what an exposure control program is (1 point)._____

_____

_____

2. List three things the program includes (3 points).

   a. _____

   b. _____

   c. _____

3. Differentiate between an IIPP, hazard communication, and exposure control (6 points). _____

_____

_____

4. Explain the health care worker's role in maintaining a safe workplace (4 points). _____

_____

_____

There are 14 possible points in this worksheet.

• WORKSHEET 8

1. Identify the 14 general safety rules by placing an *X* next to each one (14 points).

_____ a. Do not use electrical cords that are frayed or damaged.

_____ b. Run in an emergency.

_____ c. Watch out for swinging doors.

_____ d. Use handrails when using the stairs.

_____ e. Report a shock you receive from equipment to your supervisor.

_____ f. Horseplay is not tolerated.

_____ g. Walk in the middle of the hall to avoid swinging doors.

_____ h. Follow instructions carefully.

_____ i. Wipe up spills only if you have time.

_____ j. Do everything you are asked to do, and do not ask questions.

_____ k. Report any injury to yourself or others to your supervisor immediately.

_____ l. Always check labels.

_____ m. Wipe up spills, and place litter in containers.

_____ n. Follow Standard Precaution guidelines.

_____ o. Report unsafe conditions to your supervisor immediately.

_____ p. Walk! Never run in hallways.

_____ q. Wait a day or two to report a minor injury; it may get better.

_____ r. Walk on the right-hand side of the hall not more than two abreast.

_____ s. Do not use malfunctioning equipment.

_____ t. Avoid using handrails on stairs so you can securely hold items you are carrying.

2. Summarize the importance of safety in a health care environment. Explain how teamwork between the employer and the employee affects safety (6 points). _____

_____

_____

There are 20 possible points in this worksheet.

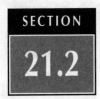

SECTION

21.2 Patient Safety

• OBJECTIVES

When you have completed this section, you will be able to do the following:

- Match key terms with their correct meaning.

- Explain how to use ambulation devices, transporting devices, postural supports, and side rails safely.

- Match descriptions and principles associated with ambulation devices, transporting devices, postural supports, and side rails.

- Explain the importance of safety measures.

- Follow safe practice guidelines when caring for patients.

• DIRECTIONS

1. Complete Worksheet 1.

2. When you are confident that you can meet each objective for this section, ask your teacher for the section evaluation.

• EVALUATION METHODS

- Worksheet

- Class participation

- Written evaluation

• WORKSHEET 1

1. Complete the following sentences (4 points).

a. Ambulation devices are used to _____

_____

b. Transportation devices are used to _____

_____

c. Postural supports are used to _____

_____

d. Side rails are used to _____

_____

2. Write each word listed below in the space next to the example or principle that illustrates it (15 points).

ambulation devices   postural supports   transporting devices   side rails

_____ a. Wheelchair.

_____ b. A release must be signed before you can leave them down.

_____ c. These must have rubber tips covering areas that touch the floor.

_____ d. Wheels must be locked when taking clients in or out of these devices.

_____ e. Walker.

_____ f. Small children always need them up.

_____ g. Vest.

_____ h. A doctor's order is required before they can be used.

_____ i. They must be loosened every two hours.

_____ j. They prevent clients from falling out of bed.

_____ k. Gurney.

_____ l. Always back these devices over indented or raised doorways.

_____ m. Lock brakes except when moving.

_____ n. Keep two fingers' width between these and the client's skin.

_____ o. Check for breaks or cracks before using.

3. Explain the importance of safety measures (2 points). _____

_____

There are 21 possible points in this worksheet.

SECTION 21.3

Disaster Preparedness

● **OBJECTIVES**

When you have completed this section, you will be able to do the following:

- Match key terms with their correct meaning.

- Identify what you are responsible for knowing and doing when a disaster occurs.

- List the three elements required to start a fire.

- Explain four ways to prevent fires.

- Summarize all safety requirements that protect the employee/student, patient, and employer.

• DIRECTIONS

1. Complete Worksheet 1 as assigned.

2. When you are confident that you can meet each objective for this section, ask your teacher for the section evaluation.

• EVALUATION METHODS

- Worksheet
- Class participation
- Written evaluation

• WORKSHEET 1

1. Define the following vocabulary words (3 points).

a. Observant _____

b. Cylinder _____

c. Potential _____

2. List five examples of disasters (5 points).

a. _____

b. _____

c. _____

d. _____

e. _____

3. Identify what you are responsible for knowing and doing when a disaster occurs. Place an *X* next to your responsibilities (9 points).

_____ a. Know who makes each type of fire extinguisher.

_____ b. Know the floor plan of your facility.

_____ c. Know what causes a tornado.

_____ d. Know the magnitude of the earthquake.

_____ e. Assess the situation and calm yourself.

_____ f. Know the nearest exit route.

_____ g. Do not place yourself in danger.

_____ h. Know the name of the nearest fire station.

_____ i. Remove those who are in immediate danger, if it is safe to do so.

_____ j. Use the stairs, not the elevator.

_____ k. Notify others of the emergency according to facility policy.

_____ l. Know the location of the alarms and fire extinguishers.

_____ m. Know your role as a health care worker when a disaster occurs.

4. List the three elements required to start a fire (3 points).

a. _____

b. _____

c. _____

5. Explain three ways to prevent a fire (3 points).

a. _____

b. _____

c. _____

6. Summarize all safety requirements that protect the employee, student, patient, and employer (5 points).

_____

_____

_____

_____

There are 28 possible points in this worksheet.

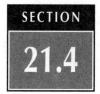

SECTION 21.4

Principles of Body Mechanics

● OBJECTIVES

When you have completed this section, you will be able to do the following:

- Match key terms with their correct meanings.
- Define body mechanics.
- List six rules of correct body mechanics.
- List six principles of body mechanics.
- Demonstrate correct lifting and moving of objects.

● DIRECTIONS

1. Complete Worksheet 1.
2. Complete Worksheet/Activity 2 as assigned.
3. When you are confident that you can meet each objective for this section, ask your teacher for the section evaluation.

● EVALUATION METHODS

- Worksheet
- Class participation
- Written evaluation

• WORKSHEET 1

1. Define the following vocabulary words (3 points).

    a. Efficiency_____

    b. Gravity _____

    c. Crouch _____

2. Define body mechanics (1 point). _____

    _____

    _____

3. List the six principles of body mechanics (6 points).

    a. _____

    b. _____

    c. _____

    d. _____

    e. _____

    f. _____

4. List the six rules of correct body mechanics, and explain why you think each one is important (12 points).

    a. _____

    b. _____

    c. _____

    d. _____

    e. _____

    f. _____

There are 22 possible points in this worksheet.

• WORKSHEET/ACTIVITY 2

Choose another student as a partner. Take turns demonstrating the process of lifting a patient. Allow other students to critique your body mechanics and suggest improvements. Then do the same for other students. As a group, discuss why it is important to evaluate coworkers in an actual healthcare environment.

There are 25 possible points in this worksheet.

SECTION 21.5 First Aid

● OBJECTIVES

When you have completed this section, you will be able to do the following:

- Match key terms with their correct meanings.
- Demonstrate the procedures for:
  - Mouth-to-mouth breathing
  - Obstructed airway
  - Serious wounds
  - Preventing shock
  - Splints
  - Slings
  - Bandaging

● DIRECTIONS

1. Complete Worksheets 1 through 8 as assigned.
2. Complete Worksheet/Activity 9 as assigned.
3. Prepare responses to each item listed in Chapter Review.
4. When you are confident that you can meet each objective for this section, ask your teacher for the section evaluation.

● EVALUATION METHODS

- Worksheets
- Class participation
- Written evaluation

● WARNINGS

- Do not make mouth-to-mouth contact with your classmate during practice.
- Remember to only pretend to do abdominal thrusts on a real person.

• WORKSHEET 1

1. Place each word listed below in the space next to the statement that best defines it (6 points).

abdominal thrust   fracture   EMS

splint   symptoms   swath

_____ a. Broken bone.

_____ b. Forceful thrust on the abdomen, between the sternum and the navel, in an upward motion toward the head.

_____ c. Emergency medical system.

_____ d. Bandage.

_____ e. Firm objects used to support an unstable body part.

_____ f. Signs that indicate a condition, usually a disorder or disease.

2. Match each definition in column B with the correct vocabulary word in column A (8 points).

Column A

_____ **1.** Cardiopulmonary

_____ **2.** Contusion

_____ **3.** Dressings

_____ **4.** Susceptible

_____ **5.** Definitive

_____ **6.** Saturated

_____ **7.** Laceration

_____ **8.** Heimlich maneuver

Column B

a. Condition in which the skin is bruised, swollen, and painful but is not broken.

b. Especially sensitive, capable of being affected.

c. Having to do with the heart and lungs.

d. Bandages, usually gauze pads that are used to cover a wound.

e. Wound or tear of the skin.

f. Clear, without question, exacting.

g. Forceful upward thrust on the abdomen, between the sternum and the navel.

h. Soaked; filled to capacity.

3. Define the following vocabulary words (3 points).

a. Impending_____

b. Priorities _____

c. Spurts_____

There are 17 possible points in this worksheet.

• WORKSHEET 2

1. What is first aid (1 point)? _____

_____

2. Write the six general principles of first aid, and explain why each is important (12 points).

a. _____

_____

b. _____

_____

c. _____

_____

d. _____

_____

e. _____

_____

f. _____

_____

3. List the life-threatening situations discussed in the text (7 points).

a. _____

b. _____

c. _____

d. _____

e. _____

f. _____

g. _____

4. Explain why these situations are life threatening (2 points). _____

_____

_____

5. Oxygen is necessary for _____ to live (1 point).

6. Permanent brain damage can occur if (a) _____ is not present for (b) _____ to (c) _____ minutes (3 points).

There are 26 possible points in this worksheet.

• WORKSHEET 3

1. List each step in the procedure for mouth-to-mouth or mouth-to-nose breathing for a victim who has stopped breathing (5 points).

   a. _____

   b. _____

   c. _____

   d. _____

   e. _____

2. Fill in the missing words to complete the following sentences (3 points).

   a. If air does not inflate the lungs when giving mouth-to-mouth breathing, you should _____ to ensure an open airway.

   b. If, after ensuring an open airway, the lungs still do not inflate, the victim should be treated for an _____.

   c. If the lungs do inflate during mouth-to-mouth breathing, give one breath every _____ seconds for an adult.

There are 8 possible points in this worksheet.

• WORKSHEET 4

1. Fill in the missing words to complete the following sentences (4 points).

   a. Obstructed airway occurs when an _____ blocks the airway.

   b. The two types of obstructions discussed are _____ and _____.

   c. Do not _____ with the victim's attempt to cough the object out.

2. List the signs of poor air exchange (5 points).

   a. _____

   b. _____

   c. _____

   d. _____

   e. _____

3. _____ occurs when there is no air exchange or there is poor air exchange (1 point).

4. List the signs of a complete airway obstruction (3 points).

   a. _____

   b. _____

   c. _____

5. List each step in the procedure to correct an obstructed airway of a conscious victim (2 points).

    a. _____

    b. _____

6. Should you begin the Heimlich maneuver if the victim is coughing (1 point)? _____

7. List each step in the procedure for obstructed airway in an unconscious victim (6 points).

    a. _____

    b. _____

    c. _____

    d. _____

    e. _____

    f. _____

There are 22 possible points in this worksheet.

• WORKSHEET 5

1. The first two hours after the onset of a heart attack are the _____ period (1 point).

2. List the early warning signs of a heart attack (3 points).

    a. _____

    b. _____

    c. _____

3. If the bleeding is pulsating in a serious wound, the _____ has been cut (1 point).

4. When an artery is cut, it is necessary to apply _____ to stop the bleeding (1 point).

5. Covering a serious wound decreases the chance of _____ (1 point).

6. When performing first aid for a serious wound, you may use a piece of (a) _____ or (b) _____ if gauze dressings are not available (2 points).

7. List the procedure for performing first aid on a serious wound (3 points).

    a. _____

    b. _____

    c. _____

8. List the procedure for performing first aid on a serious wound when direct pressure does not control the bleeding (4 points).

a. _____

b. _____

c. _____

d. _____

There are 16 possible points in this worksheet.

● WORKSHEET 6

1. Fill in the missing words to complete the following sentences (4 points).

a. Shock after a serious injury can be _____.

b. Shock _____ body functions and keeps the _____ from functioning normally.

c. A victim can be treated correctly for a wound and still _____ from shock.

2. List the procedure for preventing shock (7 points).

a. _____

b. _____

c. _____

d. _____

e. _____

f. _____

g. _____

3. While following the procedure to prevent shock, you find an open fracture of the right leg. Should you elevate the right leg (1 point)? _____

4. How should you position a victim you are treating for shock if he or she is vomiting or bleeding from the mouth (1 point)?_____

5. Should victims with breathing problems, head injury, or neck injury have their feet elevated (1 point)?_____

There are 14 possible points in this worksheet.

● WORKSHEET 7

1. Poisoning often causes (a) _____ , (b) _____, and (c) _____ (3 points).

2. List the first aid procedure for a conscious poison victim (5 points).

a. _____

b. _____

c. _____

d. _____

e. _____

3. List the first aid procedure for an unconscious poison victim (6 points).

a. _____

b. _____

c. _____

d. _____

e. _____

f. _____

4. Fill in the missing words to complete the following sentences (8 points).

a. Burns around the mouth or nose may indicate that the
_____ is burned.

b. Always check a mild burn _____ to _____
hours after it occurs. _____ and _____
may not appear until then.

c. When performing first aid on a burn victim, you strive to
_____, _____, and _____.

There are 22 possible points in this worksheet.

• WORKSHEET 8

1. What are the two main types of bone fractures (2 points)?

a. _____

b. _____

2. Bandages are necessary to prevent _____ from entering a
wound (1 point).

3. List the principles of bandaging (6 points).

a. _____

b. _____

c. _____

d. _____

e. _____

f. _____

There are 9 possible points in this worksheet.

• WORKSHEET/ACTIVITY 9

Practice and then demonstrate the following procedures as your instructor directs you. Check each one off as you complete it.

_____ a. Rescue breathing

_____ b. Obstructed airway in a conscious victim

_____ c. Obstructed airway in an unconscious victim

_____ d. Stopped breathing in an infant

_____ e. Obstructed airway in a conscious infant

_____ f. Obstructed airway in an unconscious infant

_____ g. How to treat serious wounds

_____ h. Identify pressure points on a diagram

_____ i. Preventing shock

_____ j. Treating a conscious poison victim

_____ k. Treating an unconscious poison victim

_____ l. Treating burns

_____ m. Applying a splint

_____ n. Applying a triangular sling

_____ o. Triangular bandaging of a head wound

_____ p. Circular bandaging of a small leg or arm wound

_____ q. Spiral bandaging of a large wound

_____ r. Bandaging of an ankle or foot wound

There are 18 possible points in this worksheet.

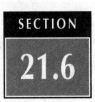

SECTION

21.6 Cardiopulmonary Resuscitation (CPR)

• OBJECTIVES

When you have completed this section, you will be able to do the following:

- Match key terms with their correct meanings.

- Demonstrate the procedures for cardiopulmonary resuscitation (CPR).

- Explain the role of a defibrillator in restoring normal heart beat.

- ## DIRECTIONS

    1. Complete Worksheet 1.

    2. Prepare responses to each item listed in Chapter Review.

    3. When you are confident that you can meet each objective listed above, ask your instructor for the section evaluation.

- ## EVALUATION METHODS

    - Worksheets
    - Class participation
    - Written evaluation

- ## WORKSHEET 1

    Match the definition in column B with the correct key term in column A (7 points).

    Column A

    _____ **1.** Cardiac

    _____ **2.** Resuscitation

    _____ **3.** Oxygenated

    _____ **4.** Defibrillator

    _____ **5.** Heel

    _____ **6.** Interlace

    _____ **7.** Compressions

    Column B

    a. The part of the hand between the palm and the wrist.

    b. Bringing back to live, revive.

    c. Put between.

    d. Pumps.

    e. A device that administers an electronic shock to restore normal heartbeat

    f. Containing oxygen.

    g. Relating to the heart.

CHECK-OFF SHEET:
21-1 How to Operate a Fire Extinguisher
Name _____ **Date** _____

Directions: Practice this procedure, following each step. When you are ready to have your performance evaluated, give this sheet to your instructor. Review the detailed procedure in your textbook.

Procedure	Pass	Redo	Date Competency Met	Instructor Initials
Student must use Standard Precautions.	☐	☐	_____	_____
1. First Response: RACE	☐	☐	_____	_____
Rescue				
Alert appropriate facility officials				
Contain Fire				
Extinguish Fire	☐	☐	_____	_____
Procedure	☐	☐	_____	_____
2. Locate fire extinguisher and check type.	☐	☐	_____	_____
3. Hold fire extinguisher upright. Pull ring pin.	☐	☐	_____	_____
4. Stand back six to ten feet and direct flow towards base of the fire.	☐	☐	_____	_____
5. Squeeze lever, sweeping side to side.	☐	☐	_____	_____
Postprocedure	☐	☐	_____	_____
6. Replace or have extinguisher recharged after use.	☐	☐	_____	_____

CHECK-OFF SHEET:
21-2 Rescue Breathing--Adult

Name _____ Date _____

Directions: Practice this procedure, following each step. When you are ready to have your performance evaluated, give this sheet to your instructor. Review the detailed procedure in your textbook.

Procedure	Pass	Redo	Date Competency Met	Instructor Initials
Student must use Standard Precautions.	☐	☐	_____	_____
1. Put on disposable gloves.	☐	☐	_____	_____
2. Check for consciousness by shaking victim's shoulder gently and asking if he or she is OK. If there is no response, activate EMS system.	☐	☐	_____	_____
Procedure	☐	☐	_____	_____
3. Open airway by placing one hand at victim's chin and the other hand on victim's forehead; gently lift chin by supporting jawbone with fingertips and lifting upward to open mouth. This is called the head tilt/chin lift.	☐	☐	_____	_____
4. Check for breathing by placing your ear near victim's mouth and nose. Turn your head so that you can see his or her chest. Look to see if chest is rising or falling. Listen for breathing. Feel for air from victim's mouth or nose on your cheek. If breathing is not present go to step 5.	☐	☐	_____	_____
5. Ventilate. Place a pocket mask over mouth and nose. Put apex (point) over bridge of nose and base between lip and chin. Give two breaths (11/2 to 2 seconds per breath) through the one-way valve. Allow lungs to empty between each breath. (If dentures obstruct the airway, remove them.) If air does not inflate lungs: retilt head to ensure an open airway and repeat the two breaths. Watch for chest to rise, allow for exhalation between breaths. (If lungs still do not inflate, treat victim for an obstructed airway; see the Obstructed Airway procedures.)	☐	☐	_____	_____
6. Check carotid pulse.	☐	☐	_____	_____
7. If breathing is absent and pulse is present, keep the airway open and give one breath to victim every 5 seconds. If there is no pulse, cardiopulmonary resuscitation (CPR) is needed to circulate oxygenated blood through body. See Section 21.6 for CPR procedures. CPR should be learned by taking a course given by a qualified instructor approved by the American Heart Association or American Red Cross.	☐	☐	_____	_____

Procedure	Pass	Redo	Date Competency Met	Instructor Initials
Postprocedure				
8. Ensure that victim has follow-up treatment or assessment by Emergency Medical Technicians or hospital personnel.	☐	☐	_____	_____
9. Discard gloves and wash hands (follow handwashing guidelines).	☐	☐	_____	_____

CHECK-OFF SHEET:
21-3 Obstructed Airway in a Conscious Victim—Adult
Name _____ Date _____

Directions: Practice this procedure, following each step. When you are ready to have your performance evaluated, give this sheet to your instructor. Review the detailed procedure in your textbook.

Procedure	Pass	Redo	Date Competency Met	Instructor Initials
Student must use Standard Precautions.	☐	☐	_____	_____

When signs of choking are present:

1. Ask "Are you choking?" Observe victim for coughing or wheezing. Do not interfere if good air exchange is present.   ☐   ☐   _____   _____

Procedure

2. Give abdominal thrust, sometimes called the Heimlich maneuver. Stand in back of victim; put your arms around victim's waist. Make a fist with one hand and put the thumb side of the fist slightly above the navel and well below the breast bone. Take your other hand and grasp list; pull into victim's abdomen with quick upward thrust. Repeat separate, rapid inward and upward thrusts until airway is cleared or patient becomes unconscious. (Use chest thrusts for a pregnant or obese victim.)   ☐   ☐   _____   _____

Postprocedure

3. Ensure that victim has follow-up treatment or assessment by Emergency Medical Technicians or hospital personnel, if needed.   ☐   ☐   _____   _____

4. Wash hands (follow hand-washing guidelines).   ☐   ☐   _____   _____

CHECK-OFF SHEET:
21-4 Obstructed Airway in an Unconscious Victim—Adult.

Name _____ Date _____

Directions: Practice this procedure, following each step. When you are ready to have your performance evaluated, give this sheet to your instructor. Review the detailed procedure in your textbook.

Procedure	Pass	Redo	Date Competency Met	Instructor Initials
Student must use Standard Precautions.	☐	☐	_____	_____
1. Activate the EMS system.	☐	☐	_____	_____
2. Put on disposable gloves.	☐	☐	_____	_____
Procedure				
3. Open airway. Place one hand at victim's chin and the other hand on victim's forehead; gently tip head back. Lift chin in head tilt/chin lift position.	☐	☐	_____	_____
4. Attempt to ventilate. Open the airway and ventilate through a pocket face mask with a one-way valve. If no air enters, retilt head and try to ventilate again. Every time you give a breath, open mouth wide and look for object. If you see an object, remove it with fingers. If you do not see an object, proceed with CPR.	☐	☐	_____	_____
Postprocedure				
5. Ensure that victim has follow-up treatment or assessment by Emergency Medical Technicians or hospital personnel.	☐	☐	_____	_____
6. Discard gloves and wash hands (follow handwashing guidelines).	☐	☐	_____	_____

CHECK-OFF SHEET:
21-5 Stopped Breathing in an Infant
Name _____ **Date** _____

Directions: Practice this procedure, following each step. When you are ready to have your performance evaluated, give this sheet to your instructor. Review the detailed procedure in your textbook.

Procedure	Pass	Redo	Date Competency Met	Instructor Initials
Student must use Standard Precautions.	☐	☐	_____	_____
1. Put on disposable gloves.	☐	☐	_____	_____
2. Check for consciousness. Shake baby's shoulders gently and speak baby's name. If no response, shout for help.	☐	☐	_____	_____
Procedure				
3. Open airway. Use head tilt/chin lift method. Do not over tilt head or neck.	☐	☐	_____	_____
4. Check for breathing. Look, listen, and feel. If not breathing:	☐	☐	_____	_____
5. Place an infant-sized barrier device on the infant's face. Ventilate through the one-way valve and give rescue breathing. Give two slow breaths using only air in your cheeks. (Too much air may overinflate an infant's lungs.) Watch for chest to rise and allow chest to fall or deflate between each breath. If air does not inflate lungs:	☐	☐	_____	_____
6. Retilt head to ensure open airway. Repeat the two breaths. If lungs still do not inflate, treat infant for an obstructed airway. If lungs do inflate:	☐	☐	_____	_____
7. Keep airway open, and give one breath to infant every 3 seconds. After 1 minute activate EMS.	☐	☐	_____	_____
8. Check pulse. Place three fingers over brachial artery/pulse. The baby's heart may have stopped. In this event, only cardiopulmonary resuscitation (CPR) will help to circulate oxygenated blood throughout the body. See Procedures 21.22, 21.23 and 21.24 for CPR procedures. CPR should be learned by taking a course offered by an instructor who is certified by the American Heart Association or the American Red Cross. We strongly recommend you complete such a program.	☐	☐	_____	_____
Postprocedure				
9. Ensure that victim has follow-up treatment or assessment by Emergency Medical Technicians or hospital personnel.	☐	☐	_____	_____
10. Discard gloves and wash hands (follow handwashing guidelines).	☐	☐	_____	_____

CHECK-OFF SHEET:
21-6 Obstructed Airway in a Conscious Infant

Name _____ Date _____

Directions: Practice this procedure, following each step. When you are ready to have your performance evaluated, give this sheet to your instructor. Review the detailed procedure in your textbook.

Procedure	Pass	Redo	Date Competency Met	Instructor Initials
Student must use Standard Precautions.	☐	☐	_____	_____
1. Put on disposable gloves.	☐	☐	_____	_____
2. Observe to determine infant's ability to cry, cough, or breathe. If there is no evidence of air exchange, shout for help.	☐	☐	_____	_____
Procedure				
3. Give five back blows. Place infant face down, supporting head and neck and tilting infant so that the head is lower than rest of body. Give five firm hits with heel of your hand over.	☐	☐	_____	_____
4. Give five chest thrusts by turning infant on its back with head lower than rest of body. Using two to three fingers, push five times on midsternum, which is about one finger's width below nipple line at midchest at a rate of about one per second.	☐	☐	_____	_____
5. Continue procedure until obstruction is clear or infant becomes unconscious. If infant becomes unconscious, stop giving black blows and start CPR.	☐	☐	_____	_____
Postprocedure				
6. Ensure that victim has follow-up treatment or assessment by Emergency Medical Technicians or hospital personnel.	☐	☐	_____	_____
7. Discard gloves and wash hands (follow handwashing guidelines).	☐	☐	_____	_____

CHECK-OFF SHEET:
21-7 Obstructed Airway in an Unconscious Infant

Name _____ Date _____

Directions: Practice this procedure, following each step. When you are ready to have your performance evaluated, give this sheet to your instructor. Review the detailed procedure in your textbook.

Procedure	Pass	Redo	Date Competency Met	Instructor Initials
Student must use Standard Precautions.	☐	☐	_____	_____
1. Put on disposable gloves.	☐	☐	_____	_____
2. Observe to determine infant's ability to cry, cough, or breathe. If there is no evidence of air exchange, shout for help.	☐	☐	_____	_____
Procedure				
3. Place infant on a firm flat surface.	☐	☐	_____	_____
4. Open infant's airway and look for an object in the pharynx. If an object is visible, remove it. Do not perform a blind finger sweep.	☐	☐	_____	_____
5. Begin CPR with one extra step–each time you open the airway, look for the obstructing object in the back of the throat. If you see an object, remove it. After about 2 minutes, activate the EMS.	☐	☐	_____	_____
6. Once the airway is clear, ventilate once every 3 seconds.	☐	☐	_____	_____
Postprocedure				
7. Ensure that victim has follow-up treatment or assessment by Emergency Medical Technicians or hospital personnel.	☐	☐	_____	_____
8. Discard gloves and wash hands (follow handwashing guidelines).	☐	☐	_____	_____

CHECK-OFF SHEET:
21-8 Preventing Shock

Name _____ Date _____

Directions: Practice this procedure, following each step. When you are ready to have your performance evaluated, give this sheet to your instructor. Review the detailed procedure in your textbook.

Procedure	Pass	Redo	Date Competency Met	Instructor Initials
Student must use Standard Precautions.	☐	☐	_____	_____
1. If patient is located in the field (not in a health care facility), contact EMS.	☐	☐	_____	_____
Procedure				
2. Provide comfort, quiet, and warmth.	☐	☐	_____	_____
3. Maintain normal body temperature by covering with blanket.	☐	☐	_____	_____
4. Keep victim calm.	☐	☐	_____	_____
5. Keep victim lying down on back if possible. Elevate feet and arms. Do not elevate an unsplinted arm or leg that is fractured.	☐	☐	_____	_____
6. If victim is vomiting, bleeding from mouth, or feels like vomiting, position victim on side. Do not move the victim if there is any possibility of a spinal injury or if the victim complains of numbness, tingling, lack of sensation, or inability to move limbs.	☐	☐	_____	_____
7. If person has a head injury, neck injury, or breathing problem, feet should not be elevated and the victim should not be turned on his or her side.	☐	☐	_____	_____
8. Do not give the victim anything to eat or drink.	☐	☐	_____	_____
9. Provide oxygen as soon as possible if you have the training and equipment to do so; otherwise, call immediately for someone who does.	☐	☐	_____	_____
Postprocedure				
10. Discard gloves and wash hands (follow handwashing guidelines).	☐	☐	_____	_____

CHECK-OFF SHEET:
21-9 Treating a Conscious Poison Victim

Name _____ Date _____

Directions: Practice this procedure, following each step. When you are ready to have your performance evaluated, give this sheet to your instructor. Review the detailed procedure in your textbook.

Procedure	Pass	Redo	Date Competency Met	Instructor Initials
Student must use Standard Precautions.	☐	☐	_____	_____
1. Put on disposable gloves.	☐	☐	_____	_____
2. Try to locate poison container (try to identify source of poisoning); do not waste time. Check victim's body and clothes for signs of poisoning.	☐	☐	_____	_____
Procedure				
3. Position victim on his side to let mouth drain.	☐	☐	_____	_____
4. Call 911 to get an ambulance as soon as possible; then call the nearest poison center, hospital, or physician.* (Directions on poison containers and for ingested substances are not always correct.) When you call, state that you have a poisoning emergency. If you have the container, be prepared to read ingredients. Follow the directions from the poison center.	☐	☐	_____	_____
5. If poison on skin, wash with water.	☐	☐	_____	_____
6. If poison is from a snakebite: Cover and wrap the affected snakebite area. Continue wrapping the entire affected limb and apply a splint. This is called the pressure immobilization technique. Remember to make sure the wound does not swell enough to make the splint a tourniquet, cutting off the blood flow. Get person to an emergency care center as soon as possible.	☐	☐	_____	_____
7. If poison is from an insect bite: Apply cold compresses. A doctor may prescribe calcium gluconate for muscle pain and an anti-anxiety drug for spasms. For any poisonous insect bite, be sure your tetanus immunization is current.	☐	☐	_____	_____
8. Be alert for breathing problems. If breathing stops, you will perform mouth-to-mask (rescue breathing) resuscitation as discussed at beginning of section.	☐	☐	_____	_____
9. Follow procedure for preventing shock.	☐	☐	_____	_____
Postprocedure				
10. Ensure that victim has follow-up treatment or assessment by Emergency Medical Technicians or hospital personnel.	☐	☐	_____	_____
11. Discard gloves and wash hands (follow handwashing guidelines).	☐	☐	_____	_____

CHECK-OFF SHEET:
21-10 Treating an Unconscious Poison Victim

Name _____ Date _____

Directions: Practice this procedure, following each step. When you are ready to have your performance evaluated, give this sheet to your instructor. Review the detailed procedure in your textbook.

Procedure	Pass	Redo	Date Competency Met	Instructor Initials
Student must use Standard Precautions.	☐	☐	_____	_____
1. Put on disposable gloves.	☐	☐	_____	_____
2. Do not give any fluids.	☐	☐	_____	_____
Procedure				
3. Position victim on his or her side in a safe place.	☐	☐	_____	_____
4. Try to identify the poison source; do not waste time.	☐	☐	_____	_____
5. Call 911 to get an ambulance as soon as possible; then call the nearest poison center, hospital, or physician. Follow their directions.	☐	☐	_____	_____
6. If chemicals have gotten on skin, wash with water. Remove clothes and jewelry that are contaminated.	☐	☐	_____	_____
7. Be alert for breathing problems.	☐	☐	_____	_____
8. Follow procedure for preventing shock.	☐	☐	_____	_____
Postprocedure				
9. Ensure that victim has follow-up treatment or assessment by Emergency Medical Technicians or hospital personnel.	☐	☐	_____	_____
10. Discard gloves and wash hands (follow handwashing guidelines).	☐	☐	_____	_____

CHECK-OFF SHEET:
21-11 Treating Burns

Name _____ **Date** _____

Directions: Practice this procedure, following each step. When you are ready to have your performance evaluated, give this sheet to your instructor. Review the detailed procedure in your textbook.

Procedure	Pass	Redo	Date Competency Met	Instructor Initials
Student must use Standard Precautions.	☐	☐	_____	_____
Preprocedure				
1. Put on disposable gloves.	☐	☐	_____	_____
Procedure				
First-Degree Burn				
2. Apply cool water to burn area, submerge burn site in cool water, or cover the area with cool damp cloths; this will reduce pain.	☐	☐	_____	_____
3. Large surface burns should never be wet as this causes shock. Large burns may be dried with sterile dressing. Apply a cold pack over dressing to reduce discomfort. Partial thickness or deeper burns (full thickness) require the following procedure.	☐	☐	_____	_____
Procedure	☐	☐	_____	_____
Second- and Third-Degree Burns				
1. Stop the burning process by smothering or dousing with water and removing smoldering or hot clothing. Remove any sources of heat such as metal jewelry, belts, etc.	☐	☐	_____	_____
2. Cover burned area with dry, sterile, nonstick dressing to help prevent infection. Do not pull away clothing that is stuck to burn site.	☐	☐	_____	_____
3. Check the patient's: **A**irway **B**reathing **C**irculation Perform CPR if necessary.	☐	☐	_____	_____
4. Contact emergency medical service.	☐	☐	_____	_____
5. Cover with a dry sterile dressing if available. A non-fuzzy clean sheet or tablecloth could be substituted if sterile dressing is not available.	☐	☐	_____	_____

Procedure	Pass	Redo	Date Competency Met	Instructor Initials
6. If you can elevate the burned area to decrease swelling, especially if head is involved and victim is having trouble breathing.	☐	☐	_____	_____
7. Follow procedure to prevent shock.	☐	☐	_____	_____

Postprocedure

8. Ensure that victim has follow-up treatment or assessment by Emergency Medical Technicians or hospital personnel.	☐	☐	_____	_____
9. Discard gloves and wash hands (follow handwashing guidelines).	☐	☐	_____	_____

CHECK-OFF SHEET:
21-12 Applying a Splint

Name _____ **Date** _____

Directions: Practice this procedure, following each step. When you are ready to have your performance evaluated, give this sheet to your instructor. Review the detailed procedure in your textbook.

Procedure	Pass	Redo	Date Competency Met	Instructor Initials
Student must use Standard Precautions.	☐	☐	_____	_____
1. Put on disposable gloves.	☐	☐	_____	_____
2. Move fractured area as little as possible.	☐	☐	_____	_____

Procedure

3. Splint area with a firm object, such as newspapers, magazines folded flat, wood, or a commercially made splint. The splint should extend from the fingertips to the elbow. Need to immobilize joints above and below injury. Pad splint with clothing or towels if possible. Place padding or roller gauze in the hand for support and comfort.	☐	☐	_____	_____
4. Secure splint in place using roller gauze, wrapping it snugly and overlapping about two-thirds each wrap, or secure splint to extremity with strips of cloth at distal and proximal ends of the arm. You can wrap roller gauze over the fracture site. Do not exert any pressure over the injury.	☐	☐	_____	_____
5. If it is an open fracture, apply dressing over wound and secure in place with tape or with roller gauze that holds splint in place.	☐	☐	_____	_____

Postprocedure

6. Ensure that victim has follow-up treatment or assessment by Emergency Medical Technicians or hospital personnel.	☐	☐	_____	_____
7. Discard gloves and wash hands (follow handwashing guidelines).	☐	☐	_____	_____

CHECK-OFF SHEET:
21-13 Applying a Triangular Sling

Name _____ Date _____

Directions: Practice this procedure, following each step. When you are ready to have your performance evaluated, give this sheet to your instructor. Review the detailed procedure in your textbook.

Procedure	Pass	Redo	Date Competency Met	Instructor Initials
Student must use Standard Precautions.	☐	☐	_____	_____
1. Put on disposable gloves.	☐	☐	_____	_____
2. Make a sling from a piece of cloth, clothing, towel, or sheet; fold or cut this material into shape of a triangle. The ideal sling is about 50 to 60 inches long at its base and 36 to 40 inches long on each side.	☐	☐	_____	_____

Procedure

Procedure	Pass	Redo	Date Competency Met	Instructor Initials
3. Position triangular material over top of patient's chest opposite the injured arm. Fold patient's arm across chest. If patient cannot hold his or her own arm, have someone assist you, or provide support for patient's arm until you are ready to tie sling. Note that one point of triangle should extend beyond patient's elbow on injured side.	☐	☐	_____	_____
4. Take bottom point of triangle and bring this end up over patient's arm. When you are finished, take this bottom point over top of patient's shoulder on the side of injured arm.	☐	☐	_____	_____
5. Draw up on ends of sling so that patient's hand is about 4 inches above elbow. Tie the two ends of the sling together, making sure that the knot does not press against back of patient's neck. Place a flat pad of dressing or a handkerchief under the knot. Leave patient's fingertips exposed so that you can see any color changes that indicate lack of circulation. Check for radial pulse. If pulse is absent, take off sling and attempt to reposition arm to regain pulse, then repeat procedure	☐	☐	_____	_____
6. Take point of material at patient's elbow and fold it forward. Pin it to front of sling. This forms a pocket for the elbow. If you do not have pin, twist excess material and tie knot in point. This will provide a shallow pocket for patient's elbow.	☐	☐	_____	_____
7. Create a swathe by folding a triangular bandage in half and then folding it to a 4-inch width. This swathe is tied around chest and injured arm, over sling. Do not place this swathe over patient's arm on uninjured side.	☐	☐	_____	_____

Procedure	Pass	Redo	Date Competency Met	Instructor Initials
Postprocedure				
8. Ensure that victim has follow-up treatment or assessment by Emergency Medical Technicians or hospital personnel.	☐	☐	_____	_____
9. Discard gloves and wash hands (follow handwashing guidelines).	☐	☐	_____	_____

CHECK-OFF SHEET:
21-14 Triangular Bandaging of an Open Head Wound

Name _____ Date _____

Directions: Practice this procedure, following each step. When you are ready to have your performance evaluated, give this sheet to your instructor. Review the detailed procedure in your textbook.

Procedure	Pass	Redo	Date Competency Met	Instructor Initials
Student must use Standard Precautions.	☐	☐	_____	_____
1. Put on disposable gloves.	☐	☐	_____	_____
2. Fold triangular bandage to make 2-inch hem along base.	☐	☐	_____	_____
Procedure				
3. Apply gauze pad over wound. With folded edge face out, position bandage on patient's forehead, just above eyes. Make certain that point of bandage hangs down behind patient's head.	☐	☐	_____	_____
4. Draw ends of bandage behind patient's head and tie them.	☐	☐	_____	_____
5. Next, pull ends to front of patient's head and tie them together.	☐	☐	_____	_____
6. Tuck in the tail at back.	☐	☐	_____	_____
Postprocedure				
7. Ensure that victim has follow-up treatment or assessment by Emergency Medical Technicians or hospital personnel.	☐	☐	_____	_____
8. Discard gloves and wash hands (follow handwashing guidelines).				

CHECK-OFF SHEET:
21-15 Circular Bandaging of a Small Leg or Arm Wound

Name _____ Date _____

Directions: Practice this procedure, following each step. When you are ready to have your performance evaluated, give this sheet to your instructor. Review the detailed procedure in your textbook.

Procedure	Pass	Redo	Date Competency Met	Instructor Initials
Student must use Standard Precautions.	☐	☐	_____	_____
1. Put on disposable gloves.	☐	☐	_____	_____
Procedure				
2. Apply dressing to wound and elevate extremity.	☐	☐	_____	_____
3. Place end of gauze roll (1 to 2 inches wide) on dressing. Anchor end of gauze roll over dressing with two initial wraps. (Place end of gauze over the dressing. Wrap gauze around the area once. Fold angled corner of gauze back over wrapped gauze.) Continue to wrap from distal (far) end of extremity to proximal (near the torso) end until entire dressing is covered. Bandage will overlap dressing on both sides. Pull bandage snug as you wrap. Overlap each wrap by about two-thirds. Cut gauze and tape end or tie gauze to secure in place.	☐	☐	_____	_____
Postprocedure				
4. Ensure that victim has follow-up treatment or assessment by Emergency Medical Technicians or hospital personnel.	☐	☐	_____	_____
5. Discard gloves and wash hands (follow handwashing guidelines).	☐	☐	_____	_____

CHECK-OFF SHEET:

21-16 Spiral Bandaging of a Large Wound

Name _____ Date _____

Directions: Practice this procedure, following each step. When you are ready to have your performance evaluated, give this sheet to your instructor. Review the detailed procedure in your textbook.

Procedure	Pass	Redo	Date Competency Met	Instructor Initials
Student must use Standard Precautions.	☐	☐	_____	_____
1. Put on disposable gloves.	☐	☐	_____	_____
Procedure				
2. Apply dressing to wound.	☐	☐	_____	_____
3. Place end of gauze roll (3 to 6 inches wide) on lower edge of dressing.	☐	☐	_____	_____
4. Anchor end.	☐	☐	_____	_____
5. Wrap gauze around arm or leg at an angle and overlap the edges.				
6. If you use up the gauze, continue the wrap with another roll.	☐	☐	_____	_____
7. Secure end by taping or tying off.				
Postprocedure				
8. Ensure that victim has follow-up treatment or assessment by Emergency Medical Technicians or hospital personnel.	☐	☐	_____	_____
9. Discard gloves and wash hands (follow handwashing guidelines).	☐	☐	_____	_____

CHECK-OFF SHEET:

21-17 Bandaging of an Ankle or Foot Wound

Name _____ Date _____

Directions: Practice this procedure, following each step. When you are ready to have your performance evaluated, give this sheet to your instructor. Review the detailed procedure in your textbook.

Procedure	Pass	Redo	Date Competency Met	Instructor Initials
Student must use Standard Precautions.	☐	☐	_____	_____
Preprocedure				
1. Put on disposable gloves.	☐	☐	_____	_____
Procedure				
2. Apply dressing to wound.	☐	☐	_____	_____
3. Place end of gauze roll (1 to 2 inches wide) on top of foot just above toes, and anchor ends.	☐	☐	_____	_____
4. On second wrap around foot, bring gauze around back of ankle and over top of foot. Bring gauze under foot and over top of foot again. Wrap around ankle and over top of foot, then under foot. Continue these steps until dressing is covered, and secure gauze by tying off or taping.	☐	☐	_____	_____
Postprocedure				
5. Ensure that victim has follow-up treatment or assessment by Emergency Medical Technicians or hospital personnel.	☐	☐	_____	_____
6. Discard gloves and wash hands (follow handwashing guidelines).	☐	☐	_____	_____

CHECK-OFF SHEET:

21-18 How to Care for a Dislocation

Name _____ Date _____

Directions: Practice this procedure, following each step. When you are ready to have your performance evaluated, give this sheet to your instructor. Review the detailed procedure in your textbook.

Procedure	Pass	Redo	Date Competency Met	Instructor Initials
Student must use Standard Precautions.	☐	☐	_____	_____

Preprocedure

1. Determine the traumatic event leading to the injury.	☐	☐	_____	_____
2. Inspect the patient's affected joint for swelling, bruising, odd configuration of joint anatomy, and altered mobility.				
3. Gently palpate the joint noting any tenderness. Palpate nearby pulses to assess the circulatory status. Obtain medical assistance right away.	☐	☐	_____	_____

Procedure

Closed Reduction

4. Provide support for the patient during the examination and any procedure that may be indicated.	☐	☐	_____	_____
5. Assist with the application of an external immobilization device.	☐	☐	_____	_____
6. Apply ice for at least the first 24 hours.	☐	☐	_____	_____
7. Monitor the patient's neurovascular status by checking for pulses, warmth, color, and sensory function of the region around the injury site. Also note any increased swelling	☐	☐	_____	_____
8. Use a pain rating scale, such as a scale of 1 to 10, to evaluate the effectiveness of the pain medication.	☐	☐	_____	_____
9. Provide education to the patient/family regarding any ongoing care necessary and any rehabilitative exercise program prescribed for after the immobilizing device is removed.	☐	☐	_____	_____

Surgical Correction

10. Monitor the patient closely in the immediate postoperative period for:

___ neurovascular status

___ pain

___ alteration in vital signs	☐	☐	_____	_____

Procedure	Pass	Redo	Date Competency Met	Instructor Initials
11. Expect the patient to have either a cast or an external immobilizer.	☐	☐	_____	_____
12. Provide pain medication as directed by the physician.	☐	☐	_____	_____
13. Apply ice as directed by the physician.	☐	☐	_____	_____
14. Use a pain rating scale, such as a scale of 1 to 10, to evaluate the effectiveness of the pain medication and other interventions provided to relieve discomfort.	☐	☐	_____	_____
15. Prepare the patient for the rehabilitation period.	☐	☐	_____	_____

CHECK-OFF SHEET:

21-19 How to Care for a Strain

Name _____ Date _____

Directions: Practice this procedure, following each step. When you are ready to have your performance evaluated, give this sheet to your instructor. Review the detailed procedure in your textbook.

Procedure	Pass	Redo	Date Competency Met	Instructor Initials
Student must use Standard Precautions.	☐	☐	_____	_____

Expect the patient to complain of pain, decreased mobility, and strength loss at the site of injury. Important points to remember when assessing the patient are:

Preprocedure

Procedure	Pass	Redo	Date Competency Met	Instructor Initials
1. Ask how the injury occurred.	☐	☐	_____	_____
2. Ask about prior joint injuries.	☐	☐	_____	_____
3. Inspect the injured joint for swelling, bruising.	☐	☐	_____	_____
4. Palpate the joint, noting any tenderness. Palpate nearby pulses to assess the circulatory status.	☐	☐	_____	_____
5. To rule out a fracture, the physician will order x-rays.	☐	☐	_____	_____

Procedure

Procedure	Pass	Redo	Date Competency Met	Instructor Initials
6. Consult with the physician for any specific instructions related to the injury.	☐	☐	_____	_____
7. Apply a compression bandage as ordered by the physician.	☐	☐	_____	_____
8. Elevate the affected joint.	☐	☐	_____	_____
9. Check with the physician. Apply ice or heat as directed. If injury is several days old the physician may order heat rather than ice to reduce pain.	☐	☐	_____	_____
10. Elevate the affected extremity.	☐	☐	_____	_____
11. Monitor the patient's neurovascular status by checking for pulses, warmth, color, and sensory function of the region around the injury site. Also note any increased swelling.	☐	☐	_____	_____
12. Medicate as directed by the physician. In most cases, analgesics, anti-inflammatory drugs, or a muscle relaxant will be prescribed. These should be dispensed by licensed heath care professionals.	☐	☐	_____	_____
13. Use a pain rating scale, such as a scale of 1 to 10, to evaluate the effectiveness of the Pain medication and other interventions.	☐	☐	_____	_____

Procedure	Pass	Redo	Date Competency Met	Instructor Initials
14. Advise the patient to rest and avoid using the strained muscle.	☐	☐	_____	_____
15. Educate the patient on prescribed exercises to follow after healing has begun.	☐	☐	_____	_____
16. Advise the patient to resume activities gradually.	☐	☐	_____	_____

CHECK-OFF SHEET:

21-20 How to Care for a Sprain

Name _____ **Date** _____

Directions: Practice this procedure, following each step. When you are ready to have your performance evaluated, give this sheet to your instructor. Review the detailed procedure in your textbook.

Procedure	Pass	Redo	Date Competency Met	Instructor Initials
Student must use Standard Precautions.	☐	☐	_____	_____

Expect the patient to complain of pain, decreased mobility, and strength loss at the site of injury. Important points to remember when assessing the patient are:

	Pass	Redo	Date Competency Met	Instructor Initials
1. Ask how the injury occurred.	☐	☐	_____	_____
2. Ask about prior joint injuries.	☐	☐	_____	_____
3. Observe the patient as he stands, walks, and sits, noting abnormalities such as change in gait or inability to bear weight on join.	☐	☐	_____	_____
4. Inspect the injured joint for swelling and bruising.	☐	☐	_____	_____
5. Palpate the joint, noting any tenderness. Palpate nearby pulses to assess the circulatory status.	☐	☐	_____	_____

Procedure

	Pass	Redo	Date Competency Met	Instructor Initials
6. Consult with the physician for any specific instructions related to the injury.	☐	☐	_____	_____
7. Immobilize the join, using a split or aircast.	☐	☐	_____	_____
8. Monitor the patient's neurovascular status by checking for pulses, warmth, color, mobility and sensory function of the region around the injury site. Also note any increased swelling.	☐	☐	_____	_____
9. Elevate the injured extremity to reduce swelling and pain.	☐	☐	_____	_____
10. Apply ice to the injury.	☐	☐	_____	_____
11. Medicate the patient with prescribed pain medication.	☐	☐	_____	_____
12. Use a pain rating scale, such as a scale of 1 to 10, to evaluate the effectiveness of the Pain medication and other interventions.	☐	☐	_____	_____
13. Provide education to the patient/family regarding any ongoing care necessary.	☐	☐	_____	_____

CHECK-OFF SHEET:
21-21 Cast Care
Name _____ Date _____

Directions: Practice this procedure, following each step. When you are ready to have your performance evaluated, give this sheet to your instructor. Review the detailed procedure in your textbook.

Procedure	Pass	Redo	Date Competency Met	Instructor Initials
Student must use Standard Precautions.	☐	☐	_____	_____

Prior to the application of the cast the nurse should establish a baseline assessment of the area to be casted.

This would include:

- Palpation of the distal pulses

- Assessment of the color, temperature, and capillary refill of the skin.

- Neurologic function, including sensation and motion in the affected area.

Special Considerations: A fiberglass cast dries immediately after application. A plaster cast dries in approximately 24 to 48 hours. During this drying period, the cast must be properly positioned to prevent a surface depression that could cause pressure areas or dependent anemia

Procedure

Procedure	Pass	Redo	Date Competency Met	Instructor Initials
1. Assess your patient frequently.	☐	☐	_____	_____
2. Check the casted area for drainage stains.	☐	☐	_____	_____
3. Elevate the extremity above patient's heart level.	☐	☐	_____	_____
4. Place absorptive pads between the moist cast and any bedding to absorb moisture.	☐	☐	_____	_____
5. Periodically check the cast for flat spots or dents. These may cause pressure areas, resulting in skin breakdown.	☐	☐	_____	_____
6. Reposition the patient every 2 hours to ensure even cast drying. Use the palm of the hand, not the fingers for repositioning in order to avoid denting the cast. Make sure bony prominences, such as heels, ankles, and elbows are pressure free.	☐	☐	_____	_____
7. Routinely assess your patient's neurovascular status. Check for swelling, pallor, numbness, tingling, loss of pulses, and cool skin areas around the cast. Notify the doctor immediately for any of these signs.	☐	☐	_____	_____
8. Notify the doctor for: drainage from the wound on the cast malodor from the cast	☐	☐	_____	_____
9. Protect the cast from getting wet.	☐	☐	_____	_____
10. Provide skin care.	☐	☐	_____	_____

CHECK-OFF SHEET:
21-22 Cardiopulmonary Resuscitation--Adult

Name _____   Date _____

Directions: Practice this procedure, following each step. When you are ready to have your performance evaluated, give this sheet to your instructor. Review the detailed procedure in your textbook.

Procedure	Pass	Redo	Date Competency Met	Instructor Initials
Student must use Standard Precautions.	☐	☐	_____	_____
1. Put on disposable gloves.	☐	☐	_____	_____
2. Check for consciousness by shaking victim's shoulder gently and asking if he or she is OK. If there is no response, activate EMS system.	☐	☐	_____	_____

Procedure

3. Check for breathing by placing your ear near victim's mouth and nose. Turn your head so that you can see his or her chest. Look to see if chest is rising or falling. Listen for breathing. Feel for air from victim's mouth or nose on your cheek. If breathing is *not* present:	☐	☐	_____	_____
4. Open airway by placing one hand at victim's chin and the other hand on victim's forehead; gently lift chin by supporting jawbone with fingertips and lifting upward to open mouth. (Do not put pressure on throat; this may block airway.) This is called the head tilt/chin lift.	☐	☐	_____	_____
5. Ventilate. Place a pocket mask over mouth and nose. Put apex (point) over bridge of nose and base between lip and chin. Give two breaths (11/2 to 2 seconds per breath) through the one-way valve. Allow lungs to empty between each breath. (If dentures obstruct the airway, remove them.) If air does not inflate lungs: retilt head to ensure an open airway and repeat the two breaths. Watch for chest to rise, allow for exhalation between breaths.	☐	☐	_____	_____
6. Check carotid pulse for 5–10 seconds.	☐	☐	_____	_____
7. If pulse is absent, begin chest compressions. Kneel on one side of the victim. Draw an imaginary line between the nipples. Place two fingers on the breast bone just below this line. Place the heel of one hand at this location. Place the other hand on top and interlace fingers. Push straight down on the chest for 30 compressions. The chest should be pushed down about 11/2 to 2 inches during each compression. Compressions should be faster than one per second, so that blood is pumped through the body at a rate of 100 pumps per minute.	☐	☐	_____	_____

Procedure	Pass	Redo	Date Competency Met	Instructor Initials
8. Give two breaths.	☐	☐	_____	_____
9. Continue to deliver 30 compressions for every two breaths until help arrives. Recheck pulse every two minutes.	☐	☐	_____	_____
Postprocedure				
10. Ensure that victim has follow-up treatment or assessment by Emergency Medical Technicians or hospital personnel.	☐	☐	_____	_____
11. Discard gloves and wash hands (follow handwashing guidelines).	☐	☐	_____	_____

CHECK-OFF SHEET:

21-23 Performing CPR, Two Person

Name _____ Date _____

Directions: Practice this procedure, following each step. When you are ready to have your performance evaluated, give this sheet to your instructor. Review the detailed procedure in your textbook.

Procedure	Pass	Redo	Date Competency Met	Instructor Initials
Student must use Standard Precautions.	☐	☐	_____	_____

1. The provider should understand that the critical concepts of quality CPR include:

     Push hard, push fast: compress at a rate of 100 compressions per minute.

     Allow full chest recoil after each compression.

     Minimize interruptions in chest compressions.

Avoid hyperventilation	☐	☐	_____	_____

Procedure

2. When a second rescuer is available to help, that second rescuer should activate the emergency response system and get the AED if available. The first rescuer should remain with the victim to begin CPR immediately.

     After the second rescuer returns, the rescuers should take turns doing chest compressions, switching after every 5 cycles of CPR. Follow the procedure for one person cardiopulmonary resuscitation assigning tasks as follows:

Actions

3. Performs chest compressions.	☐	☐	_____	_____
4. Counts out loud.	☐	☐	_____	_____
5. Switches duties with rescuer 2 every 5 cycles, taking less than 5 seconds to switch.	☐	☐	_____	_____
6. Maintains an open airway.	☐	☐	_____	_____
7. Give breaths, watching for chest rise.	☐	☐	_____	_____
8. Encourages rescuer 1 to perform compressions that are fast and deep enough to allow full chest recoil between compressions.	☐	☐	_____	_____
9. Switches duties with rescuer 1 every 5 cycles taking less than 5 seconds to switch.	☐	☐	_____	_____

CHECK-OFF SHEET:
21-24 Cardiopulmonary Resuscitation--Infant

Name _____ Date _____

Directions: Practice this procedure, following each step. When you are ready to have your performance evaluated, give this sheet to your instructor. Review the detailed procedure in your textbook.

Procedure	Pass	Redo	Date Competency Met	Instructor Initials
Student must use Standard Precautions.	☐	☐	_____	_____
1. Put on disposable gloves.	☐	☐	_____	_____
2. Check for consciousness. Shake the infant's foot for reflex action gently and speak baby's name. If no response, shout for help.	☐	☐	_____	_____
Procedure				
3. Open airway. Use head tilt/chin lift method. Do not overtilt head or neck.	☐	☐	_____	_____
4. Check for breathing. Look, listen, and feel. If not breathing:	☐	☐	_____	_____
5. Place an infant-sized barrier device on the infant's face. Ventilate through the one-way valve and give rescue breathing. Give two slow breaths using only air in your cheeks. (Too much air may overinflate an infant's lungs.) Watch for chest to rise and allow chest to fall or deflate between each breath. If air does not inflate lungs:	☐	☐	_____	_____
6. Retilt head to ensure open airway. Repeat the two breaths. If lungs still do not inflate, treat infant for an obstructed airway.	☐	☐	_____	_____
If lungs do inflate:				
7. Check pulse. Place three fingers over brachial artery/pulse. The baby's heart may have stopped.	☐	☐	_____	_____
8. If pulse is absent, begin chest compressions. Place two or three fingers near the center of the chest, just below the nipples. Push down gently on the chest for 30 compressions. The chest should be pushed down about 1/3 of its depth during each compression. Compressions should be faster than one per second, so that blood is pumped through the body at a rate of 100 pumps per minute.	☐	☐	_____	_____
9. Give two breaths and deliver 30 more compressions.	☐	☐	_____	_____
10. After two minutes of breaths and compressions, activate EMS system.				
11. Continue cycle of breaths and compressions until help arrives.	☐	☐	_____	_____

Procedure	Pass	Redo	Date Competency Met	Instructor Initials
Postprocedure				
12. Ensure that victim has follow-up treatment or assessment by Emergency Medical Technicians or hospital personnel.	☐	☐	_____	_____
13. Discard gloves and wash hands (follow hand-washing guidelines).	☐	☐	_____	_____

CHECK-OFF SHEET:

21-25 Demonstrating the Use of AED (Automated External Defibrillator)

Name _____ Date _____

Directions: Practice this procedure, following each step. When you are ready to have your performance evaluated, give this sheet to your instructor. Review the detailed procedure in your textbook.

Procedure	Pass	Redo	Date Competency Met	Instructor Initials
Student must use Standard Precautions.	☐	☐	_____	_____

Once the AED arrives, put it at the victim's side, next to the rescuer who will operate it. This will allow a second rescuer to perform CPR from the opposite side of the victim without interfering with AED operation. The following are four universal steps for operating an AED:

1. Power on the AED:

   Open the carrying case.

   Turn the power on. ☐ ☐ _____ _____

2. **ATTACH** electrode pads to the victim's bare chest:

   Choose correct pads for size/age of victim. Child pads will be used for children less than 8 years of age. Adult pads are used for the victim who is over 8 years of age.

   Peel the backing away from the electrode pads.

   Quickly wipe the victim's chest dry if covered with sweat or water. If the chest is covered with hair and electrode pads will not stick, pull the pad away from chest. This should take the hair with it. If still will not stick, shave area with razor included in the AED Kit.

   Attach the adhesive electrode pads to the

   victim's bare chest.

   — Place one electrode pad on the upperright side of the bare chest to the right of the breastbone, directly below the collarbone.

   — Place the other pad to the left of the nipple, a few inches below the left arm pit. Attach the AED connecting cables to the AED box (some are preconnected). ☐ ☐ _____ _____

Procedure	Pass	Redo	Date Competency Met	Instructor Initials

3. "Clear" the victim and **ANALYZE** the rhythm.

Always clear the victim during the analysis. Be sure that no one is touching the victim, not even the person in charge of giving breaths.

Some AEDS will tell you to push a button to allow the AED to begin analyzing the heart rhythm; others will do that automatically. The AED may take about 5 to 15 seconds to analyze.

The AED then tells you if a shock is needed. Remember if the victim has an unshockable rhythm there will be no advice to shock.

4. If the AED advises a shock, it will tell you to be sure to clear the victim.

Clear the victim before delivering the shock; be sure no one is touching the victim to avoid injury to rescuers.

— Loudly state a "clear the patient" message, such as "I'm clear, you're clear, everybody's clear."

— Perform a visual check to ensure that no one is in contact with the victim.

Press the **SHOCK** button.

The shock will produce a sudden contraction of the victim's muscles. ☐ ☐ _____ _____

5. As soon as the AED gives the shock, begin CPR starting with chest compressions. ☐ ☐ _____ _____

6. After 2 minutes of CPR, the AED will prompt you to repeat steps 3 and 4. ☐ ☐ _____ _____

Chapter 22 Dental Assistant Skills

SECTION 22.1 Responsibilities of a Dental Assistant

• OBJECTIVES

When you have completed this section, you will be able to do the following:

- Match key terms with their correct meanings.
- Describe the responsibilities of dental assistants.
- Differentiate between posterior and anterior teeth and their functions.
- Identify the following:
  — Deciduous and permanent teeth by name on a diagram.
  — Surfaces of a tooth.
  — Dental office equipment and instruments by name
- Label the following:
  — Parts of the oral cavity on a diagram
  — Teeth on a diagram using the universal method
  — Anatomical structure of a tooth on a diagram
- Teach the following:
  — How to use disclosing tablets/solutions
  — The Bass toothbrushing technique
  — Dental flossing techniques

• DIRECTIONS

1. Complete Worksheets 1 and 2.
2. Complete Worksheets 3 and 4 as assigned.
3. Complete the three parts of Worksheet 5.

4. Complete Worksheets/Activities 6 through 8.

5. When you are confident that you can meet each objective, ask your teacher for the section evaluation.

6. Prepare responses to each item listed in Chapter Review.

• EVALUATION METHODS

- Worksheets/Activities
- Class participation
- Written evaluation
- Demonstrations

• WORKSHEET 1

Match each definition in column B with the correct vocabulary word in column A.

Column A

_____ 1. Apex
_____ 2. Ala
_____ 3. ADA
_____ 4. Deciduous
_____ 5. Posterior
_____ 6. Visible
_____ 7. erupt
_____ 8. Caries
_____ 9. Proximal
_____ 10. Restorative
_____ 11. Rheostat
_____ 12. Aspirate
_____ 13. Exposure
_____ 14. Mandible
_____ 15. Cusp
_____ 16. Accessory
_____ 17. Dentition
_____ 18. Intraoral
_____ 19. Apical foramen
_____ 20. Functional stress

Column B

a. American Dental Association.
b. Intended to help.
c. Destined to fall out.
d. Natural teeth in the dental arch.
e. The outer side of the nostril.
f. Within the oral cavity.
g. Stress to tooth caused by its normal function.
h. An opening in the apex.
i. To the back.
j. Nearest or next to.
k. To return to as close to normal conditions as possible.
l. Decay.
m. Contact with radiation.
n. Able to be seen.
o. Soaking.
p. Material for making impressions.
q. Push through.
r. Jawbone.
s. Pointed or rounded raised area on the surface of the tooth.
t. Examination by feeling for unusual or abnormal conditions.
u. Control for flow of electric current.
v. Remove substances.
w. Area at the end of the tooth root.

There are 20 possible points in this worksheet.

● WORKSHEET 2

Fill in the crossword puzzle using the vocabulary words from Chapter 22 and the clues on the next page.

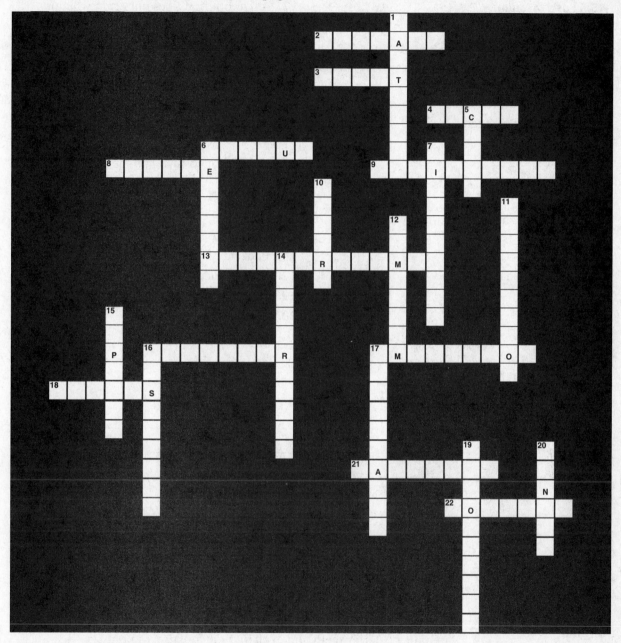

Clues

Across

2. First.
3. Push through.
4. Breaking down, rot.
6. Soft deposit of bacteria and bacteria products on teeth.
8. Calm.
9. Tissue around the apex of the tooth.
13. Sides between teeth.

Down

1. Chew.
5. Pointed or rounded, raised areas on the surface of the tooth.
6. At regular times, with time in between.
7. Ability to clearly see structures in the mouth.
10. Moving in a circular motion.
11. Removal.

16. Toward the front.
17. Any tooth that does not erupt when it normally should.
18. Depression, groove, area where gingival tip meets tooth enamel.
21. Same direction and at a distance so two points do not touch.
22. Indented.

12. Hard, thin covering or shell that covers the root.
14. Returning to as close to normal as possible.
15. Applied to surface.
16. Pockets of pus in a limited area.
17. Type of medication given by needle.
19. Loss of substance or bone.
20. Raised.

There are 25 possible points in this worksheet.

• WORKSHEET 3

1. Write the three ways teeth are identified (3 points).

   a. _____

   b. _____

   c. _____

2. Name two arches in the mouth (2 points).

   a. _____

   b. _____

3. Name the anterior teeth and explain their function (4 points).

   a. _____

   b. _____

4. Name the posterior teeth and explain their function (4 points).

   a. _____

   b. _____

5. There are _____ teeth in the deciduous dentition (1 point).

6. There are _____ teeth in the permanent dentition (1 point).

   There are 15 possible points in this worksheet.

• **WORKSHEET 4**

Identify the teeth listed below as deciduous, permanent, or both by placing the appropriate letter next to each tooth name (9 points).

a. deciduous   b. permanent   c. both deciduous and permanent

_____ **1.** Central incisors

_____ **2.** Lateral incisors

_____ **3.** Cuspids

_____ **4.** Bicuspids

_____ **5.** 1st premolar

_____ **6.** 2nd premolar

_____ **7.** 1st molar

_____ **8.** 2nd molars

_____ **9.** 3rd molars

Label the following teeth by the universal method (52 points).

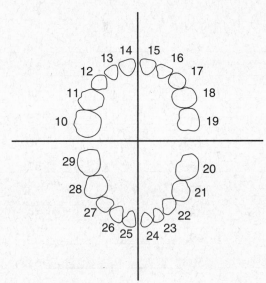

10. _____   **20.** _____

11. _____   **21.** _____

12. _____   **22.** _____

13. _____   **23.** _____

14. _____   **24.** _____

15. _____   **25.** _____

16. _____   **26.** _____

17. _____   **27.** _____

18. _____   **28.** _____

19. _____   **29.** _____

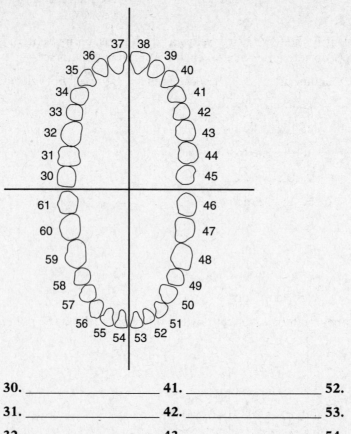

30. _____	41. _____	52. _____
31. _____	42. _____	53. _____
32. _____	43. _____	54. _____
33. _____	44. _____	55. _____
34. _____	45. _____	56. _____
35. _____	46. _____	57. _____
36. _____	47. _____	58. _____
37. _____	48. _____	59. _____
38. _____	49. _____	60. _____
39. _____	50. _____	61. _____
40. _____	51. _____	

There are 61 possible points in this worksheet.

• WORKSHEET 5

Part 1

Label the three main sections of a tooth on the following diagram (3 points).

1. _____

2. _____

3. _____

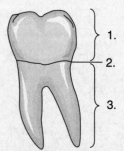

Label the structures in the following diagram (11 points).

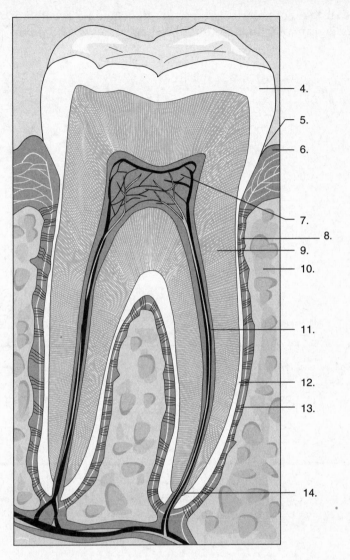

4. _____

5. _____

6. _____

7. _____

8. _____

9. _____

10. _____

11. _____

12. _____

13. _____

14. _____

Part 2

The surfaces of anterior crowns are indicated below. Photocopy the diagram, cut diagram out, and fold into the shape of a tooth (5 points). See Figure 22.8.

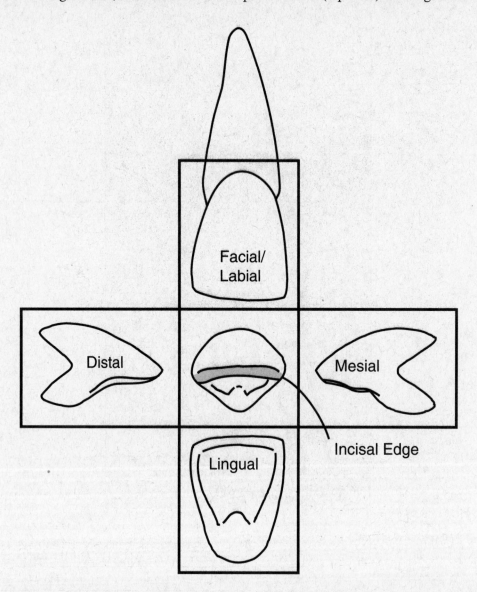

Part 3

The five surfaces of the posterior crown are indicated below. Photocopy the diagram, cut diagram out, and fold into the shape of a tooth (5 points). See Figure 22.8.

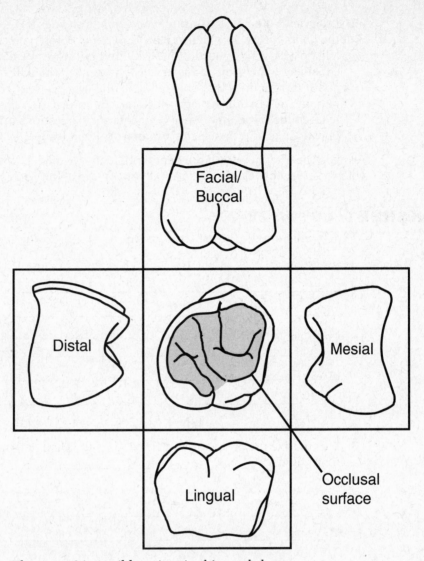

There are 24 possible points in this worksheet.

● WORKSHEET/ACTIVITY 6

1. List nine responsibilities of a dental assistant.

_____

_____

_____

_____

_____

_____

_____

_____

_____

2. Interview a dental assistant in your area. Consider the dental assistant at the dental office at which you are a patient. Before your interview, make up a list of five or six questions to ask. Find out what the dental assistant considers to be some of his or her most important skills. You might ask about the qualities that enable the dental assistant to work well with patients by providing them with accurate information and calming their fears at the same time. Keep your interview questions brief. Present your questions to your instructor for approval in advance.

Arrange the interview with the dental office in advance. If possible, conduct your interview by telephone. Present your findings to the class.

• WORKSHEET/ACTIVITY 7

1. Why might a dentist ask an assistant to use disclosing tablets or solution?

_____

_____

_____

2. Summarize the Bass brushing technique. Then demonstrate it on a tooth model. _____

_____

_____

_____

3. Summarize the procedure for flossing teeth. Then demonstrate it on a tooth model. _____

_____

_____

_____

• WORKSHEET/ACTIVITY 8

Find a partner and ask your instructor if you may organize a class spelling bee when you are close to finishing the dental assisting chapter. Get a list of dental terms:

- Read out a term.
- Have your partner select a volunteer to spell the term and write it on the board.
- Select another volunteer to define the term.
- Keep a list on the board of the people who correctly spelled or defined terms.

There are 10 possible points for each organizer of the worksheet/activity.

Volunteers get 1 point for each correct spelling or definition.

CHECK-OFF SHEET:
22-1 Bass Toothbrushing Technique

Name _____ Date _____

Directions: Practice this procedure, following each step. When you are ready to have your performance evaluated, give this sheet to your instructor. Review the detailed procedure in your textbook.

Procedure	Pass	Redo	Date Competency Met	Instructor Initials
Student must use Standard Precautions.	☐	☐	_____	_____
Preprocedure				
1. Wash hands.	☐	☐	_____	_____
2. Assemble equipment:	☐	☐	_____	_____
a. Tooth model (if using a model for teaching)	☐	☐	_____	_____
b. Protective wear (if brushing patient's teeth or if there is contact with saliva), including gloves, mask, and goggles	☐	☐	_____	_____
c. Toothbrush	☐	☐	_____	_____
Procedure				
3. Explain importance of toothbrushing.	☐	☐	_____	_____
4. Demonstrate correct brushing using model or on patient. NOTE: Put on gloves if demonstrating on patient.	☐	☐	_____	_____
a. Place soft brush on upper right molars (maxillary).	☐	☐	_____	_____
b. Position brush at 45° angle to teeth.	☐	☐	_____	_____
c. Gently move bristles into gingival sulcus.	☐	☐	_____	_____
d. Move brush in short strokes at least 10 to 20 times, keeping brush in place (wiggle-jiggle motion).	☐	☐	_____	_____
e. Move brush to next two or three teeth and repeat until all buccal/labial surfaces are brushed. NOTE: Place brush in vertical or horizontal position for anterior teeth.	☐	☐	_____	_____
f. Repeat technique beginning at upper right molars until all maxillary teeth are brushed.	☐	☐	_____	_____
g. Use short, vibrating motion to scrub occlusal surfaces.	☐	☐	_____	_____
h. Repeat this procedure for lower teeth (mandibular).	☐	☐	_____	_____
5. Ask client if he or she has any questions.	☐	☐	_____	_____

Procedure	Pass	Redo	Date Competency Met	Instructor Initials
Postprocedure				
6. Remove and clean equipment.	☐	☐	_____	_____
7. Remove protective wear.	☐	☐	_____	_____
8. Wash hands.	☐	☐	_____	_____
9. Chart TBI (toothbrushing instruction).	☐	☐	_____	_____

CHECK-OFF SHEET:
22-2 Dental Flossing

Name _____ Date _____

Directions: Practice this procedure, following each step. When you are ready to have your performance evaluated, give this sheet to your instructor. Review the detailed procedure in your textbook.

Procedure	Pass	Redo	Date Competency Met	Instructor Initials
Student must use Standard Precautions.	☐	☐	_____	_____
Preprocedure				
1. Wash hands.	☐	☐	_____	_____
2. Assemble equipment:	☐	☐	_____	_____
a. Tooth model (if using a model for teaching)	☐	☐	_____	_____
b. Gloves, mask, and goggles (if flossing patient's teeth or if there is contact with saliva)	☐	☐	_____	_____
c. Dental floss (waxed or unwaxed according to policy)	☐	☐	_____	_____
Procedure	☐	☐	_____	_____
3. Explain importance of flossing.				
4. Demonstrate correct flossing technique using model or patient. NOTE: Put on protective wear if demonstrating onpatient.	☐	☐	_____	_____
a. Cut floss 18 inches (measure from finger to elbow).	☐	☐	_____	_____
b. Wrap floss around middle or index finger of both hands, leaving 1 to 2 inches between fingers	☐	☐	_____	_____
c. Stretch floss between fingers and gently guide	☐	☐	_____	_____
d. Pass floss through contacts (where teeth touch) and wrap it around tooth in a C shape	☐	☐	_____	_____
e. Move floss up and down several times on sides of each toot	☐	☐	_____	_____
f. Unroll new floss from one hand and wrap used floss around middle finger of other hand.	☐	☐	_____	_____
g. Repeat for each tooth until all teeth in maxilla and mandible are completed.	☐	☐	_____	_____
5. Explain that there may be some bleeding of the gingiva/gums the first few times the patient does this procedure.	☐	☐	_____	_____
6. Ask patient if he or she has any questions.	☐	☐	_____	_____

CHECK-OFF SHEET:
22-3 Mounting Dental Films

Name _____ Date _____

Directions: Practice this procedure, following each step. When you are ready to have your performance evaluated, give this sheet to your instructor. Review the detailed procedure in your textbook.

Procedure	Pass	Redo	Date Competency Met	Instructor Initials
Student must use Standard Precautions.	☐	☐	_____	_____
Preprocedure				
1. Wash hands.	☐	☐	_____	_____
2. Assemble equipment:	☐	☐	_____	_____
a. Developed x-rays	☐	☐	_____	_____
b. X-ray mounts	☐	☐	_____	_____
c. View box	☐	☐	_____	_____
Procedure	☐	☐	_____	_____
3. Turn on view box.	☐	☐	_____	_____
4. Lay out x-rays. (Make certain that raised dot is facing upward.)	☐	☐	_____	_____
5. Arrange film on view box before placing into mount.	☐	☐	_____	_____
6. Mount the two or four bite-wing films.	☐	☐	_____	_____
Postprocedure				
7. Mount two central (CI) and lateral (LI) incisor films. Place mandibular films with roots downward and maxillary films with roots upward.	☐	☐	_____	_____
8. Mount the four cuspid (C) films. The two longest cuspids are maxillary teeth.	☐	☐	_____	_____
9. Mount the four bicuspid (BC) films.	☐	☐	_____	_____
10. Mount the four molars (M) films. The molars with three roots are the maxillary molars.	☐	☐	_____	_____
11. Review the anatomical charts to check mount for accuracy.	☐	☐	_____	_____
12. Turn off view box.	☐	☐	_____	_____